Foreword

I have the pleasure of being the daughter of Joseph Boyes, MD, a well-educated man—a man of many talents with a superior mind and the distinctive values of humility, loyalty and integrity. He was a straightforward family man, full of strength and vision who touched and influenced our lives immensely and was a mentor to those who knew him. I grew to understand that this gifted man was destined to leave a legacy for more admirers than I could imagine.

Challenging times were many in his life, and he rose to each occasion. During World War II, he opened a hospital in Kweilin, China for the wounded pilots of the Flying Tigers who were shot down. He served at that field hospital for three-and-a-half years.

My father designed this book to be read by those in the medical profession, but everyone can enjoy and appreciate the personal aspects of these legendary figures since he never lost sight of his plan to enlighten the reader. As he transitions from one physician to the next, his writing reflects lasting details of these pioneers in their respective fields.

As we experience challenging times let us remember the courage, determination, perseverance and wisdom of these giants from the sixteenth century to the late nineteenth century so eloquently portrayed in this book. Through the efforts and diligence of Roy A. Meals, MD, UCLA, who spearheaded the reprinting of this book, a new generation of physicians will enjoy my father's work and see first-hand the imprint Joseph Boyes, MD has left on the field of hand surgery.

Marlowe Boyes Hanlon

Preface

The use of proper names is common in medicine, especially in the surgical specialties. Syndromes, signs, and tests are given the names of discoverers or elaborators; operative procedures, incisions, or even systems of treatment come to be known simply by a proper name.

Surgery of the hand, actually that of the upper extremity, is a field of special interest, a combination of general surgery, plastic surgery, orthopaedics, and neurosurgery. All types of tissue are in the upper extremity and many diseases and abnormalities can be manifested in the hand. Thus, in this field of surgery, there are many sources for the use of persons' names. We have the syndromes of Erb, Duchenne, and Klumpke; Tinel's sign; and Weber's test. Steindler and Bunnell are remembered for operative procedures, and Dupuytren and Volkmann for deformities resulting from contractures.

Use of names in this way conserves time in conversation and words in writing, providing that the speaker and listener and the author and reader are agreed as to their meaning. Herein lies the danger, and many will therefore only grudgingly condone the use of eponyms. To be useful, the meaning must be defined, and the original source, if possible, be read and understood by all.

This collection tries to bring to our attention the sources for the eponyms that are used in surgery of the upper extremity.

There is another aspect to the use of persons' names. Should we not know something of them as individuals? How and under what circumstances did they do what they did to justify such recognition? Who or what provided the stimulus? Pliny said that no man possesses such genius that he can become commanding unless a subject suited to his talents presents itself and an opportunity occurs for their development. Dupuytren had the talents, in abundance, but the opportunity was there also. A fortuitous reporting of his lectures spread his name throughout the surgical world, and it now survives in several eponyms. Yet we hear very little of his students or those he trained. How different is the case of the German surgeon B. R. K. Langenbeck. Although he worked in the same time period as Dupuytren, and only a border away, Langenbeck's name is seldom used today, only because of a periodical he once edited; however, his students included Billroth, Esmarch, and Trendelenburg, and, in the next generation, Kocher, Kirschner, and Perthes, names all in common use today.

The selection of names in this collection is based on those commonly used in surgery of the hand, with others related historically, or by the availability of material, or of current interest. Many others should probably be presented, but the ones in this collection are offered with the hope that the reader may become better acquainted with the principal historical figures in our field and may receive some stimulus to emulate them not by seeking to follow in their footsteps, but by seeking what they sought (Basho).

As a practical matter, some end point had to be set; therefore, all names of major subjects are those whose work is completed and who have died. It is too difficult to evaluate those still living. Time has a way of putting things into perspective, and some names used so freely today will disappear; whereas others less well-known now will later be recognized for some valuable contribution. After all, it was 200 years before those in the field of surgery recognized that Guy de Chauliac had delayed the progress of the study of wound healing by adopting the "laudable pus" theory. The clean-wound practices of his predecessors, Bishop Theodoric and Henri de Mondeville, then took their rightful place. Chauliac's judgments were always weighty, but not always true.

The use of a name implies the discovery or first reporting of some sign, syndrome, or procedure, but we know that often this was the development of another's idea or some modification which improved or clarified the original. Similarly, the collateral development or discovery of a new method, such as the microscope, the x-ray, or antisepsis, may have played an important part in the discovery. One must look at the reports of those in the past in the light of the times in which they worked. Colles had been dead 50 years when Röntgen discovered the x-ray, yet Colles's description of the fracture bearing his name was clearly correct. By reviewing the lives and works of these persons chronologically, it will become clearer that, considering the conditions under which they worked, with the available facilities and the then-current state of knowledge, they were truly giants.

When Sir Isaac Newton was complimented on his discovery of the law of gravity, he answered, "If I have seen further . . . it is by standing upon the shoulders of giants." We have all stood upon someone's shoulders to enable us to see further, so this brief backward glance at these giants will, I hope, increase our appreciation of them.

My thanks go to the many Fellows in Hand Surgery, for their suggestions and their tolerance in listening to "history." I am especially grateful to Lt. Commander Ted Dupuy, U.S.N., for his many hours of labor in the stacks.

Biographical material has been obtained from sources such as dictionaries, anthologies, obituary notices, and, in some cases, personal reminiscences. We are all indebted to the unsung heroes and heroines of our craft, the medical librarians, who unstintingly give of their time and skill. I owe much to those of the Los Angeles County Medical Association Library: Mr. John M. Connor, chief librarian, and Mrs. Elizabeth S. Crahan, assistant librarian, for their time and efforts in seeking out available data.

To the editors at the J. B. Lippincott Company goes all credit for the difficult task of retrieving the original articles and portraits of this group of scientists. Only through their skill and persistence could the material have been collected and put together in attractive form.

JOSEPH H. BOYES, M.D.

Contents

The Beginning 1

The Sixteenth Century 3
Würtz

The Seventeenth Century 7
de Lapeyronie, Albinus, Camper

The Early Eighteenth Century 15
Heberden, Roland Martin

The Late Eighteenth Century 23
Cooper, Colles, Bell, Dupuytren, Delpech

The Early Nineteenth Century 38
Weber, Duchenne, Stromeyer, Little, Adams, Denonvilliers, William Horner, Schwann, Pacini, Gruber, Paget, Waller, Langer, Garrod, Poland, Thiersch, Wolfe, Esmarch, Langenbeck, Henry Martin

The Mid-Nineteenth Century 89
Mitchell, Meissner, Volkmann, Ollier, Guyon, Johann Horner, Recklinghausen, Raynaud, Ranvier, Cleland, Bennett, Erb, Parona, Reverdin, Merkel, Madelung, Nicoladoni, Sprengel, Ramón y Cajal, Marie, Beevor, Secrétan, Jones, Thomas, Klumpke, Stiles

The Late Nineteenth Century 157
Apert, de Quervain, Cushing, Perthes,
Kienböck, Kanavel, Filatov, Darrach,
Froment, Steindler, Kirschner, Tinel, Bunnell,
Gillies, Mayer, Finochietto, Mason

Postscript 212

Index 215

On the Shoulders of Giants

THE BEGINNING

The story of the persons whose names we most often use in the special field of surgery of the hand begins in the sixteenth century. This period, said to mark the beginning of modern medicine, was a time of many important changes. Vesalius, a pupil of Jacobus Sylvius, made anatomy a study of the human body, instead of that of the pig and the ape, as Galen had taught. Epidemics of syphilis and the plague, the Black Death, had ravaged Europe in the previous century. Gunpowder had been introduced, adding a new factor to the causes of wounds and compounding the treatment. The Augustinian friar, Martin Luther, made his break with Rome to start the Reformation. Gutenberg's invention had made possible the wide dissemination of knowledge.

The treatment of wounds at this time was based on the teachings of Vigo, whose textbook had gone through fifty editions, or on those of Guy de Chauliac, who considered all wounds to be poisoned and used styptics, caustics, and plasters of many types. Ambroise Paré, in France, and Brunschwig, the authority at Strassburg, were followers of this school.

Surgery for hernia and bladder stone was done by the itinerant surgeons, whose skills often were passed on from father to son. In Italy the Branca family became famous for reconstruction of missing parts, especially noses, using the old Hindu flap method.

Surgery in France was outside of the academic sphere. The most famous medical school, St. Côme, would not allow a surgeon to teach there. Paré's skill as a wound surgeon made him invaluable to the king, but he published his work in the vernacular rather than in the classical Latin of the physicians.

In England surgery had no academic standing at Cambridge or Oxford, but in 1511, Henry VIII had forbidden "irregular" surgeons to practice in

London. One had to obtain permission from the bishop and then pass an examination to qualify. By 1540, this Fellowship of Surgeons had established instructional courses and issued limited licenses.

Although in this era we do not find a man whose name has become an eponym, there was one, a Swiss, who does merit our attention.

THE SIXTEENTH CENTURY

Felix Würtz (1514–1575) was a member of the "barber's guild" and called attention to the positioning of a part that is nonfunctional. He said

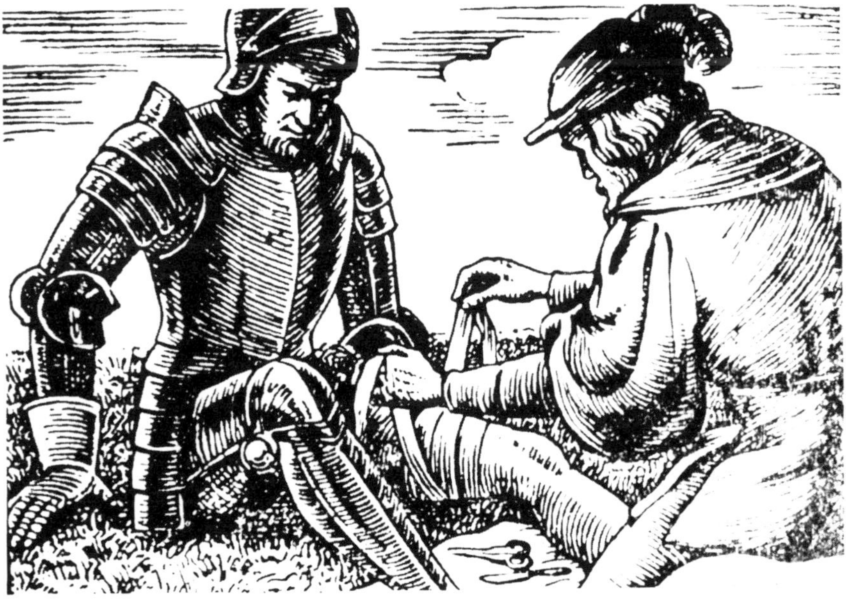

Felix Würtz applying a tourniquet to the thigh of a wounded soldier. (From Gordon, B. L.: The Romance of Medicine; the Story of the Evolution of Medicine from Occult Practices and Primitive Times. Philadelphia, F. A. Davis, 1944. Courtesy of the Library of the College of Physicians of Philadelphia)

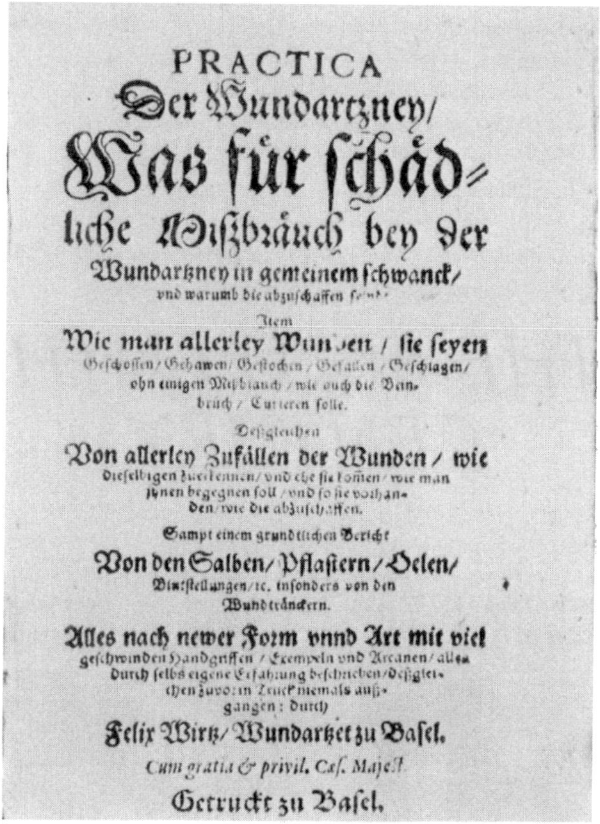

PRACTICA
Der Wundartzney/
Was für schäd-
liche Mißbräuch bey der
Wundartzney in gemeinem schwanck/
vnd warumb die abzuschaffen seind.
Item
Wie man allerley Wunden / sie seyen
Geschossen/Gehawen/Gestochen/Gefallen/Geschlagen/
ohn einigen Mißbrauch/wie auch die Bein-
brüch/Curieren solle.
Desgleichen
Von allerley Zufällen der Wunden/wie
dieselbigen zuerkennen/vnd ehe sie komen/wie man
jhnen begegnen soll/vnd so sie vorhan-
den/wie die abzuschaffen.
Sampt einem grundtlichen Bericht
Von den Salben/Pflastern/Oelen/
Dinstellungen/rc. insonders von den
Wundträncken.
Alles nach newer Form vnnd Art mit viel
geschwinden Handgriffen/Exempeln vnd Arcanen/alles
durch selbs eigene Erfahrung beschrieben/desgleichen
zuvor in Truck niemals auß-
gangen: durch
Felix Würtz/Wundartzet zu Basel.
Cum gratia & privil. Cæs. Maiest.
Getruckt zu Basel.

Felix Würtz: Practica der Wundartzney. Basel, S. Henricepetric, 1596. (Courtesy of the Library of the New York Academy of Medicine)

that if a part, such as a finger, is to become stiff and useless, it should be placed in that position which will interfere *the least* with the function of the remaining digits. This concept, of course, might be said to be the antithesis of the modern position of function that Kanavel described.

Würtz, the son of a surgeon, was born in Basle and studied at Nürnberg, Padua, and Rome. He then settled in Zurich, where he was made a member of the barber's guild in 1553. Six years later he was in Strassburg, but he finally settled in Basle, where in 1563, he published his textbook on the treatment of wounds, *Practica der Wundarzney*. He advised keeping the wounds clean, was against the use of caustics or the cautery, and recommended conservative amputations. His treatment of firearm wounds was against all tradition, which had taught that firearm wounds were "poisoned" and therefore required the cautery or hot oil. Würtz must have been a strong character, for he said that he had written no book copied from those of his forerunners, for "naught will still be naught though practiced for a thousand years." He said that he trimmed himself with no strange feathers, that he wrote only what he had made trial of, and that he had concealed nothing of what was known to him.

How much he influenced the treatment of wounds is not known, but his book, in fourteen or more editions, was used for 100 years. He struck out against the blind dogmatism of the past and boasted, "How much do you suppose I care whether Galen's or Avicenna's or Guy de Chauliac's opinion does or does not agree with mine?"

THE SEVENTEENTH CENTURY

In the seventeenth century, the one following Würtz, the surgeons, as the German word *Wundarzt* indicates, were primarily wound doctors. It was war that provided them with the experience of treating trauma. Wilhelm Fabry (1560–1624), considered to be the father of German surgery, did the first amputation above the level of gangrene, using a self-designed tourniquet. He is said to have done the first amputation of the thigh. He removed a gall stone, but he still cauterized firearm wounds in spite of Würtz's recommendations.

In the latter part of the seventeenth century, a change was taking place in the relationship of surgeons to physicians, but it was many years before there would be a real association of the two. One man, our first eponym, would make it possible for King Louis XV of France, in 1724, to force St. Côme to accept professors of surgery.

François Gigot de Lapeyronie (1678–1747) was chief surgeon to the king and chief surgeon at l'Hôpital de la Charité. De Lapeyronie, of course, is remembered for his description of penile strabismus, which is associated with Dupuytren's contracture of the palmar fascia in some 10 per cent of those patients. De Lapeyronie first reported this condition in 1743 as being one of the causes of obstruction of the "natural ejaculation of the semen," and he described three cases of what today we call Peyronie's disease, to differentiate it from other forms of plastic induration from infections, such as lymphogranuloma venereum. Peyronie's disease is a nodular thickening of the fascia of the cavernous sheaths, usually on the dorsum; the overlying skin does not become involved, as in that of the hand. Pain on erection and angulation toward the side of

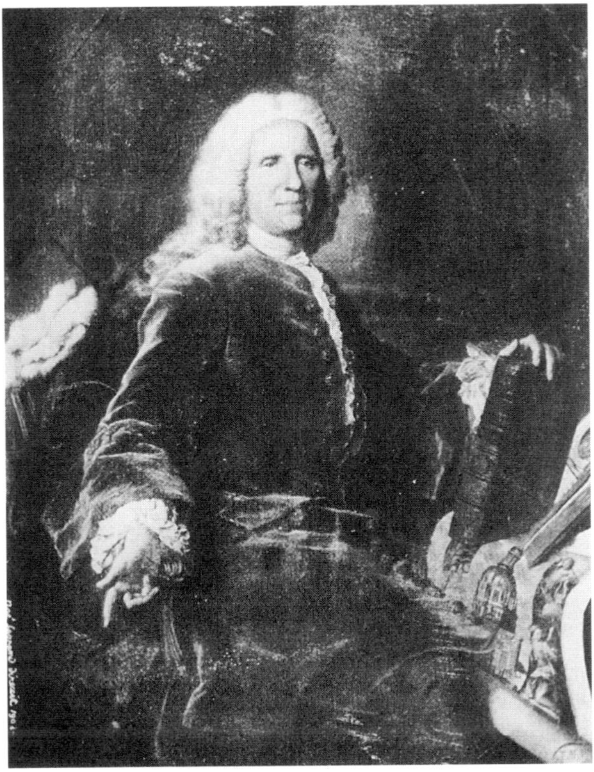

François Gigot de Lapeyronie. (From Binet, L., and Vallery-Radot, P.: La Faculté de Médecine de Paris. Cinq Siècles d'Art et d'Histoire. Paris, Masson et Cie, 1952. Courtesy of the Library of the College of Physicians of Philadelphia)

the lesion are common complaints. De Lapeyronie had called it a strabismus; but in 1903 a doctor in Pittsburgh was consulted by a patient who described his problem as being a "squint of the cock," a more graphic term illustrating well the force of the Anglo-Saxon root words. Many and varied forms of treatment have been tried, with conflicting reports of results.*

De Lapeyronie was born on January 15, 1678, in Montpellier. He was the son of a surgeon and was destined to become one of France's greatest surgeons. He spent 2 years studying philosophy and the natural sciences, and when he was 19 years old, he received his degree of Master of Surgery from the University of Montpellier. One of his professors

*For a good review, see McRoberts, J.W.: Peyronie's disease. Surg. Gynecol. Obstet., *129:*1291–1294, 1969.

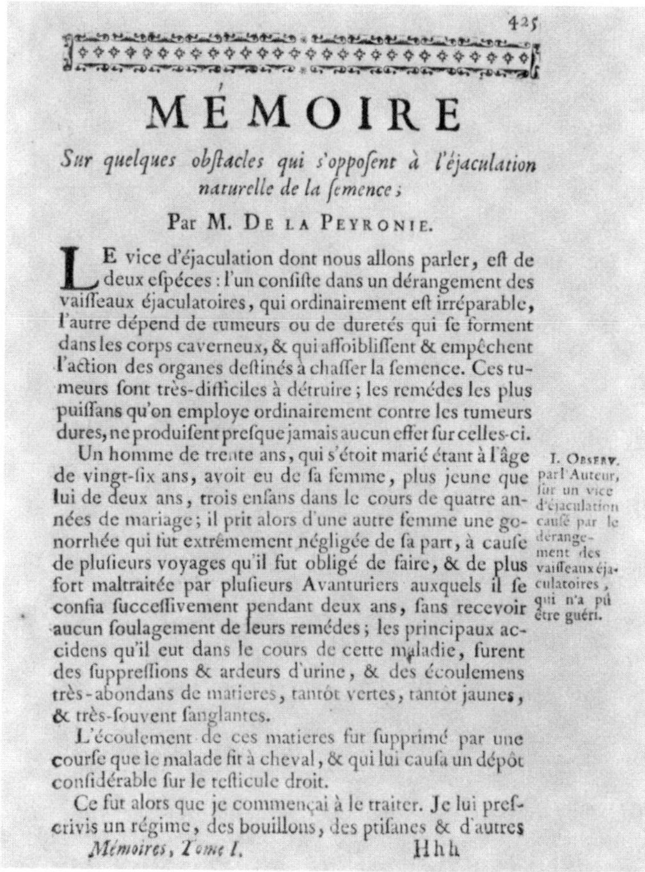

425

MÉMOIRE

Sur quelques obſtacles qui s'oppoſent à l'éjaculation naturelle de la ſemence;

Par M. De la Peyronie.

LE vice d'éjaculation dont nous allons parler, eſt de deux eſpéces : l'un conſiſte dans un dérangement des vaiſſeaux éjaculatoires, qui ordinairement eſt irréparable, l'autre dépend de tumeurs ou de duretés qui ſe forment dans les corps caverneux, & qui affoibliſſent & empêchent l'action des organes deſtinés à chaſſer la ſemence. Ces tumeurs ſont très-difficiles à détruire; les remédes les plus puiſſans qu'on employe ordinairement contre les tumeurs dures, ne produiſent preſque jamais aucun effet ſur celles-ci.

I. Observ. par l'Auteur, ſur un vice d'éjaculation cauſé par le dérangement des vaiſſeaux éjaculatoires, qui n'a pû être guéri.

Un homme de trente ans, qui s'étoit marié étant à l'âge de vingt-ſix ans, avoit eu de ſa femme, plus jeune que lui de deux ans, trois enfans dans le cours de quatre années de mariage; il prit alors d'une autre femme une gonorrhée qui fut extrêmement négligée de ſa part, à cauſe de pluſieurs voyages qu'il fut obligé de faire, & de plus fort maltraitée par pluſieurs Avanturiers auxquels il ſe confia ſucceſſivement pendant deux ans, ſans recevoir aucun ſoulagement de leurs remédes; les principaux accidens qu'il eut dans le cours de cette maladie, furent des ſuppreſſions & ardeurs d'urine, & des écoulemens très-abondans de matieres, tantôt vertes, tantôt jaunes, & très-ſouvent ſanglantes.

L'écoulement de ces matieres fut ſupprimé par une courſe que le malade fit à cheval, & qui lui cauſa un dépôt conſidérable ſur le teſticule droit.

Ce fut alors que je commençai à le traiter. Je lui preſcrivis un régime, des bouillons, des ptiſanes & d'autres

Mémoires, Tome I. Hhh

François Gigot de Lapeyronie: Mémoire sur quelques obstacles qui s'opposent à l'éjaculation naturelle de la semence. Mem. Acad. R. Chir., *1*:425–434, 1743. (Courtesy of the Library of the New York Academy of Medicine)

suggested to de Lapeyronie's father that his son should be sent to Paris to study under Mareschal, chief surgeon at l'Hôtel Dieu. When this term was completed, de Lapeyronie returned to Montpellier, practiced surgery, and taught anatomy with such success that he was soon made professor and chief of surgery. A prominent duke became his patient, and when de Lapeyronie successfully cured his fistula-in-ano, the patient, who was a friend of Louis XIV, urged him to move to Paris. He became an associate of his former preceptor, Mareschal, taught anatomy again, and became well known. Because of de Lapeyronie's influence, Louis XV set up five new teaching positions in anatomy and surgery. De Lapeyronie personally provided the money to pay the seven extra demonstrators. He did the same for his own school, Montpellier, paying for eight new teachers there and donating an amphitheater.

De Lapeyronie and Mareschal founded the Royal Academy of Surgery in Paris in 1731, to bring together and correlate the experiences of others in the surgical profession. They were able to obtain an order that severed the Society of Barbers from the Society of Surgeons and that set up standards of training and education, which allowed the use of the title "surgeon" and the practice of surgery in Paris.

De Lapeyronie wrote little, but he influenced surgical education by bequeathing funds for libraries, scholarships, lectureships, and buildings. A special bequest was made "to assure the delivery of cadavers for anatomical demonstration."

He died in 1747, in his seventieth year. His heart was inurned in a

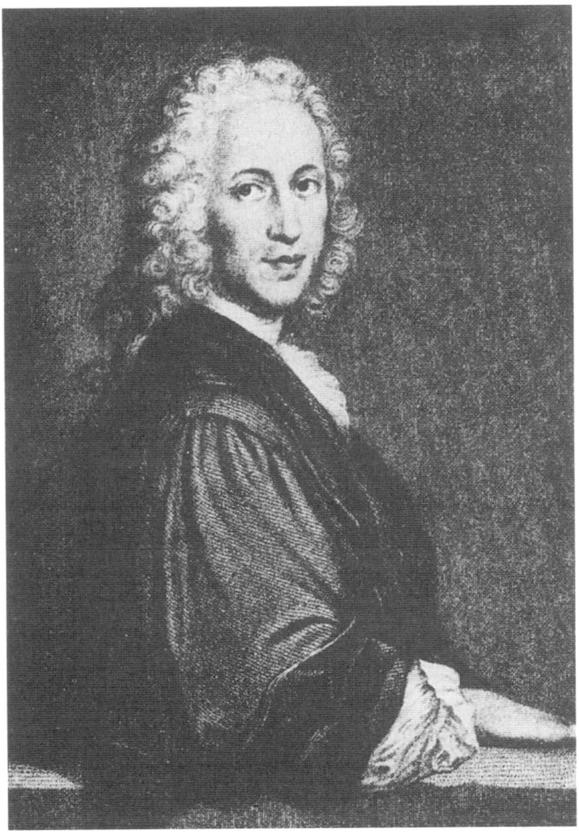

Bernhard Siegfried Albinus. (From Garrison, F. H.: An Introduction to the History of Medicine. ed. 4. Philadelphia, W. B. Saunders, 1929)

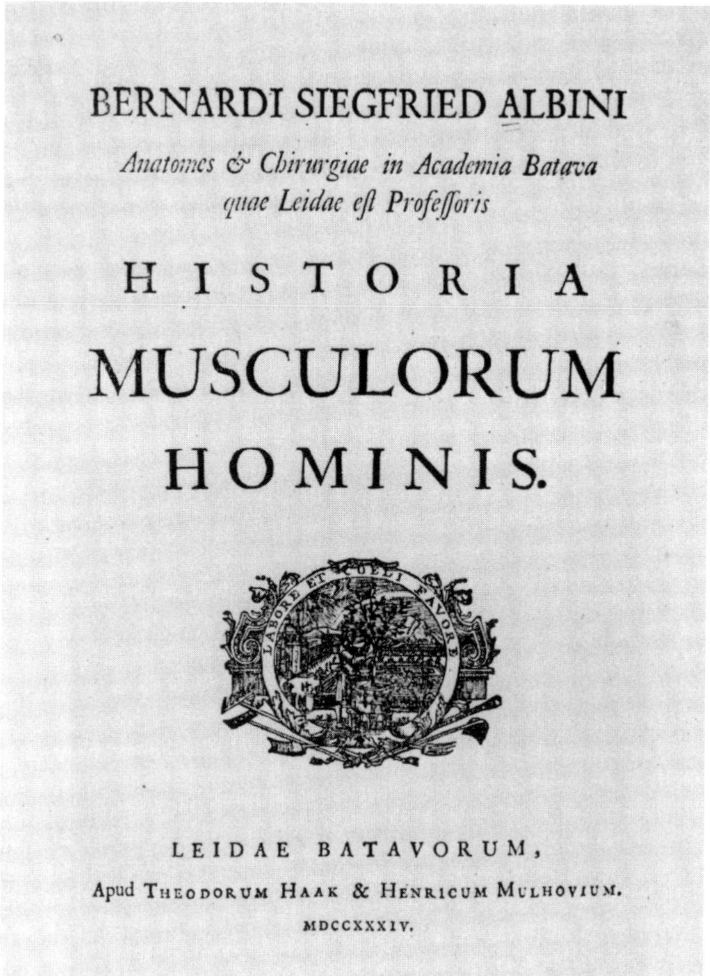

BERNARDI SIEGFRIED ALBINI

Anatomes & Chirurgiae in Academia Batava quae Leidae est Professoris

HISTORIA

MUSCULORUM

HOMINIS.

LEIDAE BATAVORUM,

Apud THEODORUM HAAK & HENRICUM MULHOVIUM.

MDCCXXXIV.

Bernhard Siegfried Albinus: Historia Musculorum Hominis. Leiden, Leidae Batavorum, Theodorum Haak & Henricum Mulhovium, 1734. (Courtesy of The Francis A. Countway Library of Medicine, Boston, Massachusetts)

monument in the church of St. Côme. The church is gone, but a bust remains in the amphitheater of the Royal Academy of Surgery. This theater was built in 1694 and has seen continuous service for more than 200 years. François Gigot de Lapeyronie can surely be listed as one of the giants of surgery upon whose shoulders others have stood to see further ahead.

In the middle of the seventeenth century, Holland was recognized as

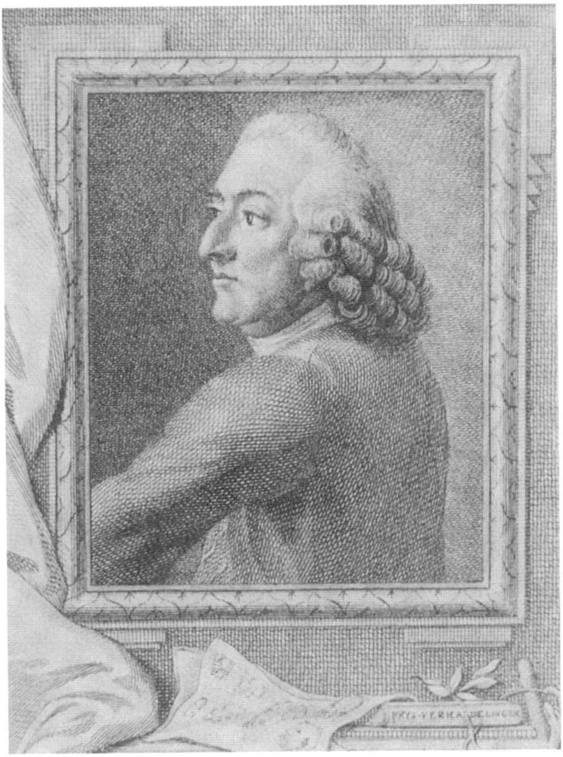

Pieter Camper. (Courtesy of the Library of the New York Academy of Medicine)

being one of Europe's most important centers of learning. It was here that Boerhaave introduced clinical teaching and that a school of anatomy became famous. The universities of Amsterdam and Leiden were best known, and we go to the latter to find two men, first associated as teacher and student, but later to be rival protagonists of a method of anatomical illustration.

The teacher, **Bernhard Siegfried Albinus** (1697–1770), has no eponym in surgery, but his anatomical studies are still quoted, especially in regard to the intrinsic muscles. He was born in Frankfort on the Oder, and, according to Billroth, the family name was Weiss. He taught first in Amsterdam, then in Göttingen, before settling in Leiden. He was professor of anatomy and surgery in 1718 and then professor of medicine in 1745. Albinus was an editor and a classifier. He edited the works of Harvey, Vesalius, and Eustachius. He published two bone atlases in 1726 and 1753, one on muscles in 1734, and others on the skeleton and skeletal muscles in 1747 and 1762. The drawings for his works were done by the artist Jan Wunderleer, directed by Albinus, and the method of projection

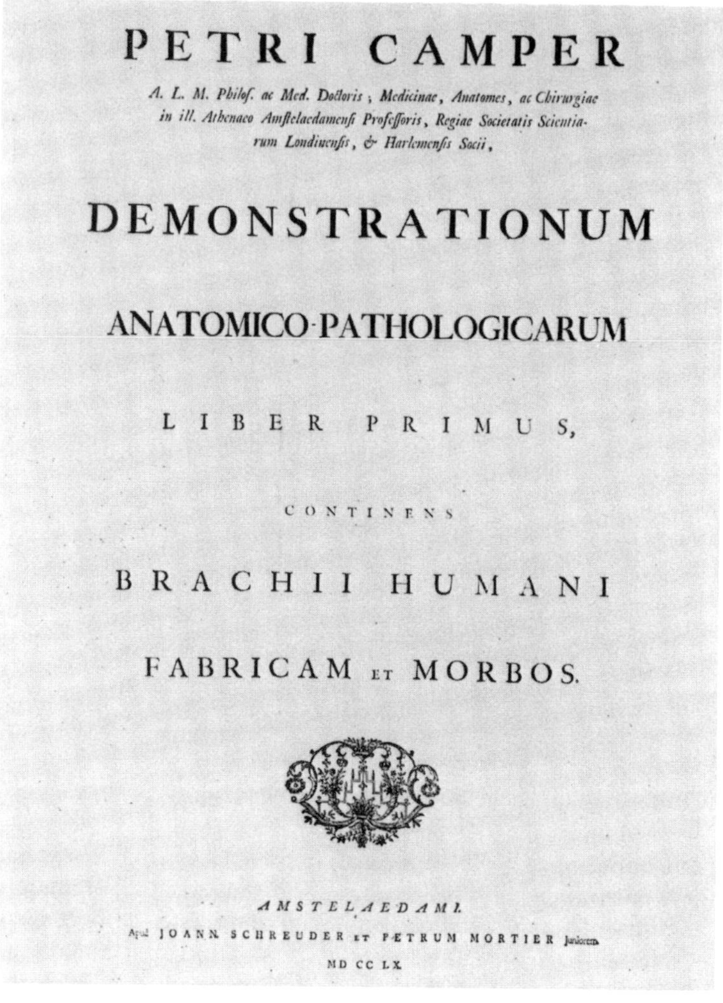

PETRI CAMPER

A. L. M. Philos. ac Med. Doctoris ; Medicinae, Anatomes, ac Chirurgiae in ill. Athenaeo Amstelaedamensi Professoris, Regiae Societatis Scientiarum Londinensis, & Harlemensis Socii,

DEMONSTRATIONUM

ANATOMICO-PATHOLOGICARUM

LIBER PRIMUS,

CONTINENS

BRACHII HUMANI

FABRICAM ET MORBOS.

AMSTELAEDAMI.

Apud JOANN. SCHREUDER ET PETRUM MORTIER Juniorem.

MD CC LX.

Pieter Camper: Demonstrationum Anatomico-Pathologicarum. vol. 1. Brachii Humani. Amsterdam, Joann. Schreuder et Petrum Mortier, 1760. (Courtesy of the Library of the College of Physicians of Philadelphia)

became the source of a bitter rivalry with his former student. The student, **Pieter Camper** (1722–1789), is the source of Camper's fascia and of the chiasm of Camper, that decussation of the superficialis tendon behind the profundus in the finger.

Camper was born in Leiden, the grandson of a physician and the son of a clergyman who had acquired great wealth in the Dutch East Indies. Extremely talented, even what today we would call a prodigy, Camper excelled in scholarship and became a capable artist in oil, aquatint, pas-

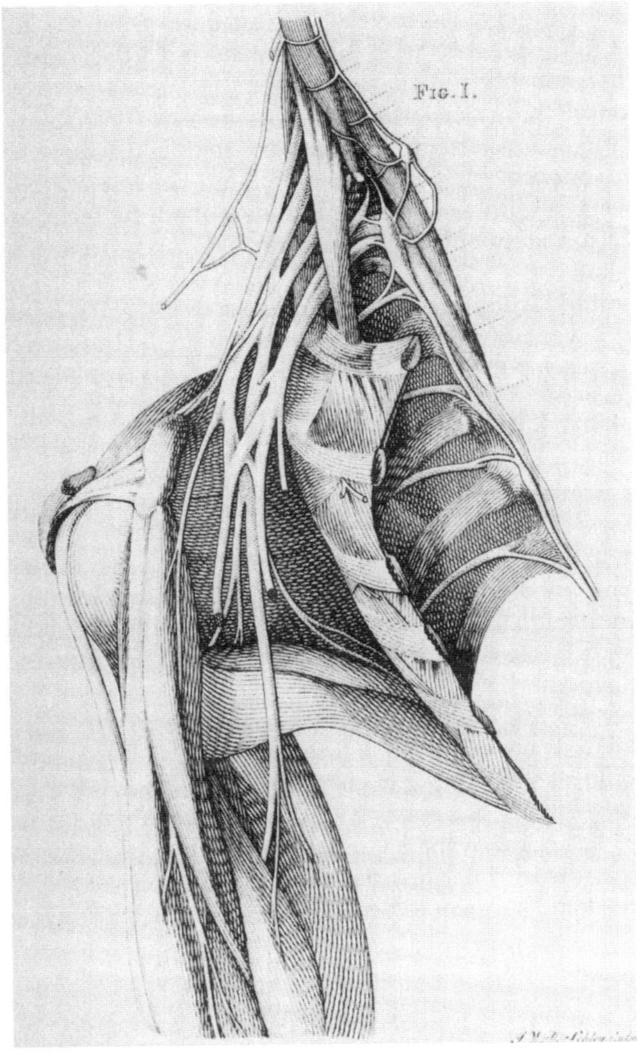

Illustration of the brachial plexus. Pieter Camper: Demonstrationum Anatomico-Pathologicarum. vol. 1. Brachii Humani. Amsterdam, Joann. Schreuder et Petrum Mortier, 1760. (Courtesy of the Library of the College of Physicians of Philadelphia)

tel, etching, and mezzotint. He was able to enter the university before he was 12 years old. He was said to be fluent in Latin, French, English, and German, and by the age of 24 he had doctorates in both philosophy and medicine. He went to England, where he studied with Smellie, the famous obstetrician, and took lessons at the Painter's Academy. Soon he was a professor of philosophy at a Dutch university, then added the chairs of medicine and surgery. He traveled a great deal, especially to England, and was on intimate terms with the scientists and artists of his time. It is said that he probably did the illustrations for Smellie's book on midwifery on one of these visits. After a term as professor of anatomy, surgery, and medicine at Amsterdam, he went to Groningen, where he took the same chairs but also included that of botany. He was a prolific writer, with interests in anthropology, and he described the facial angle as an index of race and popularized the term *Caucasian* from a study of a Georgian skull.

In anatomical illustration he insisted on an architectural aspect, that is, the part is viewed not as if from one particular angle, but as if the axes of vision struck each part from the same distance. This type of orthographic representation had been used by da Vinci, but Albinus, with his drawings, had followed Vesalius in viewing the parts in perspective. The argument between Camper and Albinus was quite serious.

Camper argued against Caesarean section and advocated symphysiotomy, performing the operation experimentally on pigs. He also wrote on fractures of the patella, congenital dislocation of the hip, and bladder stone. He dissected a rhinoceros, an orangutan, and an elephant. Retiring from medicine, he spent 17 years as a politician and served on the state council. He died in April, 1789, of exudative pleurisy and was buried in Leiden.

Whenever we use the term "chiasm of Camper," we are paying our respects to a most unusual man, a brilliant mind, and a giant of his time. But we should also remember his teacher and his rival, Albinus, because his school of anatomy has persisted. Today, Albinus's successor, J. M. F. Landsmeer, has clarified the anatomy and function of many parts of the hand, such as the intrinsic muscles and the mechanics of the wrist joint, to enable the hand surgeon to become more knowledgeable in his field.

THE EARLY EIGHTEENTH CENTURY

In Italy the doctors of this period were primarily physiologists and pathologists, and their names are not in common use among surgeons. Valsalva (1666–1723) was a pupil of Malpighi, and he in turn taught Morgagni (1682–1771). In France there was Nicolas Andry of Lyon (1658–1742), a clergyman who coined the word *orthopaedics,* and who, as dean of the medical faculty in Paris, was antisurgery. Jean-Louis Petit (1674–1750) was the first to amputate at different levels, that is, not a guillotine division. He used a screw tourniquet and was also the first to open the mastoid.

In Germany the itinerant surgeons were still busy, but the 1700s brought many changes in medical education. The Berlin Charité opened in 1727, and Vienna's famed Allgemeine Krankenhaus, in 1784. Lorenz Heister (1683–1758) published his textbook in 1718, a work that was to be used for 120 years. The university medical school at Göttingen was opened in 1736, and through its successive professors of surgery, was to influence German surgery for the next 200 years. Albrecht von Haller (1708–1777) was its first professor of surgery, but he never performed an operation on a living body.

Our next eponym comes from England. **William Heberden** (1710–1801) should be remembered for more than calling attention to the nodes in the fingers that bear his name. He was a scholarly, keen observer who made careful notes of all the important cases that he saw in his practice, and when he was more than 70 years of age, he began to compile these into a

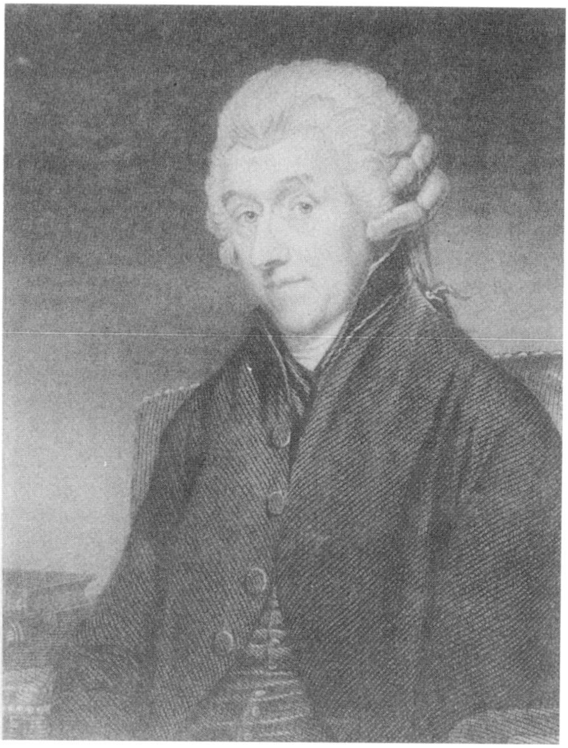

William Heberden. (Courtesy of the Library of the New York Academy of Medicine)

Commentaries on the History and Cure of Diseases. Written in classical Latin, they were translated into English by his son and published simultaneously the year after Heberden's death. Of the 102 short chapters, one of less than 100 words describes the "little hard knobs" on the fingers almost as a casual observation, yet his name is perpetuated for this rather than for other more important observations that he made.

In these commentaries and other writings, Heberden gave what was probably the first clear description of angina pectoris, the autopsy done by John Hunter, and an early account of chickenpox, distinguishing it from smallpox. He had noted the relationship of the development of stones to urinary-tract infection and was consulted by Benjamin Franklin for a bladder stone. Heberden and Franklin then collaborated on a paper concerning the success of smallpox inoculation in America and England. Heberden described nyctalopia and anaphylactic purpura, long before Schönlein and Henoch. All this work was done before the stethoscope was invented, and before the use of the clinical thermometer, laboratory

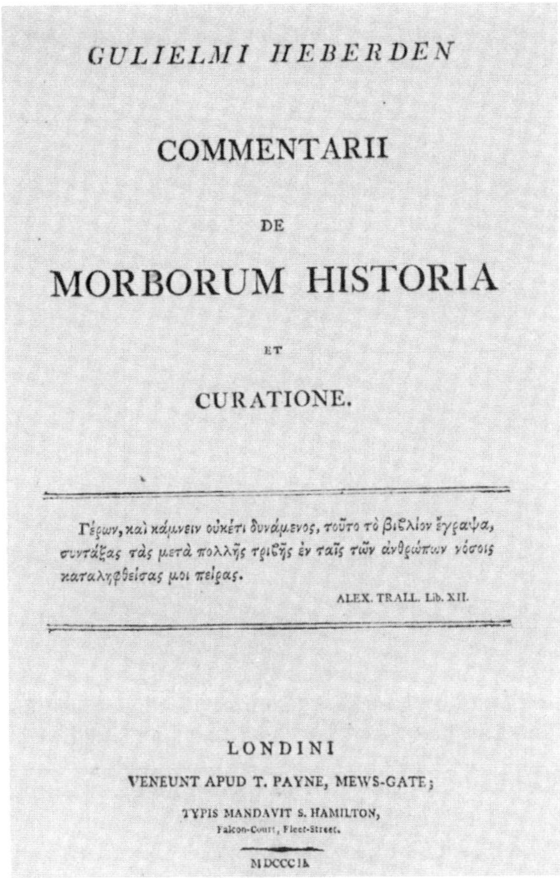

GULIELMI HEBERDEN

COMMENTARII

DE

MORBORUM HISTORIA

ET

CURATIONE.

Γέρων, καὶ κάμνειν οὐκέτι δυνάμενος, τοῦτο τὸ βιβλίον ἔγραψα, συντάξας τὰς μετὰ πολλῆς τριβῆς ἐν ταῖς τῶν ἀνθρώπων νόσοις καταληφθείσας μοι πείρας.

ALEX. TRALL. Lib. XII.

LONDINI

VENEUNT APUD T. PAYNE, MEWS-GATE;

TYPIS MANDAVIT S. HAMILTON,

Falcon-Court, Fleet-Street.

MDCCCII.

William Heberden: Commentarii de Morborum Historia et Curatione. London, T. Payne, 1802. (Courtesy of the Library of the College of Physicians of Philadelphia)

examinations, x-ray, or the microscope in the study of disease. A true follower of Hippocrates's dictum, "observe and record," he used his senses and portrayed what he saw, heard, and felt in simple, clear terms. He was probably the last of the writers in classical Latin, although Latin, particularly in medical theses, was still used in the middle of the nineteenth century in Germany, where Volkmann's doctoral dissertation was given in what was described as fluent Latin.

Heberden was born in London. He was graduated from Cambridge and then studied medicine at London Hospital. He practiced for 10 years in Cambridge before returning to London. Heberden became a prominent member of the College of Physicians. He spent his summers at Windsor, where he was later buried.

CAP. 28.

De Nodis Digitorum.

NUNQUAM rite intellexi naturam tumorum, qui interdum nascuntur, ad pisi magnitudinem, prope tertium digitorum articulum. Nihil certe illis commune est cum arthritide; quoniam in multis reperiuntur, quibus morbus ille est incognitus. Per hominis ætatem manent; vacant omni dolore, neque spectant ad exulcerationem. Proinde deformitas major est, quam incommodum: quanquam motus digitorum aliquantulum impeditur.

William Heberden: De nodis digitorum. *In* Commentarii de Morborum Historia et Curatione. London, T. Payne, 1802. (Courtesy of the Library of the College of Physicians of Philadelphia)

William Heberden's son, known as the younger, was born of the second wife, who was a member of a well-known family, the Wollastons. The son became a physician, graduating from Oxford and studying at St. George Hospital. A classical scholar, as was his father, he translated the commentaries into English. He became a physician to King George III, but retired from practice after a series of family tragedies. One son died from a wound received in the dissecting room, and soon afterwards, another son and a daughter died.

One of the Wollastons, William Hugh (1766–1828), a grandnephew of Heberden senior, was also a physician, but he failed in practice. However, he made a fortune by inventing a welding process for platinum, as well as discovering the metals palladium and rhodium. He was the one who suggested the standardization of the imperial gallon as the volume of 10 pounds of water at 62° F. He also wrote a paper describing the semidecussation of the optic tracts, a condition that was first hypothesized by Newton.

Surgery in England during this period was dominated by Percival Pott (1714–1788), who in 1736 gave a systematic course of lectures at St. Bartholomew's Hospital. At St. Thomas's Hospital, William Cheselden (1688–

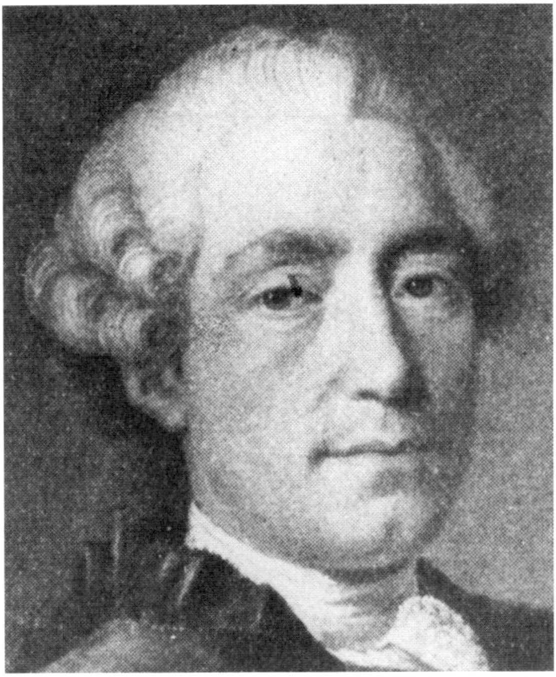

Roland Martin. (From Svenska Män Och Kvinnor: Biografisk Uppslagsbok. Stockholm, Albert Bonniers Förlag, 1949. Reproduced by permission of Svenska Porträttarkivet, Nationalmuseum, Stockholm. Courtesy of Kungliga Biblioteket, Stockholm, Sweden)

1752) was lecturing and becoming famous for his lithotomies; it is recorded that the time of operation varied from 30 to 120 seconds! John Hunter (1728–1793) had come from Edinburgh, where Alexander Monro I (1697–1767), the first professor, never practiced as an operating surgeon.

In the early 1700s, one of the students at Leiden was Peter Martin, who came from the university at Uppsala to take his degree in medicine. When he returned to Sweden, a son, **Roland Martin** (1726–1788), was born who was to be the first to describe the interesting cross connection of median and ulnar nerves in the forearm, now known as the Martin-Gruber anastomosis. His description was made in 1763 while he was professor of anatomy in Stockholm. Roland Martin studied at Uppsala under Linné, took his degree in 1751, and practiced medicine for a few years. He then went to Paris, where in 1754, he was a prosector to Antoine Petit and did anatomical dissections of the chorda tympani. When he returned to Stockholm he concentrated on the anatomy of the nervous

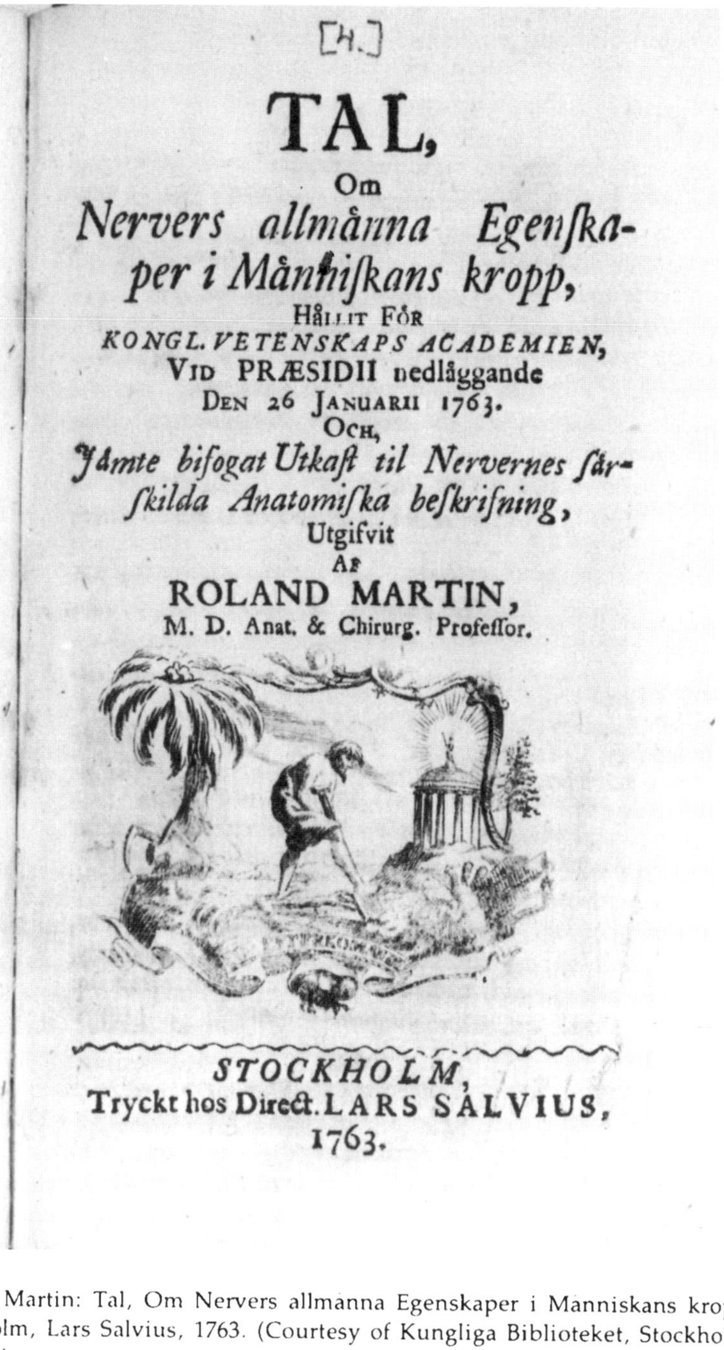

[H.]

TAL,

Om

Nervers allmänna Egenſka-
per i Månniſkans kropp,

Hållit För

KONGL. VETENSKAPS ACADEMIEN,

Vid PRÆSIDII nedläggande

Den 26 Januarii 1763.

Och,

Jämte bifogat Utkaſt til Nervernes ſär-
ſkilda Anatomiſka beſkrifning,

Utgifvit

Af

ROLAND MARTIN,

M. D. Anat. & Chirurg. Profeſſor.

STOCKHOLM,

Tryckt hos Direct. LARS SALVIUS,

1763.

Roland Martin: Tal, Om Nervers allmänna Egenskaper i Manniskans kropp. Stockholm, Lars Salvius, 1763. (Courtesy of Kungliga Biblioteket, Stockholm, Sweden)

system. He died in 1788, leaving not only a record of many anatomical papers but of many essays on varied subjects.

When present, this interconnection from median to ulnar nerve in the forearm can be the cause of some confusion in the diagnosis of ulnar nerve lesions in the elbow region. Since these fibers crossing over from median to ulnar nerves in the forearm are motor fibers, even if the ulnar nerve is cut at the elbow, the nerve supply to the adductor pollicis and first dorsal interosseus will still be intact. Only the interossei on the ulnar side of the hand and the profundi of the ring and little fingers will be paralyzed. Since this occurs in a significant number of people, it should be thought of as a possible explanation of what might appear to be a bizarre set of physical findings.

In the *Acta Orthopaedica Scandinavica* appeared a supplemental monograph on ulnar paralysis by Lennart Mannerfelt,* which explains in great detail the various phenomena seen in lesions of the ulnar nerve (see Gruber, Froment).

*Mannerfelt, L.: Studies on the hand in ulnar nerve paralysis. Acta Orthop. Scand., Suppl., *87*:1–176, 1966.

THE LATE EIGHTEENTH CENTURY

Reaching the end of the eighteenth century, there are now only a few years left before we will find other persons whose names have come down to us as eponyms. There were others, however, who, although not remembered specifically for something related to hand surgery, were important and deserving of some recognition.

Sir Astley Paston Cooper (1768–1841) was one of these persons. Although we do not have a lesion or operation in our field to remember him by, he did describe the contracture of the palmar fascia 10 years before Dupuytren. He distinguished this fascial contracture from the deformities that result from scarred tendon sheaths, and he treated the contracture by subcutaneous fasciotomy long before Adams made the procedure popular. Cooper's name, of course, is used by anatomists and abdominal surgeons in referring to a specific fascial layer, a type of hernia, and so forth.

Incidentally, in references concerning Dupuytren's contracture, we often find one to an article by Felix Plater of Basle (1614), who has been credited with an early description of this condition of the palmar fascia; however, Talbott's translation of the Latin original seems to show clearly that Plater's patient, developing a "contracture" after a sudden, extreme force was applied to the fingers, really had a rupture of the pulleys over the flexor tendons, rather than the typical contracture of the fascia, with its insidious onset and characteristic appearance.

Cooper was a most remarkable man, said to have been the greatest and most popular surgeon of his day. He was born in Norfolk County. His

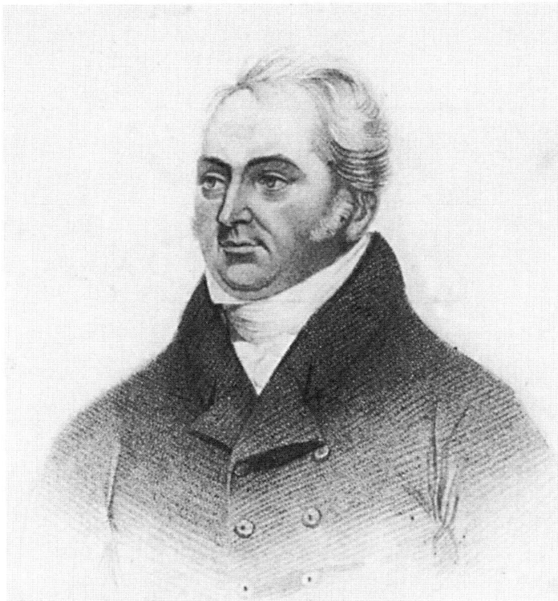

Astley Paston Cooper. (Courtesy of the Library of the College of Physicians of Philadelphia, Sturgis Collection)

father was a minister and a scholar, his mother an authoress. When he was 15 years old, he was sent to be an apprentice to his uncle, William Cooper, at that time a surgeon at Guy's Hospital. For some reason, after a few months he transferred his apprenticeship to a Henry Cline at St. Thomas's Hospital. These two hospitals were then associated under the name of the United Borough Hospitals.

Cooper's passions were the dissecting room and teaching. He spent a year in Edinburgh and returned to share lectures with Cline; Cooper lectured in surgery and Cline in anatomy. The lectures were very popular, drawing as many as 400 persons at one sitting. Cooper married a distant cousin of Cline's, who brought with her a large dowry which permitted him to continue his dissections and lectures without the worry of practice. It is said that he was so devoted to his course of lectures that he gave the customary evening lecture on his wedding day, unbeknownst to the audience. A belated honeymoon was spent in Paris, where he attended the lectures of Desault and Chopart and listened to the oratory of Danton, Marat, and Robespierre. He was present on August 10, 1792, when the Tuileries was attacked.

Later, when Cline retired from St. Thomas's and Cooper did not get the appointment, there was a breakup in the association of the two hospitals.

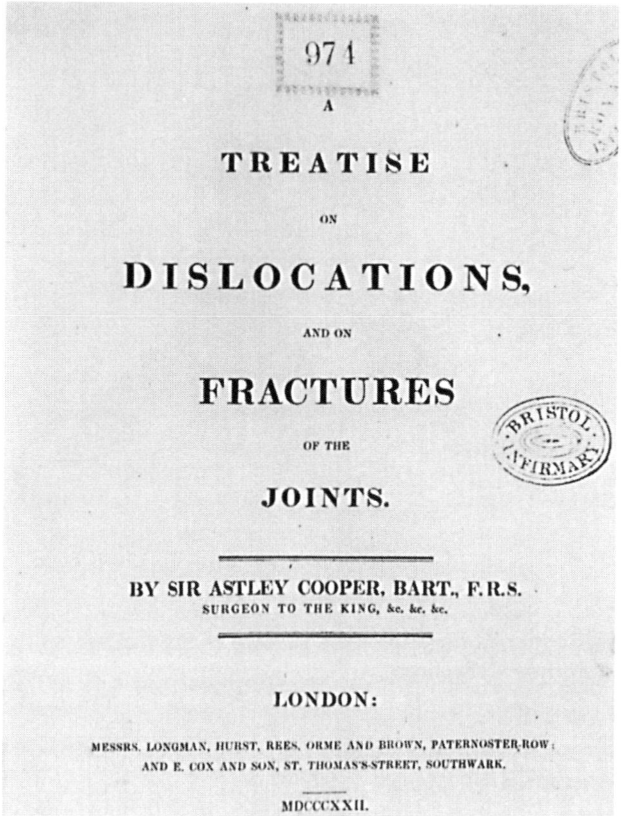

A

TREATISE

ON

DISLOCATIONS,

AND ON

FRACTURES

OF THE

JOINTS.

BY SIR ASTLEY COOPER, BART., F.R.S.
SURGEON TO THE KING, &c. &c. &c.

LONDON:

MESSRS. LONGMAN, HURST, REES, ORME AND BROWN, PATERNOSTER-ROW;
AND E. COX AND SON, ST. THOMAS'S-STREET, SOUTHWARK.

MDCCCXXII.

Astley Paston Cooper: A Treatise on Dislocations, and on Fractures of the Joints. ed. 1. London, Longman, Hurst, Rees, Orme and Brown, 1822. (Courtesy of the Library of the New York Academy of Medicine)

Cooper became a surgeon at Guy's Hospital, succeeding his uncle William, his first preceptor. Guy's Hospital in these years saw men such as Bright, Addison, and Hodgkin. Cooper was an equal in his field.

Cooper developed a large practice, said to be the largest and most lucrative of anyone before or since his time. He was made a baronet by George IV for removing a wen from the royal scalp, a reward for something which today seems but a minor bit of surgery. But members of royalty often demanded special attention of their surgeons, although the reward was not often so out of proportion to the deed. Cooper's knighthood should rather be seen as a reward for the years of study, teaching, and example he set for British surgery.

When Franklin Roosevelt was President, he had a wen on the back of

524 ON DISLOCATIONS OF

and the first and second phalanges are, consequently, drawn up and projected against the shoe, so as to prevent the patient being able to take his usual exercise.

Amputation required. I have frequently seen young ladies the subject of this inconvenience in the toe, and attribute it to the tightness of their shoes; it appears an extremely harsh measure, on the part of the surgeon, to amputate a toe under such circumstances, yet it is sometimes absolutely necessary, as it deprives the person of exercise, and of many of the enjoyments of life. In the first person I saw with this state of the toe, I refused to amputate, fearful of tetanus being produced by the operation; but the lady went to another surgeon, who complied with her request, and she did very well. In consequence of the perfect recovery of this lady, and the comfort which she derived from the loss of this annoyance, I was induced at the request of Mr. Toulmin, of Hackney, to remove for Miss T——, a patient of his, one of her toes, which was constantly irritated by the pressure of her shoe in walking, and prevented her taking that exercise necessary to the preservation of her health; she did very well, perfectly recovering the use of her foot.

The fingers are sometimes contracted in a similar manner, by a chronic inflammation of the thecæ, and aponeurosis of the palm of the hand, from excessive action of the hand, in the use of the hammer, the oar, ploughing, &c. &c. When the thecæ is

Astley Paston Cooper: A Treatise on Dislocations, and on Fractures of the Joints. ed. 1. p. 524. London, Longman, Hurst, Rees, Orme and Brown, 1822. (Courtesy of the Library of the New York Academy of Medicine)

his head; it was removed at Bethesda Naval Hospital in Maryland. Two surgeons were required, one a neurosurgeon, Craig, to excise the offending mass from the VIP skull, and a plastic surgeon, George Webster, to close the wound. Such is the age of specialization! Neither received a medal for their work.

Cooper wrote on hernia, fractures and dislocations, and diseases of the breast. He received many honors from French, German, Dutch, and Russian societies. He died in 1841; his attending physician had been Richard Bright. Autopsy findings showed a healed tuberculosis of the lungs and the granular kidneys of Bright's disease.

While Cooper was at Guy's Hospital, one of the students was John Keats, who had been licensed as an apothecary in 1816. He became a

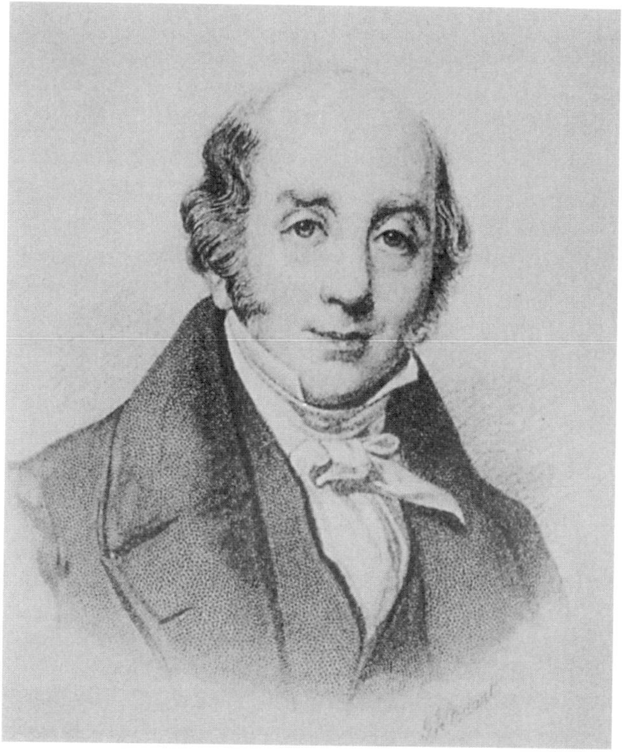

Abraham Colles. (From Kelly, E. C.: Selections from the writings of Abraham Colles. Med. Classics, 4:1027, 1940. Courtesy of the Library of the New York Academy of Medicine)

surgical dresser under Cooper but left to practice with one William Lucas. Lucas's reputation as a surgeon was not good; even Cooper referred to him as being "rash in the extreme," and Keats, no doubt, was influenced by this in giving up medicine for poetry. Severely criticized for his poetry, Keats was dubbed "Pestleman Jack" and was advised to go back to his plasters and pills. Keats died within a few years of tuberculosis, but his poetry is still one of the glories of the English language, thanks to Lucas, whose bungling surgery turned Keats away from medicine, and to Keats's indomitable spirit in writing, despite the early critics.

Another of Cooper's students, more advanced than a surgical dresser, was the Irish surgeon **Abraham Colles** (1773–1843). Only a few years younger than Cooper, Colles had attended Trinity College in Dublin and graduated in medicine at Edinburgh under Monro II. He then studied for a short time with Cooper in London. Colles's grandfather was a physician, but his father ran a marble quarry.

Colles's description of the fracture of the lower radius, which goes by

V.

On the Fracture of the Carpal extremity of the Radius. By A. Colles, M. D. one of the Professors of Anatomy and Surgery in the Royal College of Surgeons in Ireland.

THE injury to which I wish to direct the attention of surgeons, has not, as far as I know, been described by any author; indeed the form of the carpal extremity of the radius would rather incline us to question its being liable to fracture. The absence of crepitus, and of the other common symptoms of fracture, together with the swelling which instantly arises in this, as in other injuries of the wrist, render the difficulty of ascertaining the real nature of the case very considerable.

Abraham Colles: On the fracture of the carpal extremity of the radius. Edinburgh Med. Surg. J., *10*:182–186, 1814. (Courtesy of the Library of the College of Physicians of Philadelphia)

his name, was published in 1814. It was a clear description of the deformity—localizing the area of injury; mentioning the lack of crepitus; and noting the backward or dorsal tilt of the articular surface of the radius, the laxity of the lower ulna, and the difficulty of maintaining the reduction. He pointed out that, if the treatment was insufficient, in time the motion would return and pain disappear, but the deformity would remain. He was clearly knowledgeable of Desault's work and differentiated that lesion from the fracture he was describing.

Colles was 41 when his report was published. He had already been professor of anatomy and surgery for 10 years, and 3 years previously had described Colles's fascia. He emphasized regional rather than systemic anatomy in his study of pathological processes. Documenting his findings with great detail, he was a lucid writer and an excellent teacher. Although surpassed by many in his operative techniques, he was a hard worker and was well thought of for his diagnostic ability and method of handling difficult problems. He was described as being of medium height and well build, with a clear eye and a dignified manner.

In addition to the description of the fracture of the radius and the perineal fascia, Colles's law is named for him. This law noted that a child born of a mother who had no obvious symptoms of syphilis may show the disease at an early age and is capable of infecting a healthy wet nurse, yet never will the child induce an infection in the mother. This work, done long before the spirochete was discovered, as well as his report of

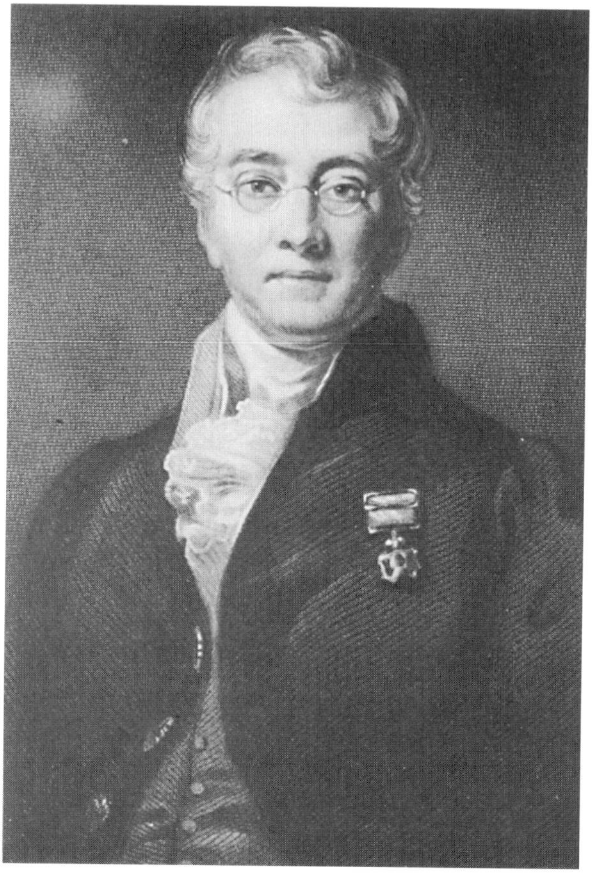

Charles Bell. (Courtesy of the Library of the College of Physicians of Philadelphia, Sturgis Collection)

the fracture, written long before Röntgen's discovery, well illustrates the careful observations and logical thinking of this Irish surgeon.

Colles was twice president of the Irish College of Surgeons. When he was 66 years of age, he declined an offer of a baronetcy, and he retired 2 years later because of ill health. He died at the age of 70 of emphysema, and his attending physician was William Stokes.

A contemporary of Cooper in England and Colles in Ireland was **Charles Bell** (1774–1842), who was born in Edinburgh but who then lived in London for many years. Bell is remembered for Bell's palsy, Bell's law, and the long thoracic nerve of Bell. Although we have nothing specific in surgery of the hand named after him, his name belongs among those having a more direct connection, because of his monograph on the

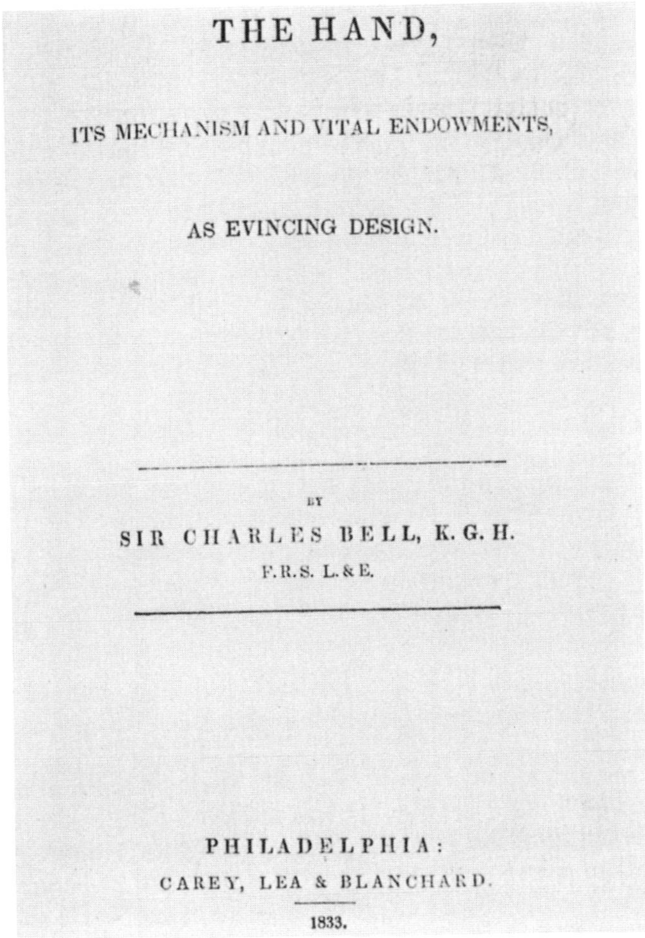

THE HAND,

ITS MECHANISM AND VITAL ENDOWMENTS,

AS EVINCING DESIGN.

BY

SIR CHARLES BELL, K. G. H.

F.R.S. L.&E.

PHILADELPHIA:

CAREY, LEA & BLANCHARD.

1833.

Charles Bell: The Hand, Its Mechanism and Vital Endowments, as Evincing Design. Philadelphia, Carey, Lea & Blanchard, 1833. (Courtesy of the Library of the College of Physicians of Philadelphia)

anatomy of the hand. Bell wrote what was called the Bridgewater Treatises, Treatise IV, titled, *The Hand, Its Mechanism and Vital Endowments as Evincing Design*, in answer to the offer of the Bishop of Bridgewater for monographs in the sciences illustrating the master plan of the Creator. In this work, Bell compared the upper extremity of man to that of the animals, and he graphically described and illustrated the principles of anatomy as related to function. It is beautifully written and well worth being used as an introductory book for young residents in reconstructive surgery. The style is a little old-fashioned, but the words are put together in a most readable fashion. For example, he wrote: "With the possession of an instrument like the hand, there must be a great part of the organization which strictly belongs to it, concealed. The hand is not a thing appended, or put on, like an additional movement in a watch; but a thousand intricate relations must be established throughout the body in connection with it." Or again, "We have seen that the system of bones, muscles, and nerves of this extremity is suited to every form and condition of vertebrated animals; and we must confess that it is in the human hand that we have the consummation of all perfection as an instrument."

This work alone would be enough to entitle him to a place in our anthology, but Charles Bell was also a surgeon, and his descriptions of gunshot wounds and of injuries to tendons and their sheaths are magnificent.

Charles Bell was the youngest of four boys; his father died when he was 5, and his early education was provided by his mother. He was skilled in drawing, painting, and etching and was self-taught in Latin and Greek. He was induced to study medicine by his older brother, John, who operated a private school of anatomy in Edinburgh and who, in his own right, was an anatomist and an artist of some note. When Charles graduated from Edinburgh, he spent most of his time doing dissections and drawings. Then there was a period of dissension between the senior and junior members of the staff of the Royal Infirmary. Both Charles and his brother were not reappointed to the staff, and Charles was not even allowed to sketch the pathological specimens. This drove him to London, where he opened a school of anatomy and attracted many students because of his skill and learning. He was offered a partnership in the famous Great Windmill Street School of John and William Hunter. Accepting this, he gained entree to the Middlesex Hospital, and he became professor of anatomy in the Royal College of Surgeons at age 50. He was knighted by William IV.

He returned to Edinburgh in 1836 to become professor of surgery and died 6 years later of coronary thrombosis, while visiting in England. He is buried in All Hallows churchyard, and a plaque in the local church commemorates the event. This scholarly, studious, and serious Scot deserves a place in the pantheon of anatomists and surgeons who have contributed to the field of surgery of the hand.

In this period of Cooper, Colles, and Bell, there appeared in France one of the most unusual men, a giant of his time, whose name is still today the source of many eponyms. **Guillaume Dupuytren** (1777–1835) is the last of our giants bridging the eighteenth and nineteenth centuries. He was a unique person, very difficult to understand, with most unusual talents. His contemporaries and his biographers have described him as being cold, ruthless, overweeningly ambitious, contemptuous of his

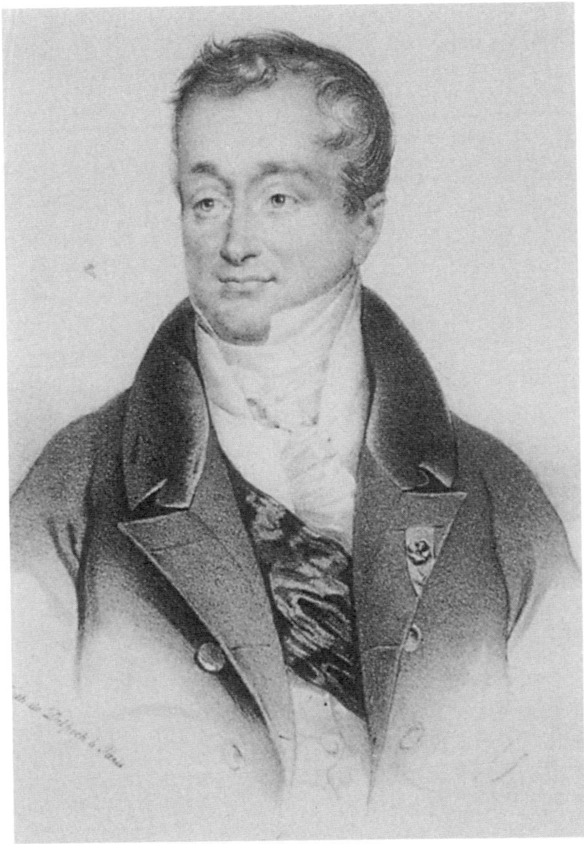

Guillaume Dupuytren. (Courtesy of the Library of the New York Academy of Medicine)

superiors as well as his subordinates, unscrupulous, overbearing, more respected than beloved, a shrewd diagnostician, an operator of unrivaled aplomb, a wonderful clinical teacher, nobody's friend, and the first of surgeons but the last of men. That he had talent and skill there is no doubt. For more than 30 years he was the most renowned surgeon in Europe. His writings are few, but his lectures were reported by students and assistants and were translated and published in England and, in 1883, even in New York. He made many contributions to surgery—a listing in medical classics covers thirty or more pages.

Our interest in this most unusual man lies in his reporting of the contracture of the palmar fascia that bears his name. He failed to credit Astley Paston Cooper with the original description—perhaps through an

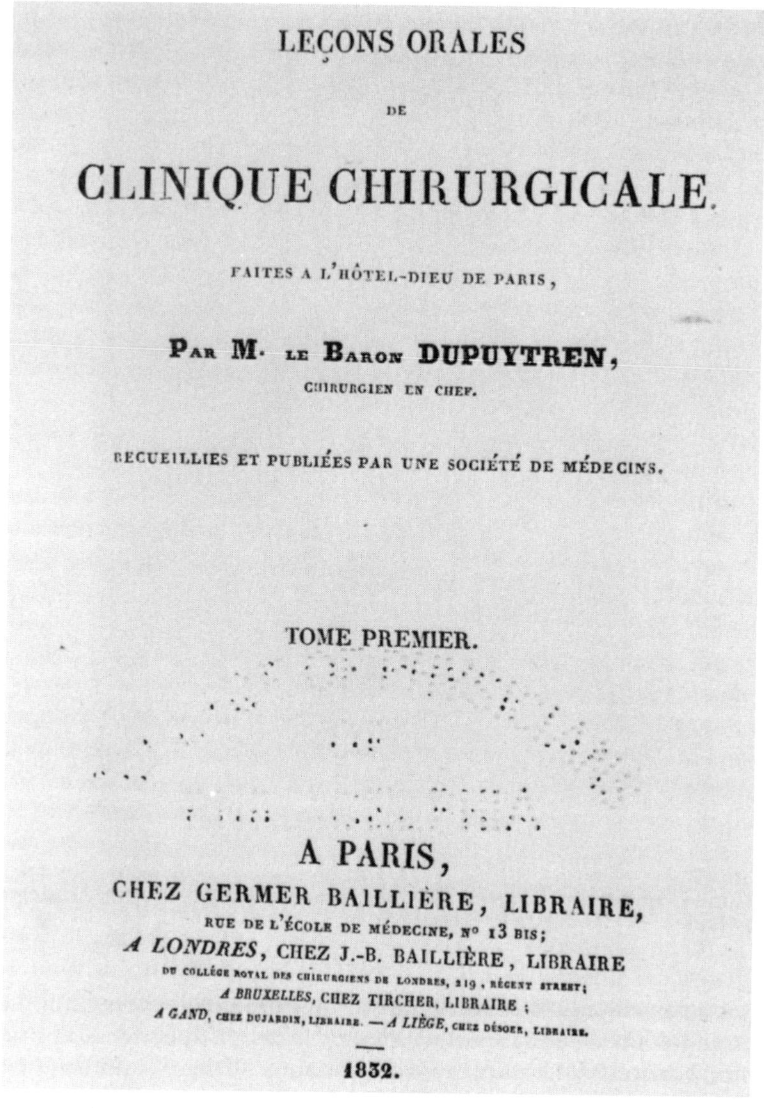

LEÇONS ORALES

DE

CLINIQUE CHIRURGICALE,

FAITES A L'HÔTEL-DIEU DE PARIS,

PAR M. LE BARON DUPUYTREN,

CHIRURGIEN EN CHEF.

RECUEILLIES ET PUBLIÉES PAR UNE SOCIÉTÉ DE MÉDECINS.

TOME PREMIER.

A PARIS,

CHEZ GERMER BAILLIÈRE, LIBRAIRE,

RUE DE L'ÉCOLE DE MÉDECINE, N° 13 BIS;

A LONDRES, CHEZ J.-B. BAILLIÈRE, LIBRAIRE

DU COLLÉGE ROYAL DES CHIRURGIENS DE LONDRES, 219, RÉGENT STREET;

A BRUXELLES, CHEZ TIRCHER, LIBRAIRE;

A GAND, CHEZ DUJARDIN, LIBRAIRE. — *A LIÈGE*, CHEZ DÉSOER, LIBRAIRE.

1832.

Guillaume Dupuytren: Leçons Orales de Clinique Chirurgicale. Paris, Germer Baillière, 1832. (Courtesy of the Library of the College of Physicians of Philadelphia)

oversight, because when he discussed the diagnosis and treatment of the fracture of the lower fibula, which also bears his name, he did refer to the works of Percival Pott and Charles Bell.

Dupuytren's treatment of the contracture of the palmar fascia consisted of open division of the palmar band; whereas Cooper had recommended doing it through a small opening in the skin. (We will see later how William Adams, based on his experiences with subcutaneous tenotomy, designed the modern subcutaneous procedure.) Both Cooper and Dupuytren regarded the contracture as being a result of trauma, the former implicating excessive use of a hammer, oar, or plough as the cause; whereas the latter said it was caused by too violent or too long continued activity.

Dupuytren was born in a small town, Pierre Buffiere. His father was a lawyer or advocate of limited means, and only through the kindness of an army officer stationed at Pierre Buffiere did Dupuytren have any chance of an education. This officer obviously noted the youngster's intelligence and arranged for young Dupuytren to be enrolled in the College of La Marche in Paris, the principal of which was the officer's brother. Their faith in the boy was proven when he became a good student and excelled in philosophy. Why he took up medicine we do not know, but as so many others, it started with anatomy and then pathology. He was only 18 when he was appointed prosector in the medical school, and in a few years he was made chief of the anatomical laboratory. He studied anatomy with Boyer at the Charité and undertook a course of study in physiology and pathology. At 23 he was giving a course of lectures in anatomy, and by the age of 26, had added a course in pathology. Laennec was his student and assistant, but they later quarreled over Dupuytren's treatment and criticism of the work of Bichat, the former chief of pathology.

In 1804, when he was 27 years old, he obtained his first surgical appointment to l'Hôtel Dieu. He was made a surgeon of the second class, and here he began the surgical career in which he would remain the rest of his life and would gain for this hospital a worldwide reputation.

Dupuytren obviously struggled against many obstacles. He was poor and could get no help from his father, who did not agree to his staying in Paris. Perhaps these hardships embittered him and were the cause of his most difficult temperament. He was constantly conniving in his struggle to get ahead; but he did have the talent, and he did apply himself to his work. Nevertheless, he certainly had few friends.

He was competitive to the utmost. A story is told that at one stage, both he and Roux were in line for some surgical appointment. Each had to deliver a thesis in public before the examiners, after being told the topic only 4 hours in advance. Dupuytren won; later when they both wanted to marry the same woman, Dupuytren was again the victor.

In 1808 he was made adjunct surgeon under Pelletan and now was only one step away from being the chief, the position for which he had struggled. Pelletan was no match for the brilliant young surgeon. Pelletan was of the old school, described as having "somewhat laissez-faire principles." Dupuytren knew his anatomy and pathology; he studied the patients carefully, and his surgery was deft, sure, and positive. He became an excellent diagnostician and completely overshadowed the old chief. The final moment came when a Russian army officer was brought in with a large mass in the inguinal region, which Pelletan diagnosed as an abscess and, upon opening it, was unable to stop the hemorrhage. The patient died, and a commission of Russian surgeons investigated the incident. Pelletan lost his position, and Dupuytren was made chief.

L'Hôtel was never to be the same. Dupuytren organized the surgical services, keeping 113 beds to himself. He was tireless, starting with rounds at 6 A.M. on the wards, discussing the patients in practically a monologue. He left no doubt that he was the chief, and though he was said to be sympathetic toward the patients, he could be cold and imperious to his assistants and others of the profession. He demanded detailed histories and records of repeated examinations. He spoke with finality. One of the sayings attributed to him was, "I have been mistaken, but I have been mistaken less than other surgeons." One is reminded of the current definition of a surgeon as one who may be wrong but is never in doubt.

After the rounds, it was customary for the chief, ensconced on a big green sofa, to discuss the problems seen in that session. At this time, notes were made by one of the house officers who was specifically designated for that purpose. After the operating session, further discussions took place and then a review of the pathology. Dupuytren was the first surgeon to make it a rule to be present at the autopsy of any patient who died on his service. An evening visit to the operated patients completed the long day.

Dupuytren developed a large private practice, but this came slowly because of his dedication to his hospital work. He accumulated a fortune, even one time offering a third to the king, who was in some financial strait. Much of his money went to endow the Musée Dupuytren (of pathology).

In 1833 he had a small stroke, resulting in some thickening of his speech. The next year he took his first vacation, traveling to Italy. He died in February, 1835.

Dupuytren was probably the best-known surgeon of his day and contributed much to surgery. But he was a "meteor in the world of science." Balzac, in 1837, published the novel *Messe de l'Athée*, in which the character Dr. Desplein is supposed to be Dupuytren. His poverty of the early years and his struggles are well described, and Balzac ends with the saying, "Like all geniuses, he was without an heir." True, he had no heirs, and few of what must have been a multitude of students have carried on his work. Laennec was one of Dupuytren's students for a short

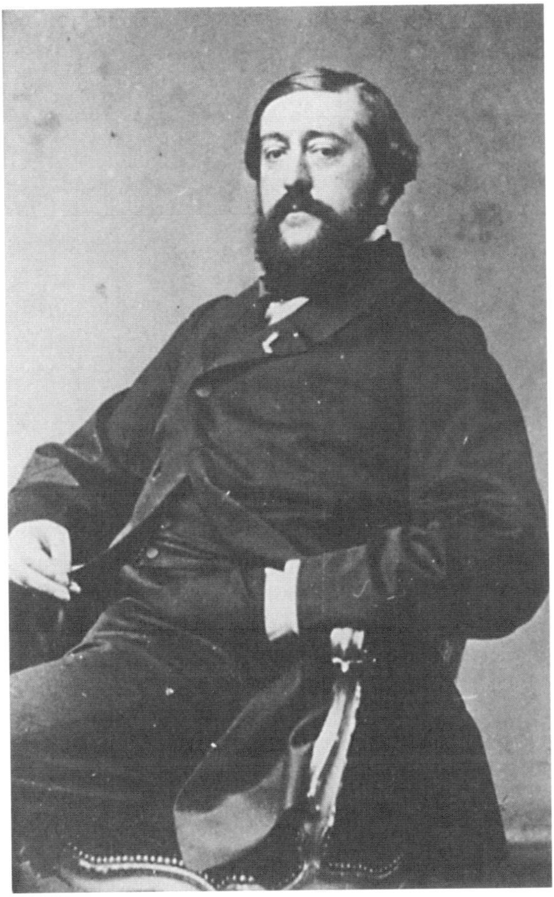

Jacques Matthieu Delpech. (From French Doctors of the 2nd Half of the 19th Century. Courtesy of the Rare Book Collection of the Library of the Los Angeles County Medical Association)

time, but he made his name in medicine, not in surgery. Some of his other students were Lembert, Nélaton, and possibly Dieffenbach, but none truly inherited his standing or carried on in his place. None of his biographers even mentions who succeeded him as chief surgeon.

Dupuytren was a genius, but a "meteor." He is well remembered in many eponymic lesions even today. We can respect his skills, his talents, and his dedication, but it is difficult to excuse his lust for power and the means he used to attain his place in the surgical world.

The seventeenth and eighteenth centuries gave us many names that have come down to us a eponyms, for these were times of individuals.

CONSIDÉRATIONS SUR LA DIFFORMITÉ APPELÉE PIEDS-BOTS.

IL est peu d'affections qui aient moins fixé l'attention des observateurs, et sur lesquelles on ait moins d'études approfondies et de principes fondés sur l'observation de la nature. Il faut peut-être rapporter à deux principaux motifs l'état stationnaire de la science à cet égard : en premier lieu, la maladie dont il s'agit est chronique, et la patience de l'homme est rarement à l'épreuve d'une longue application et de la lenteur des découvertes; en second lieu, une maladie qui altère pour jamais les formes extérieures, et qui peut rendre très-défectueuse l'une des plus importantes fonctions, devait tenter la cupidité des empiriques, en raison de l'empressement des malades. Il faut même convenir, à la honte de l'art, que, à l'occasion de cette difformité, plusieurs médecins se sont montrés aussi dépourvus de délicatesse et d'humanité que les empiriques; en sorte que la science est restée privée d'un grand nombre de faits importans, dont la

Jacques Matthieu Delpech: Considérations sur la difformité appelée pieds-bots. Chir. Clin. Montpellier, *1*:147–473, 1823. (Courtesy of the National Library of Medicine, Bethesda, Maryland)

The outstanding surgeons were anatomists first and were also knowledgeable in pathology. Many of the principles they followed were empirical, handed down by tradition or developed as the result of their own observations. Experimental surgery was not common, though Camper had done his symphysiotomy on pigs to demonstrate the feasibility of the procedure, and John Hunter was performing his experiments. They were the exceptions.

There was another surgeon of this time whose name has no connection with surgery of the upper extremity, but who should be mentioned because of the relationship of his work to the development of subcutaneous fasciotomy for Dupuytren's contracture.

Jacques Matthieu Delpech (1777–1832) was the pioneer orthopaedist of France. In 1816 he did the first subcutaneous tenotomy of the Achilles tendon for clubfoot. Knowing of this work, William J. Little, in search of relief of his deformity, would consult him and later, after Stromeyer's operation on him, would bring the operation to England and then influence Adams to try it for the palmar fascia contracture.

Delpech was shot and killed by a patient upon whom he had operated for a varicocele. The patient claimed that he was left "unfit for marriage."

THE EARLY NINETEENTH CENTURY

The nineteenth century saw many new medical discoveries and developments. It was a time of tremendous change in the thinking of men, with advances in communication, mechanics, and applied science. Fielding H. Garrison* has summarized the changes in medicine in this period as being the discovery of anesthetics, the development of antiseptic surgery by Lister and aseptic surgery (steam sterilization) by Ernst von Bergmann, the change to conservative surgery of the extremities, and the rise of the surgical specialties (e.g., plastic, orthopaedic, abdominal, and intracranial surgery). Important endeavors during this period were the beginning of medical education in the United States and Russia, the founding of surgical societies and associations, and the transmission of information and rapid interchange of ideas by means of special periodicals and journals.

Also in this era were the Napoleonic Wars; Faraday's discovery of the induced current of electricity, which led to the works of Duchenne and Erb; and the cell theory of Schleiden and Schwann, which focused the attention of anatomists and pathologists on the detailed structure of organs. The use of the microscope followed improvements in the making of lenses, and the Weigert's stains brought out the ultrastructure. Koch's discovery of the tubercle bacillus was the stimulus for a whole new field.

*An Introduction to the History of Medicine. With Medical Chronology, Suggestions for Study and Bibliographic Data. Philadelphia, W. B. Saunders, 1929.

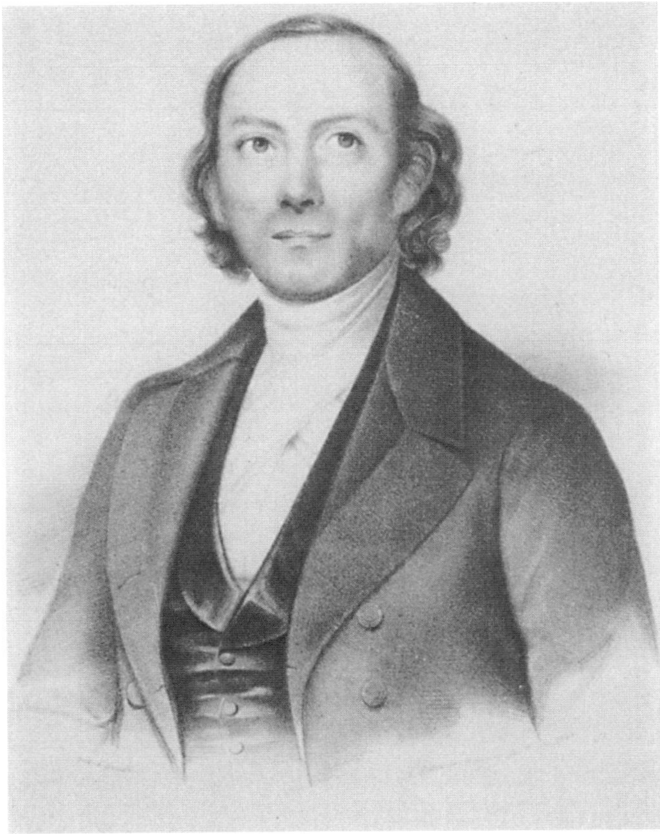

Ernst Heinrich Weber. (Courtesy of the Library of the New York Academy of Medicine)

Pasteur's work, of course, set the stage for Lister and, later, Bergmann. The Civil War in the United States saw the first use of battlefield ambulances and a planned system of evacuation through the work of the surgeon general, Letterman. The pavilion system of hospital construction developed from the experiences of this war and the Franco-Prussian War of 1870. Röntgen's discovery came in the last decade of this marvelous century, and the first vascular suture bridged the nineteenth and twentieth centuries.

The first names we come across in this nineteenth century era are those of two men whose work helped to clarify the function of the peripheral nerves.

Ernst Heinrich Weber (1795–1878) gave us Weber's law—the intensity of a sensation is dependent on the mode of application of the

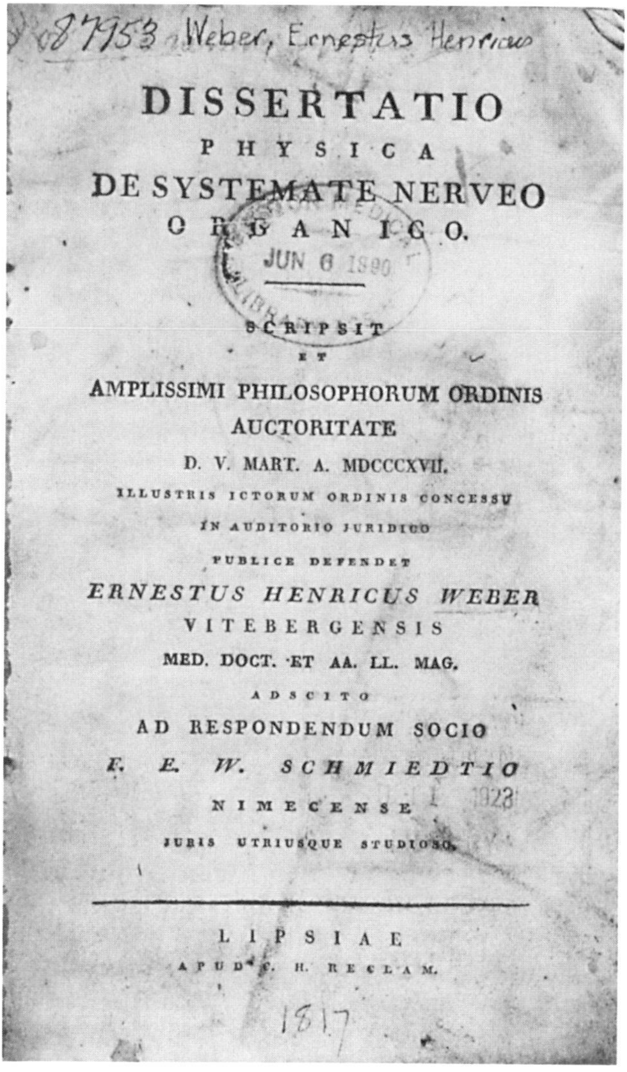

DISSERTATIO
PHYSICA
DE SYSTEMATE NERVEO
ORGANICO.

SCRIPSIT
ET
AMPLISSIMI PHILOSOPHORUM ORDINIS
AUCTORITATE
D. V. MART. A. MDCCCXVII.
ILLUSTRIS ICTORUM ORDINIS CONCESSU
IN AUDITORIO IURIDICO
PUBLICE DEFENDET
ERNESTUS HENRICUS WEBER
VITEBERGENSIS
MED. DOCT. ET AA. LL. MAG.
ADSCITO
AD RESPONDENDUM SOCIO
F. E. W. SCHMIEDTIO
NIMECENSE
IURIS UTRIUSQUE STUDIOSO.

LIPSIAE
APUD C. H. RECLAM.

Ernst Heinrich Weber: Dissertatio Physica de Systemate Nerveo Organico. Leipzig, C. H. Reclam, 1817. (Courtesy of the Library of the New York Academy of Medicine)

stimulus—and the Weber-Fechner law—the intensity of sensation varies with the log of the stimulus. The Weber test (or the two-point discrimination popularized by Moberg) was described in 1834 as being a tactile illusion, occurring when two compass points kept equidistant are applied to the skin over similar surfaces of varying sensitivity and cause the subject to experience a converging sensation as one goes from an area of increased sensitivity to one of lesser sensitivity. The illusion involves the relative location and the estimation of the intervening distance, the latter being the basis for the present method of use.

Ernst was the oldest of three boys and acted as a preceptor for his younger brothers, Eduard Friedrich Weber (1806–1871) and Wilhelm Eduard Weber (1804–1891). They collaborated in various studies, Ernst and Eduard on a study of the inhibitory action of the vagus nerve. With Wilhelm, Ernst was the first to study and measure the pulse wave, and in 1836 these two (Wilhelm was professor of physics at Göttingen) published an important work on the physiology of motion and the mechanism of joints. Wilhelm is credited with having built the first electromagnetic telegraph in 1833.

Their father was professor of theology at Wittenberg, where the boys were born and went to school. Ernst took his medical degree there in 1815 and then practiced for 2 years in Leipzig. He returned to Wittenberg as privatdocent until 1821, when he was appointed professor of anatomy and physiology, succeeding his former teacher, Rosenmüller. He remained as chief of both for 45 years before giving up the chair of physiology to Ludwig. Five years later he retired, and William His took the chair of anatomy.

Weber's major interest was in the field of sensation, measuring the senses of pain, heat, pressure, and smell. The rotary electromagnetic apparatus was used in the vagal stimulation experiments.

When we use the two-point discrimination test as a measure of tactilegnosis (Moberg), we are paying tribute to an illustrious family of investigators whose early work set the stage for much of the work on peripheral nerves that was to follow.

The second name we come across in the early nineteenth century is that of **Guillaume Benjamin Amand Duchenne** (1806–1875)—or as he preferred to call himself, Duchenne de Boulogne. Born of generations of seafaring people, he carried the traits of these stubborn, determined people with him to overcome many difficulties and eventually, but belatedly, to become one of the giants of our profession. His life presents an extraordinary example of a person working against all odds, in spite of the disregard of most of his confreres. Except for Trousseau, who spoke in his behalf, and for Charcot, much of his work would have been lost, for he had difficulty in expressing his ideas. Not having a hospital appointment or a teaching position, he made his way through the wards of the Paris hospitals, examining patients, recording his findings, and following through to the autopsy to verify his hypotheses. He was a joke to the interns and was ridiculed by most of the staff, but this man of medium height and build, with broad shoulders and a deep chest, was indepen-

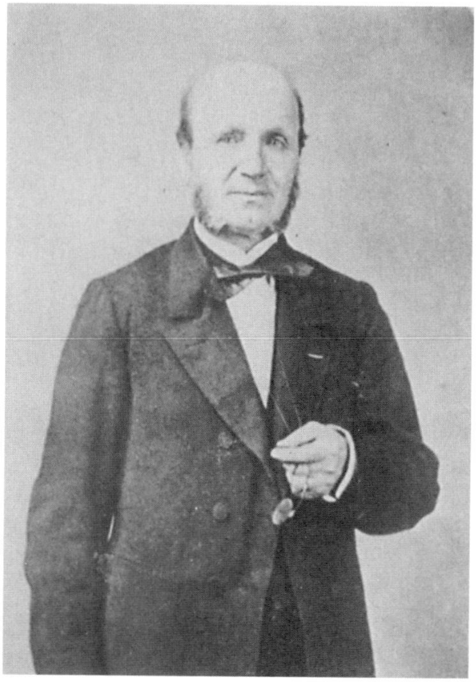

Guillaume Benjamin Amand Duchenne. [From Scrapbook of portraits of physicians and surgeons. New York?, 18—?] (Courtesy of the Library of the New York Academy of Medicine)

dent and tenacious, and he persevered through all trials. He sometimes appeared to be absentminded, but he could be jolly or brusque, yet cordial. He was never to be discouraged. He said he wanted to live in his works, that honors won today might be forgotten tomorrow, but his work would still live. And it has lived, for he was a keen observer who recorded his findings, carried out his tests with care, and honestly reported what he found. His writings were well received in other countries, and when he died—though only a few close friends attended the funeral—his name was familiar to workers in neurology in Rome, St. Petersburg, Geneva, and Leipzig. Yet it was 20 years before the neurologists in France granted him recognition and gave him his rightful place, with Charcot and Marie, as one of the giants of neurology.

Duchenne's name is known to us for his descriptions of pseudohypertrophic muscular dystrophy; poliomyelitis, locomotor ataxia, and progressive bulbar paralysis. He was accurate in his descriptions, and he carefully delineated the various clinical entities. He is best known for the

L'ÉLECTRISATION LOCALISÉE

ET DE SON APPLICATION

A LA PHYSIOLOGIE, A LA PATHOLOGIE ET A LA THÉRAPEUTIQUE,

PAR LE DOCTEUR

DUCHENNE DE BOULOGNE,

Lauréat de l'Institut de France et de la Société de médecine de Gand,
Membre titulaire de la Société de médecine de Paris, correspondant des Académies
ou Sociétés de médecine de Bordeaux, Lyon, Strasbourg,
Dresde, Florence, Genève, Leipzig, Stockholm, Würzbourg, etc., etc.

Accompagné de 108 Figures intercalées dans le texte.

A PARIS,

CHEZ J.-B. BAILLIÈRE,

LIBRAIRE DE L'ACADÉMIE IMPÉRIALE DE MÉDECINE,
RUE HAUTEFEUILLE, 19;

A LONDRES, CHEZ H. BAILLIÈRE, 219, REGENT-STREET;
A NEW-YORK, CHEZ H. BAILLIÈRE, 290, BROADWAY;
A MADRID, CHEZ BAILLY-BAILLIÈRE, CALLE DEL PRINCIPE, N° 11.

1855.

L'auteur et l'éditeur se réservent le droit de traduction à l'étranger.

Guillaume Benjamin Amand Duchenne: L'électrisation Localisée. Paris, J. B. Baillière, 1855. (Courtesy, Library of the College of Physicians of Philadelphia)

description of progressive muscular atrophy—though Aran published the case reports, giving credit to Duchenne. Duchenne believed that poliomyelitis was a disease of the spinal cord, agreeing with Heine, and he studied the paralyses of lead poisoning. Erb-Duchenne paralysis gets its name from the publication in 1877 by Erb, who quoted Duchenne's observation of similar paralyses in the newborn.

Duchenne was graduated in medicine from the University of Paris in 1831, during the time of Laennec, Dupuytren, Magendie, Velpeau, and Cruveilhier. He returned to Boulogne, married, and had a son. After 2 years his wife died, and he became depressed and failed to keep up his practice. He read, played the violin, and spent hours at the waterfront with the local fishermen. His wife's family took the son, and after some years Duchenne decided to return to Paris. He had become interested in electricity as a method of treatment (Faraday had discovered the induced current in 1831) and, urged by a friend and classmate, Dr. Charles Gros, he made the break and spent the rest of his life in Paris.

One cannot imagine what the study of nervous diseases was at that time. There was no separation of functional from organic lesions; all patients with motor problems were classified as having "paralysis." There was no systematic examination of the nervous system; that was developed later by Erb in Germany. Waller's work on degeneration was not yet done. A country doctor, with his battery and electrodes, lacking any official position, was not very welcome by the monarchs of the wards.

Duchenne apparently had great difficulty in expressing his ideas; it was said that it would have been impossible for him to lecture on any subject, and it was Trousseau who expressed his ideas for him. His writings, however, were well received, and his publications were frequent. There is a question as to how familiar he was with the work of others, especially in the German and English literature, although in those times there was little interchange in any field. It was the time of the revolution, the siege of Paris, and the rise and fall of the Paris commune.

His first publication was on the stimulation of muscles by the faradic current (1855). Eventually, a complete work, the *Physiology of Motion*, came out. Emmanuel Kaplan has translated this most interesting study, one of the classics of medicine. It is in this work that one finds the first studies of the effects of paralysis of the intrinsic muscles of the hand.

Duchenne's son was graduated as a physician, and they were finally reunited in Paris. Unfortunately, the son died of dementia praecox at the age of 25. The young man's wife, Mlle. Julie Bonnel, was a great comfort to Duchenne in his last years, when, within 1 year, his second wife, a brother, his son, and a number of other relatives died. It was the year of the siege of Paris and a most depressing period. Duchenne began to

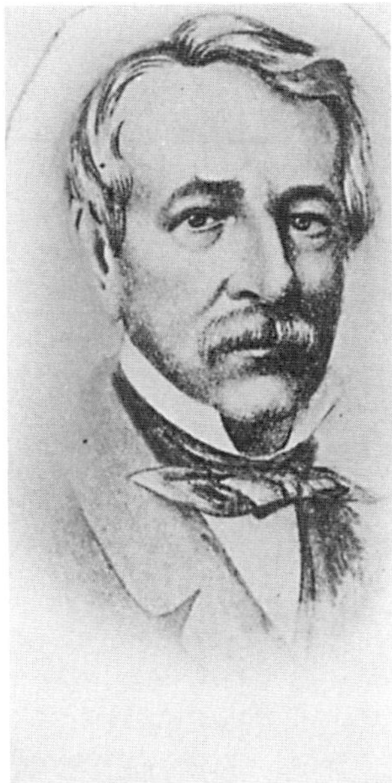

Georg Friedrich Louis Stromeyer. (From Keith, Sir Arthur: Menders of the Maimed. London, Oxford University Press, 1919)

show signs of cerebral arteriosclerosis, and after 4 years of steady suffering, he died of a cerebral hemorrhage. He was buried at Boulogne. Finally, in 1897, a monument to his memory was placed in the Hospital of the Salpêtrière.

Duchenne became "commanding" because there was a subject suited to his talents and an opportunity present for their development. But he made the subject, and he created the opportunity, in spite of overwhelming obstacles.

In Germany during this early part of the nineteenth century, much was happening in surgery. Langenbeck went from the professorship at Kiel to Berlin, where he succeeded Dieffenbach. He had trained Billroth, Esmarch, and Trendelenburg. Stromeyer took the chair at Kiel.

Georg Friedrich Louis Stromeyer (1804–1876) was born in Hanover and studied in Göttingen and Berlin. His father, Christian F. Stromeyer, was also a surgeon who had spent a year of study in England; later he would bring Jenner's cowpox inoculation method to Germany. He influenced his son to travel to France and England. Georg Stromeyer was a professor, first at Erlangen, then at Munich and Freiburg before settling in Kiel, where he was also the surgeon general of the Hanoverian army. He wrote extensively on war wounds and field sanitation. In 1870 he was

VI.

Die Durchschneidung der Achillessehne, als Heilmethode des Klumpfuſses, durch zwei Fälle erläutert.

Von

Dr. Louis Stromeyer,

Königl. Hann. Hofchirurgen und Lehrer der Chirurgie an der chirurgischen Schule zu Hannover.

Mit einer Abbildung.

Obgleich schon von andern Wundärzten die Durchschneidung verkürzter Sehnen als Heilmethode einzelner Verkrümmungen empfohlen worden ist, so gebührt doch unstreitig Delpech, der leider vor kurzem als Opfer seines Berufes und seines Erfindungsgeistes durch die Hand eines verruchten Mörders gefallen ist, das Verdienst, diese Operation wissenschaftlich begründet zu haben, indem er die Bildung einer fibrösen Zwischensubstanz als das eigentliche Heilbestreben dabei aufstellte, eine Verbesserung, wodurch der Methode erst ihr Werth gesichert wird, indem man auf diese Weise nicht die Muskeln, deren Sehnen man durchschneidet, für immer

N 2

Georg Friedrich Louis Stromeyer: Die Durchschneidung der Achillessehne, als Heilmethode des Klumpsusses, durch zwei Fälle erläutert. Mag. Gesamte Heil, Berlin, pages 195–218, 1833. (Courtesy of the National Library of Medicine, Bethesda, Maryland)

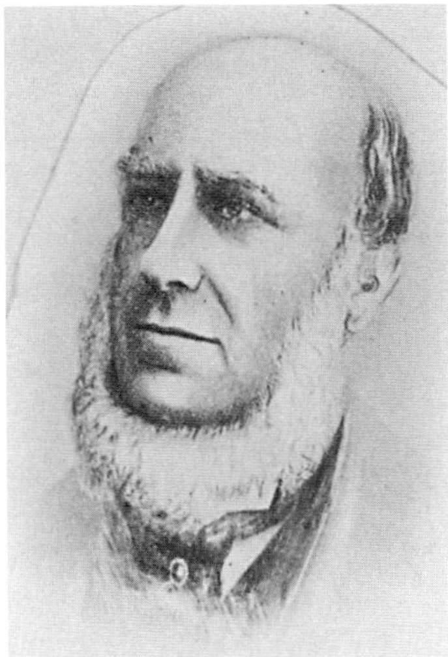

William John Little. (From Keith, Sir Arthur: Menders of the Maimed. London, Oxford University Press, 1919)

in the Prussian army for the battle of Sedan and the siege of Paris, where Volkmann was a surgeon at headquarters. Esmarch and Thiersch trained under Stromeyer.

It was in 1836 that Stromeyer operated on **William John Little** (1810–1894), doing a subcutaneous tenotomy of the Achilles for talipes equinovarus. Delpech, at Montpellier, had done this operation some years before, but when Little consulted him he was not very encouraging, because of the fear of infection.

Little was born in East London. At 2 years of age, he had a febrile disease, with resulting palsy of the left foot. At the age of 16, having gone to early school in France, he was apprenticed to an apothecary. Two years later, he enrolled as a student at London Hospital.

The relief of his deformity was uppermost in his mind and, being familiar with French, he knew of Delpech's work. Delpech advised him not to have the operation because of the fear of infection, so Little returned to England to study for his surgical qualification at Guy's Hospital, with Hodgkin in the autopsy room and with Robert Grant in anatomy. He failed in practice as a surgeon and believed that his only solution was to qualify as a physician, but this meant 2 more years of study. He decided to go to Germany, to Johannes Müller's laboratory in Berlin.

Müller was one of the leading anatomists and had the faculty of attract-

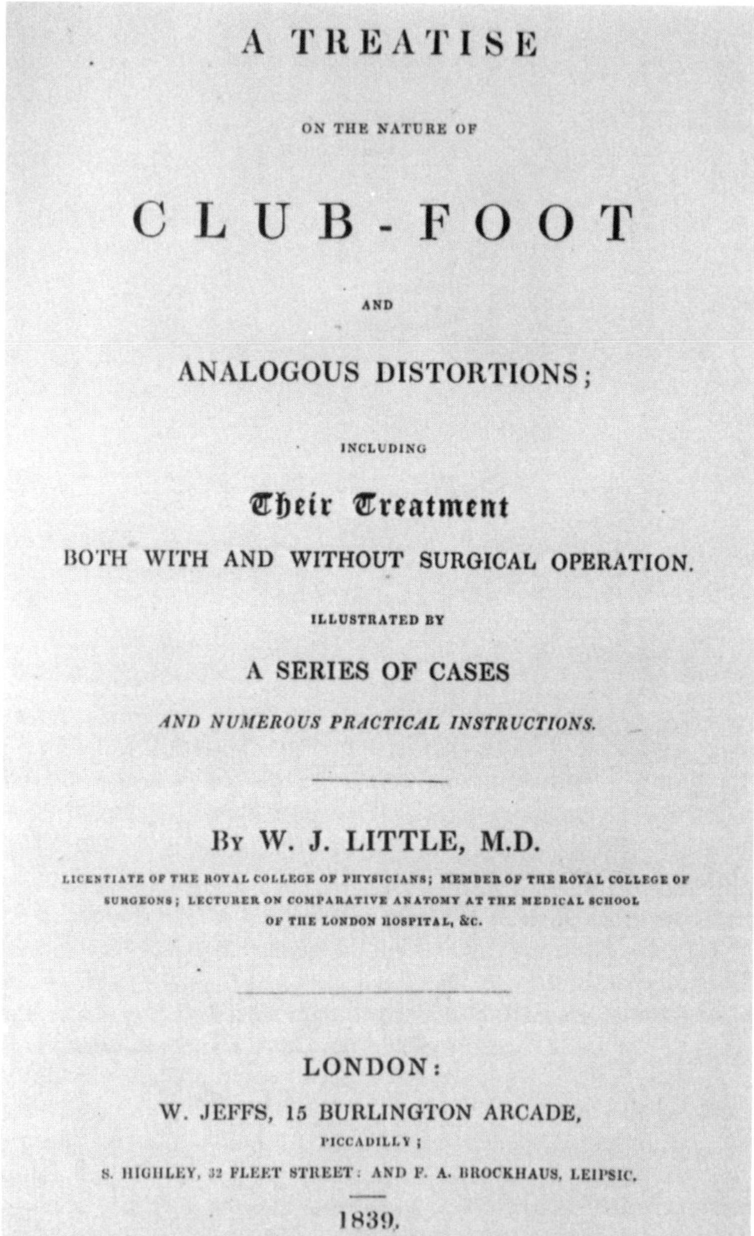

A TREATISE

ON THE NATURE OF

CLUB-FOOT

AND

ANALOGOUS DISTORTIONS;

INCLUDING

Their Treatment

BOTH WITH AND WITHOUT SURGICAL OPERATION.

ILLUSTRATED BY

A SERIES OF CASES

AND NUMEROUS PRACTICAL INSTRUCTIONS.

BY W. J. LITTLE, M.D.

LICENTIATE OF THE ROYAL COLLEGE OF PHYSICIANS; MEMBER OF THE ROYAL COLLEGE OF SURGEONS; LECTURER ON COMPARATIVE ANATOMY AT THE MEDICAL SCHOOL OF THE LONDON HOSPITAL, &c.

LONDON:

W. JEFFS, 15 BURLINGTON ARCADE,

PICCADILLY;

S. HIGHLEY, 32 FLEET STREET: AND F. A. BROCKHAUS, LEIPSIC.

1839.

William John Little: A Treatise on the Nature of Club-foot and Analogous Distortions. London, W. Jeffs, 1839. (Courtesy of the Library of the College of Physicians of Philadelphia)

ing students who later became famous in their own right. At this time, Schwann, Henle, and Remak were there, and Adams joined them. Hearing of Stromeyer's work, Little went to Kiel and had the operation, which was successful. Little became engrossed in the subject, wrote his doctoral thesis on the treatment of clubfoot, and introduced the operation into England. He wrote on all aspects of foot deformity. Whereas Delpech and Stromeyer had tenotomized only the Achilles, Little cut any tendon that added to the deformity. Also, Stromeyer had applied splints after operation, to correct the deformity gradually, whereas Little attempted to obtain an immediate correction.

Little became the pioneer orthopaedist in London and founded the Royal Orthopaedic Hospital, which later became the Royal National Orthopaedic Hospital. He described the spastic disease that is named for him in a paper given before the obstetrical society, and he also pioneered the use of intravenous saline. Some years later, he became less enthusiastic about the tenotomies. He retired in 1884 and died 10 years later.

While Little was active, Paget, who was only 25 years old, was working at St. Bart's Hospital, studying the blood supply of tendons. But an associate of Little, William Adams was doing the same work and made a major contribution to the subject.

William Adams (1820–1900) was born in London and went to medical school at St. Thomas's. He studied anatomy and physiology at a private school, called Webb, under a man named Grainger. When, in a few years, this school was taken over by St. Thomas's Hospital, Adams was named curator of the museum and demonstrator of anatomy.

His association with Little and the Royal Orthopaedic Hospital stimulated his interest in the healing of tendons. He published a monograph on it in 1860, in which he disagreed with Paget. Adams believed that the sheath had an essential role in the healing process, and he based his ideas on the study of human material; over a 9-year period he was able to study fifteen instances of tendon sections done from 4 days to 3 years before. Adams wrote a prize-winning essay on clubfoot in 1866, and he developed an ingenious splint that was used for many years.

It was Adams's use of the principle of subcutaneous surgery that led to his monograph on its use for Dupuytren's contracture, in which he also described a method of relieving depressed scars, such as those from old tuberculous sinuses in the neck. For his fasciotome, Adams designed a knife and pointed out the technique of multiple small openings in the skin, and the importance of undermining the skin first and then dividing the contracted band, with the knife edge *away* from the skin, thus avoiding the possibility of damaging one of the neurovascular bundles. Adams used a splint to keep the finger extended.

Adams was also interested in scoliosis and problems in the hip. He

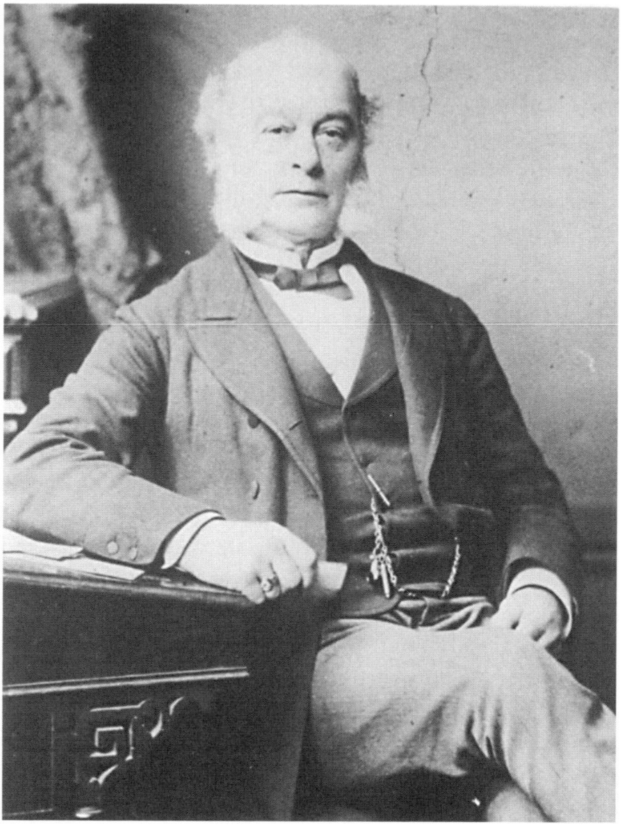

William Adams. (Courtesy of the Library of the College of Physicians of Philadelphia, Sturgis Collection)

was probably the first in England to perform the Langenbeck subcutaneous osteotomy of the femur for the hip ankylosed in flexion. He reported a series of sixty cases of congenital dislocation of the hip; he regarded the condition as being a defect of the acetabulum, and because he was unable to maintain the reduction, he considered the deformity to be incurable.

Adams visited the United States in 1876, when he and Lister were observers at an operation done by Sayre. He was made an honorary member of the American Orthopaedic Association in 1895.

William Adams should have his name coupled with the operation of subcutaneous fasciotomy for Dupuytren's contracture. His surgery in this and other areas was the best of his day; it was built on a solid foundation of anatomy and pathology. He made some of the early observations on healing in human tendons and, with the equipment and

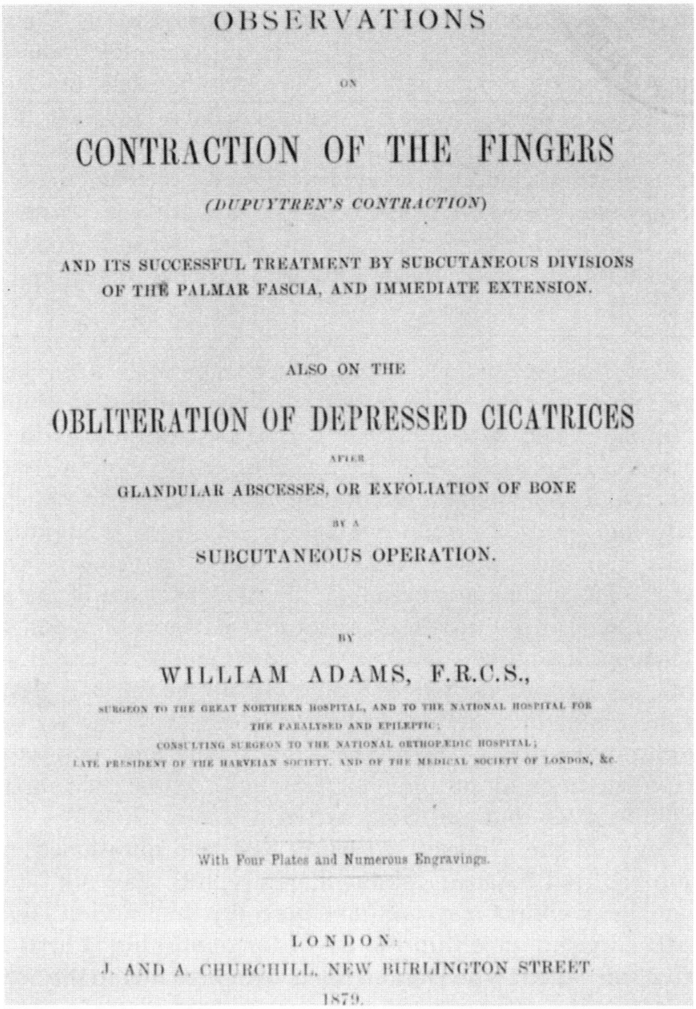

OBSERVATIONS

ON

CONTRACTION OF THE FINGERS

(DUPUYTREN'S CONTRACTION)

AND ITS SUCCESSFUL TREATMENT BY SUBCUTANEOUS DIVISIONS OF THE PALMAR FASCIA, AND IMMEDIATE EXTENSION.

ALSO ON THE

OBLITERATION OF DEPRESSED CICATRICES

AFTER

GLANDULAR ABSCESSES, OR EXFOLIATION OF BONE

BY A

SUBCUTANEOUS OPERATION.

BY

WILLIAM ADAMS, F.R.C.S.,

SURGEON TO THE GREAT NORTHERN HOSPITAL, AND TO THE NATIONAL HOSPITAL FOR THE PARALYSED AND EPILEPTIC;
CONSULTING SURGEON TO THE NATIONAL ORTHOPÆDIC HOSPITAL;
LATE PRESIDENT OF THE HARVEIAN SOCIETY, AND OF THE MEDICAL SOCIETY OF LONDON, &c.

With Four Plates and Numerous Engravings.

LONDON:
J. AND A. CHURCHILL, NEW BURLINGTON STREET
1879.

William Adams: Observations on Contraction of the Fingers. London, J. and A. Churchill, 1879. (Courtesy of the Library of the College of Physicians of Philadelphia)

methods then available, came to conclusions regarding this process that have continued to be valid.

Adams's surgical career covered the major part of the nineteenth century. He saw the change from the subcutaneous method of surgery to open operation when Listerism was introduced. He retired the year Ernst von Bergmann introduced steam sterilization and the era of aseptic surgery began. The principal aim of subcutaneous surgery also had been the prevention of contamination, but by excluding the air. The carbolic acid spray, of course, was an attempt to do the same, by "cleaning" the air. Some operating rooms still use the ultraviolet light for this same purpose, but only when the room is not in actual use; however, the use of these rays during operation was promoted for many years at Duke University. Interestingly enough, when the original Lane Hospital was built in San Francisco, the walls of the one operating room were plastered with a mixture of bichloride of mercury and the usual lime and cement! Today we have Charnley's "greenhouse," the laminar flow rooms, and special masks, all efforts to exclude the "bad" air from the open wounds.

The story of what is now an accepted procedure of treatment for some of the palmar fascial contractures has taken us through many years and the work of many men. Cooper described the lesion and divided the bands through small skin incisions; Dupuytren called attention to the disease and made it recognizable by his descriptions, but he divided the skin and bands, leaving the wound open. Little, because of his own deformity and the good result obtained by Stromeyer, brought the subcutaneous methods into general use; Adams, working with Little, adapted the subcutaneous methods to the specific lesion of the palm.

In the middle of the nineteenth century, a French surgeon, **Charles Pierre Denonvilliers** (1808–1872), transposed some skin flaps in what we today call the Z-plasty maneuver, though he did not call it by that name, nor did he apparently recognize it as a new method. (Perhaps it is one of those techniques that is "discovered" repeatedly, and only when it is brought to our attention in some publication do we feel that some priority should be given that particular writer.)

This origin of the Z-plasty procedure has been questioned, and the confusion occurred because Denonvilliers's reports were not illustrated. Although Denonvilliers may not have been the first, Robert Henry Ivy, the plastic surgeon, gave him the credit for publishing it first. Ivy believed that the patient who Denonvilliers demonstrated to the Société de Chirurgie in 1854, before operation and again that same year after operation, was the source for a drawing that was done to illustrate the procedure in a textbook that was published in 1911. This same drawing was copied into John Staige Davis's work in 1919.

One of Denonvilliers's students, Cazelles, in his thesis, added that the same shifting of flaps in the Z fashion was used by Denonvilliers to correct a scar at the corner of the mouth as well as the ectropion that resulted from the extension of this scar to the eye. Cazelles's work illustrated the before and after condition in a drawing.

Denonvilliers was born in Paris, took his medical degree there in 1837, and became an accomplished anatomist and surgeon. He taught descrip-

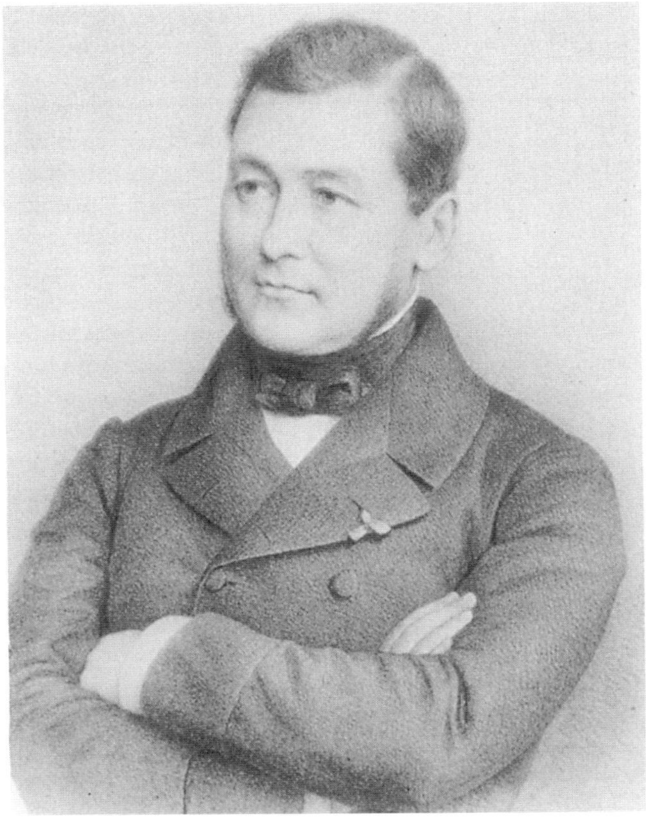

Charles Pierre Denonvilliers. (Courtesy of the Library of the New York Academy of Medicine)

tive and surgical anatomy for many years and succeeded Breschet in the chair of anatomy. He had the reputation of being an excellent operator, especially in plastic procedures.

He was very active in teaching and performing surgery, and, he was a prolific writer for 20 years. In 1858, he suddenly stopped these activities. He became inspector general of public instruction for medicine and took an active part in the development of medical education. When his only son died prematurely in 1864, he never again appeared in public. Death followed a stroke in 1872. Two years later a memorial service was held by the surgical society, and its secretary, Felix Guyon, said, "He (Denonvilliers) was dying for 8 years."

— 35 —

COMITÉ SECRET.

Prix fondé par J.-B. Duval. — La Société de chirurgie de Paris, après une donation de M. Duval, fonde à titre d'encouragement un prix annuel de la valeur de 100 francs, en livres, pour l'auteur de la meilleure thèse de chirurgie publiée en France dans le courant de l'année. Autant que possible, les recherches doivent porter sur un seul sujet, et s'appuyer sur des observations recueillies par l'auteur lui-même dans un service d'hôpital.

Tous les auteurs anciens ou modernes qui ont traité le même sujet devront être indiqués, ainsi que la source précise des citations.

Sont admis seuls à concourir les docteurs ayant rempli les fonctions d'internes définitifs dans les hôpitaux civils, ou ayant un grade analogue dans les hôpitaux militaires ou de la marine.

Les auteurs qui voudront concourir devront adresser *franco*, avant le 15 mai 1855, deux exemplaires de leur thèse au secrétaire général de la Société, et indiquer dans la lettre d'envoi les hôpitaux où ils ont fait leurs études.

Le secrétaire de la Société : E. FOLLIN.

Séance du 19 juillet 1854.

Présidence de M. HUGUIER.

PRÉSENTATION DE MALADES.

M. DENONVILLIERS fait voir à la Société un jeune homme qui, en exerçant sa profession de rémouleur, reçut au visage un éclat d'une meule qui se brisa en plusieurs fragments. Il y eut un décollement assez considérable des parties profondes; mais le malade guérit, en conservant toutefois une bride cicatricielle qui s'étend de l'angle externe de l'œil droit à la commissure de la lèvre du même côté. Le tiraillement exercé par cette cicatrice sur la paupière inférieure est plus grave que celui de la lèvre, car l'œil ne peut pas se fermer. De plus, les cils déviés se rapprochent de la conjonctive et y entretiennent un état inflammatoire. Cette fâcheuse difformité engage M. Denonvilliers à pratiquer ici une opération; mais avant d'entreprendre quelque chose, il a voulu présenter ce malade à la Société, qui appréciera plus tard le résultat opératoire.

Summary of a case which Charles Pierre Denonvilliers presented to the Society of Surgery, Paris. Bull. Soc. Chir., 5:35–36, 1854–1855. (Courtesy of the Library of the College of Physicians of Philadelphia)

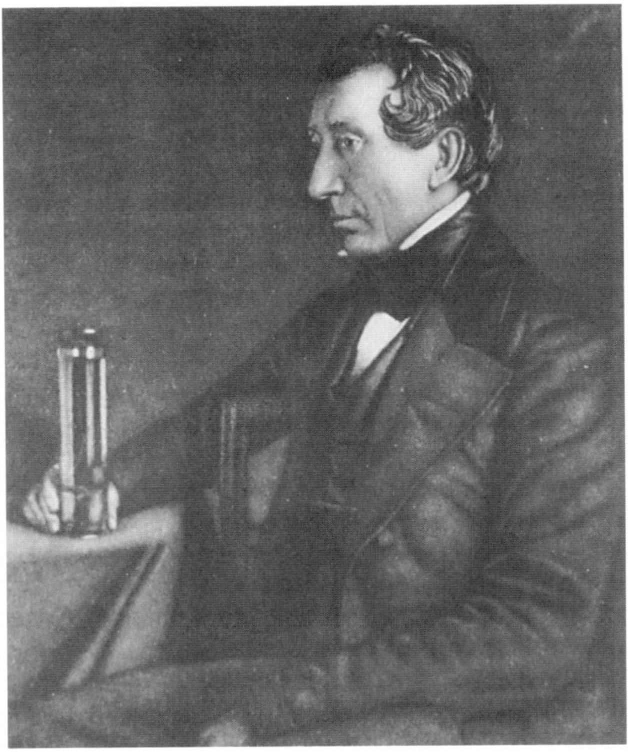

William E. Horner. (Courtesy of the Library of the College of Physicians of Philadelphia, Sturgis Collection)

A. F. Borges and T. Gibson* have recently found evidence of a prior use of the Z-plasty procedure by the American surgeon and anatomist, **William E. Horner** (1793–1853). In 1837 Horner described a procedure in the right lower eyelid, and his diagram of the operation (Figure 2 of Borges and Gibson's paper) leaves no doubt that this was the procedure that today would be called a Z-plasty.

Neither Horner nor Denonvilliers used the term Z-plasty, and it was not until 1913 that an article with that title appeared in the literature. S. L. McCurdy† used the term "Z-plastic" surgery and showed an example of an operation done in 1904 using what he called a Z-incision, and of others done later using typical Z-plasties on burn scars of the neck, axilla, and hand.

*The original Z-plasty. Brit. J. Plast. Surg., *26:*237–246, 1973.

†Z-plastic surgery. Plastic operations to elongate cicatricial contractions of the neck, lips, and eyelids, and across joints. Surg. Gynecol. Obstet., *16:*209–212, 1913.

Warren on *Stammering.* 99

this power by imitation where it is possible, and where it is not—where he cannot obtain assistance, he will find directions in books on elocation, for the articulation of the elementary sounds. His practice should be conducted before a glass.

The rapid results produced by the system called Mrs. Leigh's, I have said were real. They were made, and can be made as speedily as I have declared. But though the cures appear perfect for the time, until they are confirmed by long habit, there is great danger of a relapse. In a few cases, they will remain permanent, but in a majority, unless the course is persisted in, the difficulty returns. Moreover, if the affection is produced, as I have said, by mental causes, as long as those causes remain in the mind unchecked, they will be constantly acting to reproduce the disease. *Causa non sublata, non tollitur effectus.*

Liability to embarrassment, or to be carried away by strong emotion, will constantly operate to produce a recurrence of stammering. Now this disease is different from all others, for the moment the patient who has imagined himself cured, hears himself stammer, he loses confidence; the fear of stammering returns, and causes him to stammer in his next attempt at utterance. Perfect self command, is, therefore, all important.

Whatever method may be employed for the relief of this affection, no permanent advantage will be gained, in the majority of cases, unless resolutely persevered in for one or two years. With this perseverance, it may be cured with as much certainty as any other chronic disorder, and this not by any new or patent method, but simply by attention to the course I have described.

Boston, August, 1837.

Art. V. *Clinical Report on the Surgical Department of the Philadelphia Hospital, Blockley, for the months of May, June, and July, 1837.* By William E. Horner, M. D., Surgeon, Professor of Anatomy in the University of Pennsylvania, &c.

As this institution presents the most extensive and complete example of a clinical establishment in the United States, the following summary of its features may be interesting to such as have not seen it. It is a portion of the Alms-house for the city and adjoining districts of Philadelphia. Its name is rather conventional than estab-

William E. Horner: Clinical report on the surgical department of the Philadelphia Hospital, Blockley, for the months of May, June, and July, 1837. Am. J. Med. Sci., *21*:99–112, 1837. (Courtesy of the Library of the College of Physicians of Philadelphia)

William Horner—not to be confused with J. F. Horner of Horner's syndrome—was also responsible for the discovery of the tensor tarsi muscle, which bears his name. He was born in Warrenton, Virginia. A local physician, an Edinburgh graduate, taught him the basic sciences, and Horner then attended two sessions at the University of Pennsylvania Medical School. The War of 1812 found him enlisting in the army, so that his graduation was delayed until 1814. His primary interest was anatomy, and he became a prosector for Wistar, whose name is com-

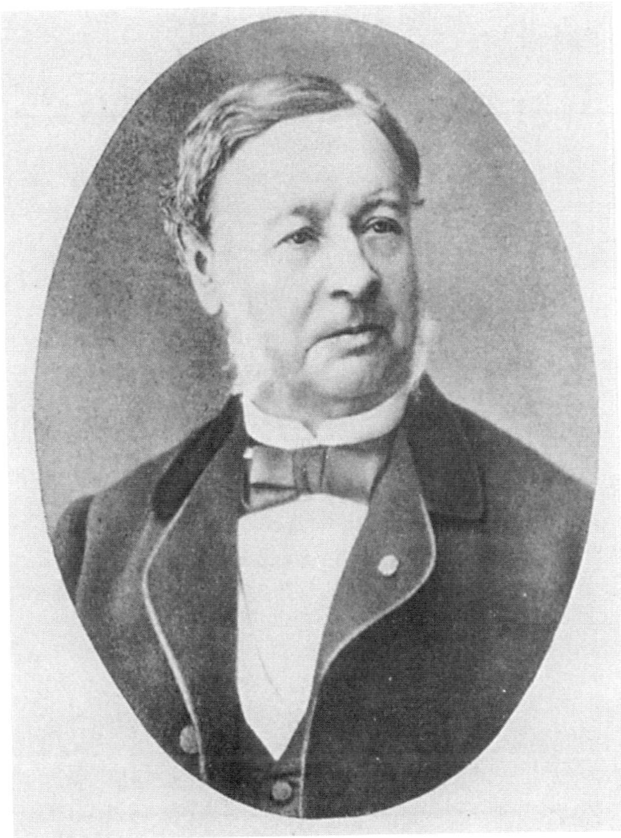

Theodor Schwann. (From Beilage Munch. Med. Wochenschr., 57[2]:279, 1910. Courtesy of the Library of the New York Academy of Medicine)

memorated in the Wistar Institute of Anatomy as well as in the Wisteria vine. Horner succeeded Philip Physick as professor of anatomy in 1831.

One of the young men in Johannes Müller's laboratory in Berlin, when Little came there, was **Theodor Schwann** (1810–1882), co-author of the cell theory and a brilliant investigator. The Schwann cell is most interesting in its structure, its relation to myelin, and its response to injury. It was described in 1838, but Schwann had made some notable discoveries before this, actually four in the 5 years he spent with Müller. His thesis (1834)—a work that was suggested by Müller—was to show that air is necessary for the development of the chick embryo. In 1836 he discovered pepsin in the stomach, and in 1837, he first described the striped muscle in the upper esophagus. He antedated Pasteur when he was able to show that putre-

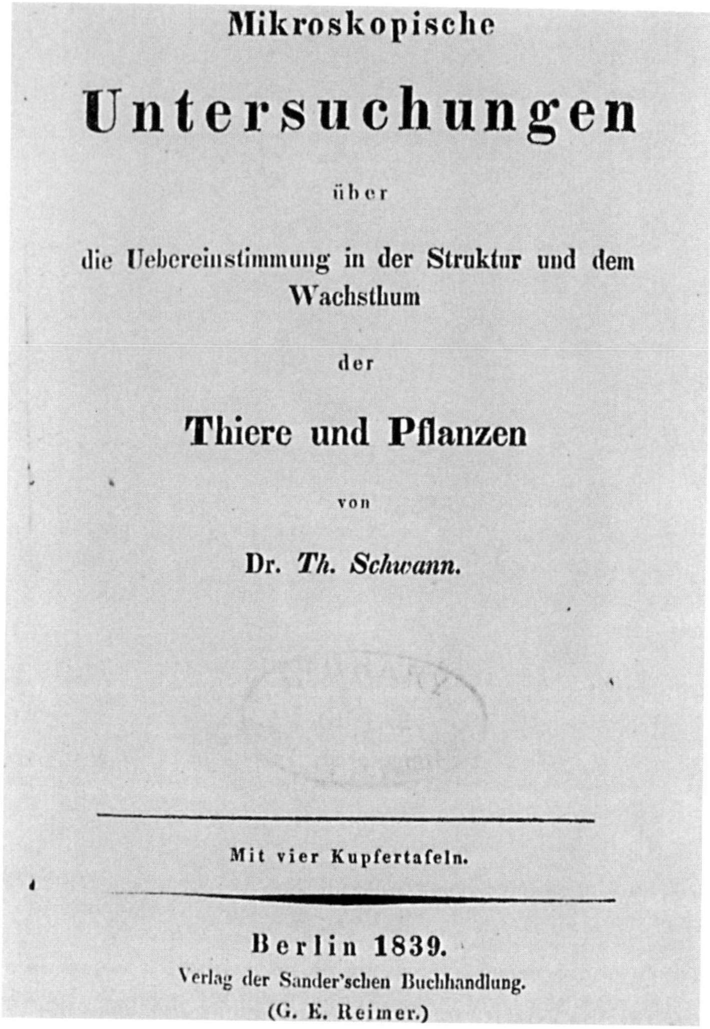

Mikroskopische

Untersuchungen

über

die Uebereinstimmung in der Struktur und dem Wachsthum

der

Thiere und Pflanzen

von

Dr. *Th. Schwann.*

Mit vier Kupfertafeln.

Berlin 1839.

Verlag der Sander'schen Buchhandlung.

(G. E. Reimer.)

Theodor Schwann: Mikroskopische Untersuchungen über die Uebereinstimmung in der Struktur und dem Wachsthum der Thiere und Pflanzen. Berlin, Verlag der Sander'schen Buchhandlung (G. E. Reimer), 1839. (Courtesy of the Library of the College of Physicians of Philadelphia)

faction was caused by living cells and that heat destroyed them, and that fermentation caused by yeast could be prevented by heating the culture.

Schwann was born in Neuss near Düsseldorf. He inherited from his father, a jeweler and printer, a skill and facility for making instruments and apparatuses that played a major part in his later laboratory experiments. He was at Würtzburg for awhile with Schönlein but then went to

Bonn, with the intention of studying theology. Here he came under the influence of Müller, who was then professor of anatomy. Schwann went to Berlin when Müller took the chair there, and he received his medical degree from the University of Berlin in 1834. Here, in the next 4 years, he did his major work—the last of which before he left was the finding that the tension of a contracting muscle varies with its length.

Müller's influence was great. In his laboratory, along with Schwann, were Remak and Henle. Schwann went on to head the departments at Liège and Louvain; Henle went to Göttingen, where he trained Merkel.

Schwann's name is coupled with that of Matthias Schleiden as co-developers of the cell theory. During dinner one evening, Schleiden, who had been trained in law but was now studying botany at the university, impressed Schwann with his hypothesis of the plant cell as being the structural unit, and Schwann began to look at his animal specimens in the same light. Schleiden's work came out in 1838, Schwann's the year following. The mere fact of seeing "cells" was not new; Hooke had described one in 1665, and in 1682 Drew, a botanist, had described the nucleus. It was the concept of the cell being as the structural unit of the living organism and plant that made Schwann and his dinner companion famous.

Schleiden went on to become a noted professor of botany at Jena. Schwann went first to Louvain and made one other discovery, that of the role of bile for proper digestion. He then spent many years at Liège, leading the quiet life of a professor. This amiable, unpretentious bachelor refused the offer of chairs at many other universities. He retired in 1880 and died in Cologne in 1882, while visiting his brother.

His major contributions were made while he was in Müller's laboratory; I am sure that Schwann would agree that he saw further because of the guidance, help, and training he received from his preceptor.

In 1835 a student presented a paper before the medical society of Florence, Italy. He described his findings and titled his presentation a "New Organ of Pacini." He was **Filippo Pacini** (1812–1883), only 23 years old, not yet qualified as a doctor, and probably a little brash. The organ of Pacini (now called the Vater-Pacini* corpuscle) is commonly seen in operations on the hand, when dissection is done in a bloodless field. Varying greatly in size, these subcutaneous corpuscles, presumably having to do with the sensation of pressure, are quite numerous. Every few years someone reports their presence in excessive numbers and relates this to the occurrence of Dupuytren's contracture, but there has never been any proven relationship.

---

*Abraham Vater (1684–1751) was born in Wittenberg and became professor of anatomy and botany there in 1719. He described the corpuscle in 1717. He is also remembered in the eponym, the ampulla of Vater.

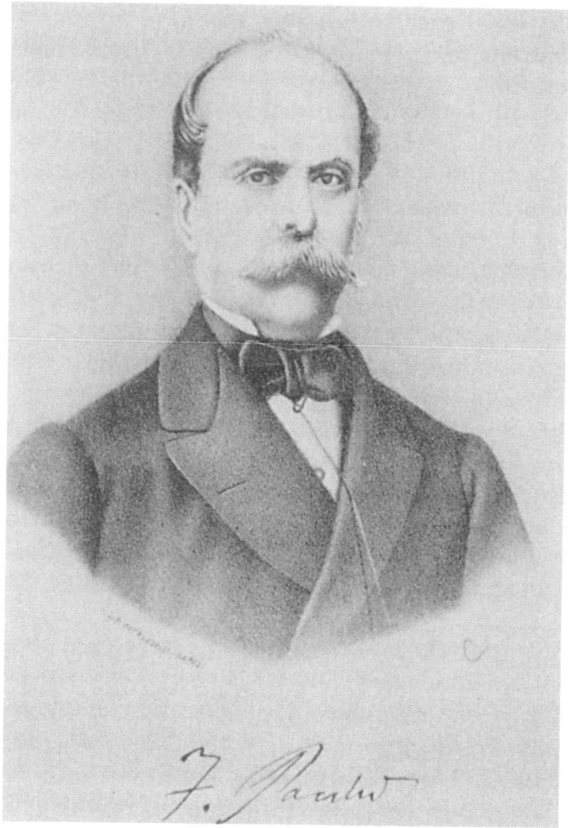

Filippo Pacini. (From Medicina Contemporanea. Naples, Supp., 1884. Courtesy of the Library of the New York Academy of Medicine)

Pacini's paper was not well received. Perhaps it was thought to be presumptuous of one so young, or maybe the method of presentation was such that objection was made. Whatever it was, Pacini returned to his medical course at Pistoja—which was also his birthplace—and continued his observations. Amici had developed an achromatic lens for the microscope, a major advance. Obtaining one of these, Pacini persisted in and published his work, with illustrations, in 1840. Curiosity and an observing mind in a young student, combined with good equipment—such is the talent, which, when combined with opportunity, produces an eponym.

He then went to Pisa as assistant to the professor, and there, with the best available equipment, he studied the human retina. He felt, however, that he had not been given proper recognition in Pisa, so he went to

Florence, where he worked in various positions but was never recognized by his confreres to the degree he thought he should have been. Most of his work was done with the microscope. He studied the electric organs of certain fish, and, in the cholera epidemic of 1854, he described and identified the bacilli as the causative organism, but did not distinguish the comma form that Koch did. He also wrote on the use of artificial respiration in the treatment of coma from overdoses of alcohol or narcotics.

He died at 71, disappointed in being denied membership in the Academy in Rome; however, his scientific achievements were recognized in other countries. An obituary notice at the time of his death described him as being modest and added that although he was often engaged in controversy, he never "sinned against urbanity or good taste."

Another man in this period also felt frustrated in his position and, thinking there was little chance of reaching the desired professorship, took a long chance and accepted a position in Russia.

Wenzel L. Gruber (1814–1890) became one of the world's most renowned anatomists for his descriptions of anomalies, malformations, and monsters. To those of us in the field of surgery of the upper extremity, he is known for the Martin-Gruber anastomosis of median to ulnar nerve in the forearm (see R. Martin). He published more than 500 articles on anatomical observations during a period of 40 years.

He was born in Deutsch-Böhmen and went to school in Prague, graduating in medicine in 1844. He was a prosector for Hyrtl and later for Bochdalek. It was in 1847 that he concluded that his chances of obtaining a professorship were poor, so he accepted an offer from Pirogoff to come to Russia, with the understanding that in 3 years he would be offered the chair of descriptive anatomy. He accepted, but had to undergo many difficulties because of academic intrigues, and the promised position was denied him. When Pirogoff left the Academie, however, Gruber was chosen to be professor of pathologic anatomy, and later added the chair of practical anatomy.

It was not unusual for scientists to be enticed to Russia. Architects, artists, engineers, and teachers of medicine had been recruited from Europe to build up the Russian empire ever since the time of Peter the Great.

Gruber stayed on in Russia, and on his twenty-fifth anniversary and again on his thirtieth, he was re-elected professor. A great ovation was rendered on his thirty-fifth year, one of such magnitude that, it was said, was not easy for a Russian, much less a foreigner.

A catalogue of his published articles was printed in 1884. Little of his personal life is known, but he must have been an industrious worker and a keen observer and recorder of his findings. He is another example of

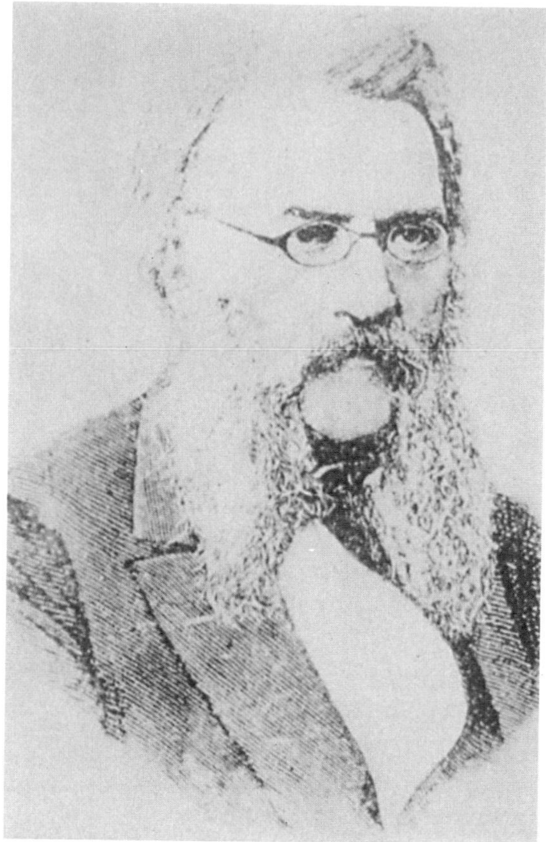

Wenzel L. Gruber. (From Ravitch, M. L.: Romance of Russian Medicine. New York, Liveright Publishing Corp., 1937. Courtesy of the Library of the New York Academy of Medicine)

one of the many anatomists to whom surgeons owe a debt of gratitude for their detailed observations. We do well to honor him and Roland Martin, the Swedish anatomist who described the interesting variation of the peripheral nerve supply of the hand.

In England there was a man whose life spanned almost all of this fascinating nineteenth century. **Sir James Paget** (1814–1899) was a young man of 25 working in the laboratory at St. Bartholomew's Hospital when Little returned from Berlin, his clubfoot corrected. This was just 2 years after Little had started the Royal Orthopaedic Hospital (now the Royal National Orthopaedic Hospital). William Adams, who later would refute some of Paget's ideas on tendon healing was in his late teens, studying anatomy.

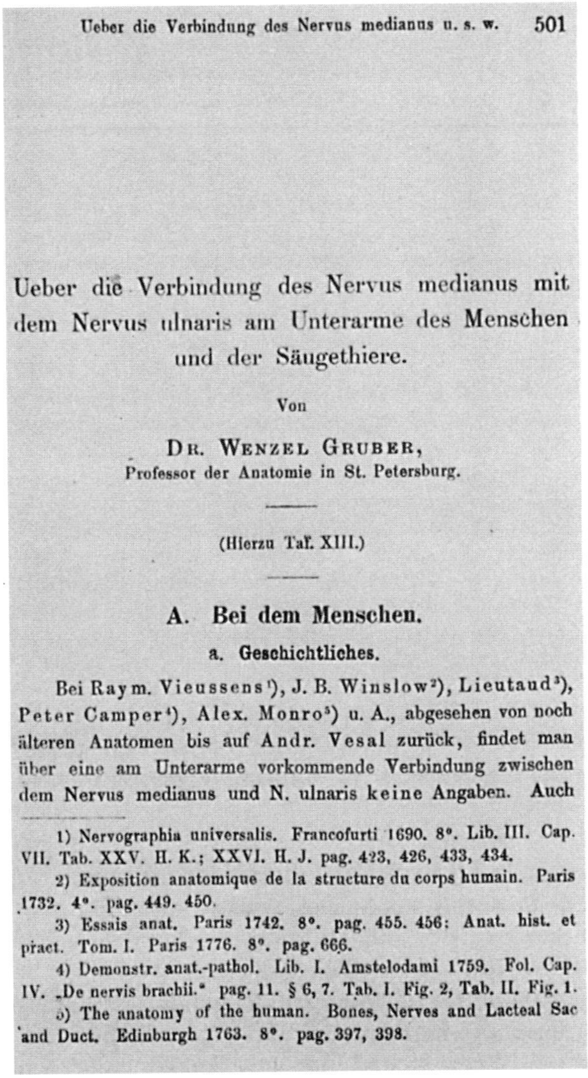
Ueber die Verbindung des Nervus medianus u. s. w. 501

Ueber die Verbindung des Nervus medianus mit dem Nervus ulnaris am Unterarme des Menschen und der Säugethiere.

Von

Dr. Wenzel Gruber,
Professor der Anatomie in St. Petersburg.

(Hierzu Taf. XIII.)

A. Bei dem Menschen.

a. Geschichtliches.

Bei Raym. Vieussens[1]), J. B. Winslow[2]), Lieutaud[3]), Peter Camper[4]), Alex. Monro[5]) u. A., abgesehen von noch älteren Anatomen bis auf Andr. Vesal zurück, findet man über eine am Unterarme vorkommende Verbindung zwischen dem Nervus medianus und N. ulnaris keine Angaben. Auch

1) Nervographia universalis. Francofurti 1690. 8°. Lib. III. Cap. VII. Tab. XXV. H. K.; XXVI. H. J. pag. 423, 426, 433, 434.
2) Exposition anatomique de la structure du corps humain. Paris 1732. 4°. pag. 449. 450.
3) Essais anat. Paris 1742. 8°. pag. 455. 456; Anat. hist. et pract. Tom. I. Paris 1776. 8°. pag. 666.
4) Demonstr. anat.-pathol. Lib. I. Amstelodami 1759. Fol. Cap. IV. „De nervis brachii." pag. 11. § 6, 7. Tab. I. Fig. 2, Tab. II. Fig. 1.
5) The anatomy of the human. Bones, Nerves and Lacteal Sac and Duct. Edinburgh 1763. 8°. pag. 397, 398.

Wenzel L. Gruber: Ueber die Verbindung des Nervus medianus mit dem Nervus ulnaris am Unterarme des Menschen und der Säugethiere. Arch. Anat. Physiol. Wiss. Med. (Leipzig), *37*:501–522, 1870. (Courtesy of the Library of the College of Physicians of Philadelphia)

Paget, using techniques from Müller's laboratory in Berlin, studied the healing of tendons, using the Achilles of the rabbit. He found that the space between the cut ends filled up with what he called "nucleated blastema," and that the sheath played no part in the repair process.

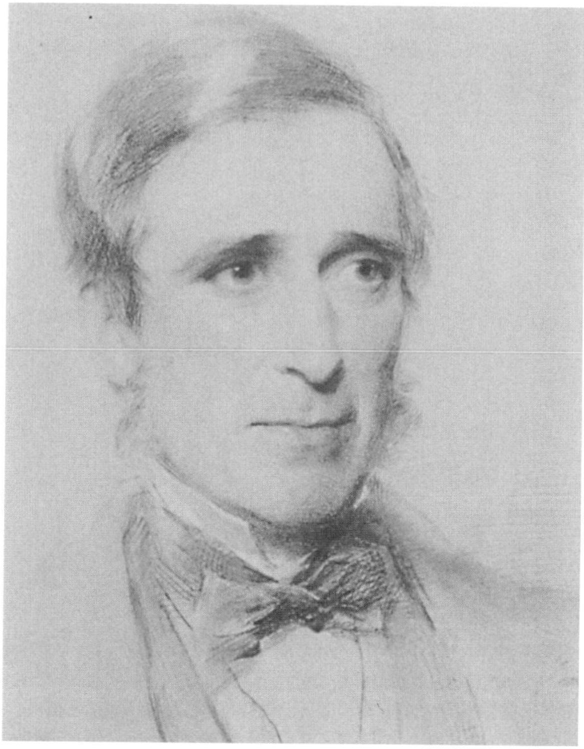

Sir James Paget. (Courtesy of the Library of the New York Academy of Medicine)

Adams, however, in his work later, considered the sheath to be an essential factor in determining the form and direction of the new tendon.

Paget, to become one of England's most honored surgeons, was called the "foremost surgical philosopher and orator of his day." We have no eponym for Paget specific to surgery of the hand, but because of his ideas on tendon healing and nerve repair, and especially because he reported one of the earliest, if not the first case of compression of the median nerve in the carpal canal, he deserves a place in our list of names.

Paget was born in Yarmouth. He was one of sixteen children of a man of varied interests: brewing, shipowning, and purveying supplies to the British navy. One of Paget's brothers later became regius professor of medicine at Cambridge.

As was the custom, Paget's early education included a foundation of Latin and Greek, and then he was apprenticed to a surgeon for 4 years. Then he was ready to study medicine. In his first year at St. Bart's, he discovered some small specks in the muscles of a cadaver. Curious, he borrowed a microscope from the botany department and discovered the *Trichina (Trichinella) spiralis*. The specimen was given to Richard Owen, who reported it and gave it its name.

Paget was obviously a good student. He was widely read, and it is said that he was able to translate from German, French, Dutch, and Italian—languages learned largely on his own. Despite his apparent talents, he was unable to obtain a surgical appointment and therefore spent many years as curator of the museum of anatomy, and, later, as a demonstrator of anatomy. It was only after a long 15 years—during which he was also a subeditor of the *London Medical Gazette*—that he finally began to practice surgery and obtained a consultant's post at St. Bart's. He was a popular lecturer; his sessions were well attended. He also developed a large private practice. But he persisted in his scientific work. Both Paget's disease of the nipple and that of the bone were reported after he had resigned his active hospital appointment.

But let us go back a few years. In 1847, after Paget—then 33 years old—had just been appointed surgeon and had done his first operation in that capacity, he described what to him were two methods of nerve healing, at a meeting of the Royal College of Surgeons. He reported two cases.

Paget said that if a nerve is cut, *immediate* union of the fibers takes place if the nerve ends are in contact. As proof, he described a patient, aged 11, who had cut his median nerve; within 1 month there had been a complete recovery! If the nerve ends were not in contact, Paget said, scar tissue would fill the gap, and new nerve fibers would develop in this gap and join to those in the divided ends. The theory was wrong, but the idea of the importance of contact made immediate suture of the divided ends advisable.

This idea of uniting the divided ends was not new. Marie Jean Pierre Flourens, a graduate of Montpellier, had gone to Paris and in 1828 studied with Cuvier and Lamarck. Flourens reportedly transposed nerves of rooster wings, crossing the nerves of extensors to flexors.

One wonders if Paget was really familiar with work that had already been done in his own country. In 1819 (28 years before Paget's lecture to the Royal College of Surgeons) the Jacksonian Prize was given to Joseph Swan (1791–1874), who was at that time a young surgeon, assistant to his father in the town of Lincoln, and a former student at Guy's and St. Thomas's Hospitals. Swan was familiar with the practices of veterinarians in the country who had cut the nerves in horses' feet. Swan knew that some recovery occurred. (Delpech, the well-known French surgeon, however, taught that recovery of nerve function never occurred through scar tissue.) Swan had shown in his work that section of the sciatic nerve in rabbits did result in recovery, under certain conditions. If there was a

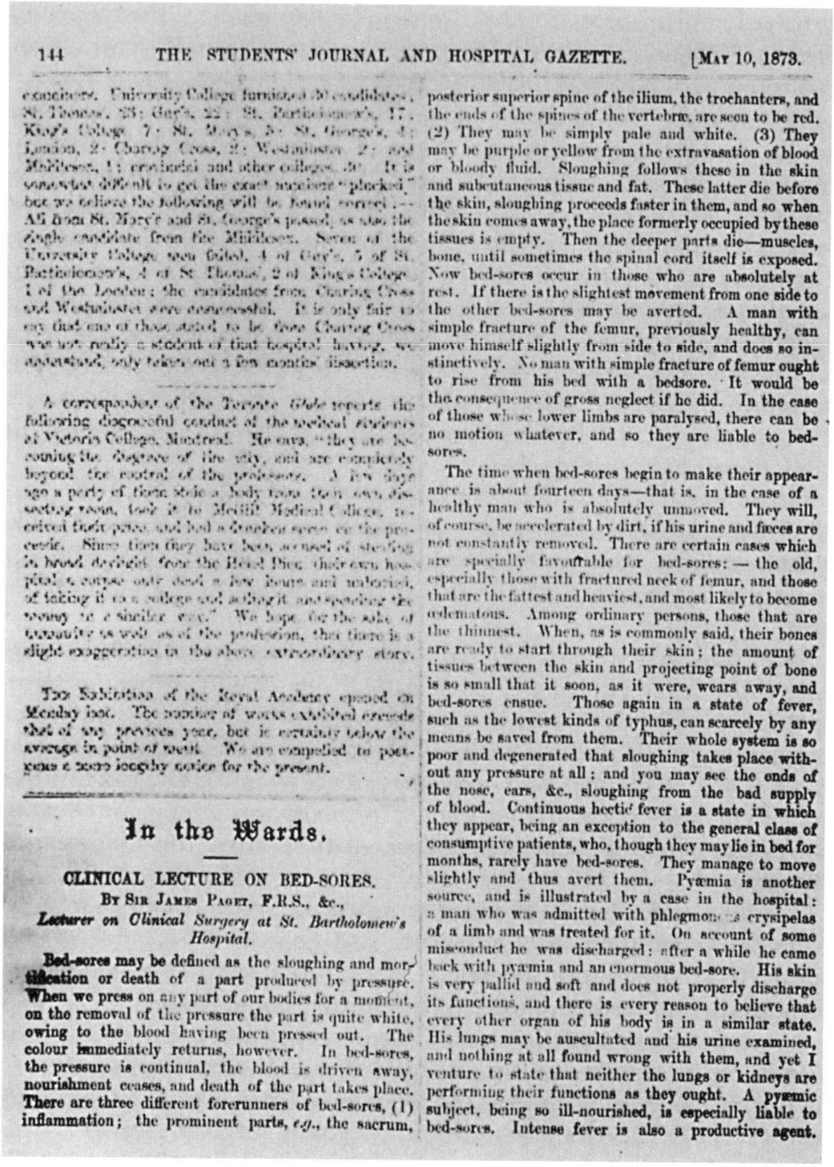

144 THE STUDENTS' JOURNAL AND HOSPITAL GAZETTE. [MAY 10, 1873.

[illegible]

In the Wards.

CLINICAL LECTURE ON BED-SORES.

By Sir James Paget, F.R.S., &c.,

Lecturer on Clinical Surgery at St. Bartholomew's Hospital.

Bed-sores may be defined as the sloughing and mortification or death of a part produced by pressure. When we press on any part of our bodies for a moment, on the removal of the pressure the part is quite white, owing to the blood having been pressed out. The colour immediately returns, however. In bed-sores, the pressure is continual, the blood is driven away, nourishment ceases, and death of the part takes place. There are three different forerunners of bed-sores, (1) inflammation; the prominent parts, *e.g.*, the sacrum, posterior superior spine of the ilium, the trochanters, and the ends of the spines of the vertebræ, are seen to be red. (2) They may be simply pale and white. (3) They may be purple or yellow from the extravasation of blood or bloody fluid. Sloughing follows these in the skin and subcutaneous tissue and fat. These latter die before the skin, sloughing proceeds faster in them, and so when the skin comes away, the place formerly occupied by these tissues is empty. Then the deeper parts die—muscles, bone, until sometimes the spinal cord itself is exposed. Now bed-sores occur in those who are absolutely at rest. If there is the slightest movement from one side to the other bed-sores may be averted. A man with simple fracture of the femur, previously healthy, can move himself slightly from side to side, and does so instinctively. No man with simple fracture of femur ought to rise from his bed with a bedsore. It would be the consequence of gross neglect if he did. In the case of those whose lower limbs are paralysed, there can be no motion whatever, and so they are liable to bed-sores.

The time when bed-sores begin to make their appearance is about fourteen days—that is, in the case of a healthy man who is absolutely unmoved. They will, of course, be accelerated by dirt, if his urine and fæces are not constantly removed. There are certain cases which are specially favourable for bed-sores:—the old, especially those with fractured neck of femur, and those that are the fattest and heaviest, and most likely to become œdematous. Among ordinary persons, those that are the thinnest. When, as is commonly said, their bones are ready to start through their skin; the amount of tissues between the skin and projecting point of bone is so small that it soon, as it were, wears away, and bed-sores ensue. Those again in a state of fever, such as the lowest kinds of typhus, can scarcely by any means be saved from them. Their whole system is so poor and degenerated that sloughing takes place without any pressure at all; and you may see the ends of the nose, ears, &c., sloughing from the bad supply of blood. Continuous hectic fever is a state in which they appear, being an exception to the general class of consumptive patients, who, though they may lie in bed for months, rarely have bed-sores. They manage to move slightly and thus avert them. Pyæmia is another source, and is illustrated by a case in the hospital: a man who was admitted with phlegmonous erysipelas of a limb and was treated for it. On account of some misconduct he was discharged: after a while he came back with pyæmia and an enormous bed-sore. His skin is very pallid and soft and does not properly discharge its functions, and there is every reason to believe that every other organ of his body is in a similar state. His lungs may be auscultated and his urine examined, and nothing at all found wrong with them, and yet I venture to state that neither the lungs or kidneys are performing their functions as they ought. A pyæmic subject, being so ill-nourished, is especially liable to bed-sores. Intense fever is also a productive agent.

Sir James Paget: Clinical lecture on bed-sores. Student's J. Hosp. Gaz., *1*:144, 1873. (Courtesy of the Library of the New York Academy of Medicine)

simple puncture of the nerve or partial section, recovery was complete; but if the section was complete, even though some function was recovered, it was never a complete and full recovery.

Swan had practiced in London since 1830 (17 years before Paget's lecture), and he was a member of the Council of the Royal College of Surgeons. He may have been present at Paget's lecture. Waller was practicing at this time in Kensington. Three years after Paget's lecture, Waller would show, by his experiments on the frog's tongue, the stages of nerve repair.

A few years later, in 1853, Paget reported a case, apparently seen in consultation with a Mr. Hilton, of a patient with a healed fracture of the lower end of the radius who had ulceration of the thumb and index and middle fingers, which was relieved by splinting the wrist in flexion. There was no record of any other treatment. This is presumably the first record of a compression of the median nerve in the carpal tunnel.

Paget was a popular surgeon, and he made friends easily. He was at the height of his career when he almost died as a result of a cellulitis of the right hand extending past the shoulder, caused by an infected laceration received while doing an autopsy. He resigned from his hospital work and was made a baronet by Queen Victoria. His writings continued, however, and both diseases known by his name were described in these later years. He also wrote a paper on bed sores, in which he recommended the use of a water bed.

He died at the age of 85, one of England's most honored surgeons. His son, the bishop of Oxford, rendered him the last rites, and a funeral service was held in Westminster Abbey. Lister was one of the pallbearers.

As so many others, Paget had spent many years in anatomy and pathology before his surgical career began. He was a keen observer and an excellent speaker, and his writings are examples of simple, clear descriptions of clinical states. He never used two words if one would do. He said, "To be brief was to be wise; to be epigrammatic was to be clever."

Augustus Volney Waller (1816–1870) was in practice in Kensington when he described the degeneration of a nerve distal to a point of division, and the regeneration of the axis cylinder and reconstitution of the nerve in the repair stage, a process which we call Wallerian degeneration. This was a major breakthrough in the study of peripheral nerves and opened up a whole new field of investigation of the nerve tracts. This process of degeneration and repair—now so well understood, with better microscopes and more advanced staining techniques—disproved Paget's theories of how divided nerves healed, but emphasized the necessity of accurate approximation of the nerve trunks in the surgical repair.

Waller's experiment on the frog's tongue showed that the process of regeneration was dependent on the presence of an axis cylinder. He even noted that the orderly progression of events varied in rate, being more

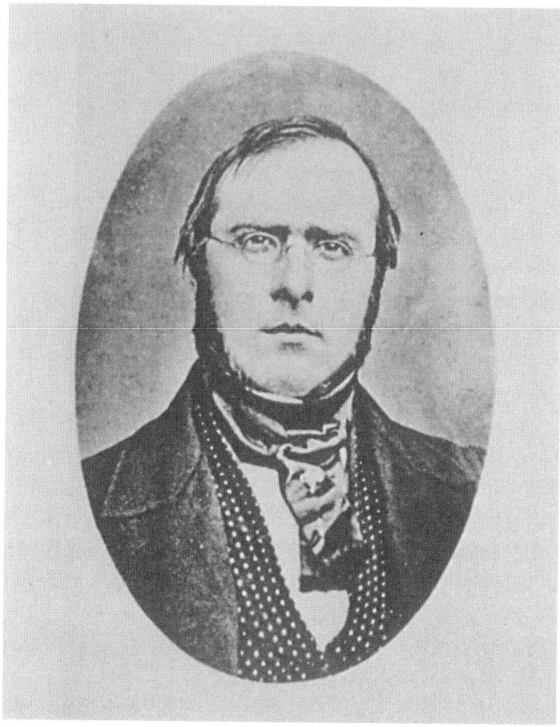

Augustus Volney Waller. (From Stirling, W.: Some Apostles of Physiology. London, Waterlow and Sons, 1902. Courtesy of the Library of the New York Academy of Medicine)

rapid in the young and during the summer, and that daily galvanic stimulation did not increase the speed of regeneration.

Clarification of the embryological development of the nerve fiber was a long time away. Balfour, in England, described what he thought were cells migrating out and laying down the nerve fiber. Wilhelm His, Sr., who succeeded Ernst Weber, was a master histologist. He invented a good microtome, and with more advanced techniques, in 1886 was able to show that the axis cylinder arose from the nerve cell. He thought that these cells Balfour described were primarily for nourishment of the fiber itself. Finally, in 1904, Harrison, working in Mall's Laboratory at Johns Hopkins, was able to show the independence of the axis cylinder or nerve fiber and the Schwann cell. Using the tadpole as a model, Harrison found that when the dorsal crest of the embryo was removed, the fiber still developed, but was then without the surrounding sheath.

Waller, with his laboratory in his home, using what today would be considered primitive equipment, set in motion a chain of studies on peripheral nerves; studies that now are being done with even more

[423]

XX. *Experiments on the Section of the Glossopharyngeal and Hypoglossal Nerves of the Frog, and observations of the alterations produced thereby in the Structure of their Primitive Fibres. By* AUGUSTUS WALLER, *M.D. Communicated by Professor* OWEN, *F.R.S.*

Received November 22, 1849,—Read February 21, 1850.

THE object of the present observations is to describe certain alterations which take place in the elementary fibres of the nerve after they have been removed from their connection with the brain or spinal marrow.

The following is a brief summary of the opinions and researches of modern physiologists on alterations of the nerve-tubes.

BURDACH* placed a ligature on the sciatic nerve of a frog, and after the lapse of a week found no alteration of the primitive fibres either above or below the ligature.

STEINRUCK† did the same, and states that in three cases the whole nerve was more slender than on the healthy side, and ascribed it to the atrophy of the neurolema.

VALENTIN‡ denies likewise that there is any alteration of the primitive fibres in the lower portion of the nerve.

GUNTHER and SCHÖN§, whose researches are most interesting, state that the primitive fibres being examined towards the end of a week, after division of the nerve when it had lost its irritability, it was perceived that they had no longer the full round appearance of the sound ones. Here and there their contents appeared as if curdled; from eight to fourteen days after section these structural changes became still more evident, and continued to increase until the fibres appeared flat, broken up, entirely losing their transparency, their contents appearing as if disjointed.

NASSE‖ states, that five months after section of the sciatic nerve of a frog, the tubes below the section were broken up into granules and small clumps; that all the nerve-tubes were strongly granulated, in some the small granules being united into oval bodies, which appeared to be surrounded by a pale cylindrical membrane, which in some was wanting, owing probably to its disorganization.

Having in a former communication to the Royal Society described the nerves of the papillæ and of the muscular fibre in the frog's tongue in their normal condition.

* Beitrag zur Mikroskopischer Anatomie der Nerven, E. BURDACH. Konigsberg, 1837, p. 42.

† De Nervorum Regeneratione. Berolini, 1838, p. 72.

‡ De Functionibus Nervor Cerebral, &c. Lib. iv. 1839, p. 127.

§ MÜLLER's Archiv, 1840, Versuche und Bemerkungen über Regeneration der Nerven, p. 276.

‖ Ueber die Veränderungen der Nerven-fasern nach ihrer Durchschneidung, MÜLLER, Arch. 1839, p. 400.

Augustus Volney Waller: Experiments on the section of the glossopharyngeal and hypoglossal nerves of the frog, and observations of the alterations produced thereby in the structure of their primitive fibres. Philos. Trans. R. Soc. Lond., *140*:423–429, 1850. (Courtesy of the National Library of Medicine, Bethesda, Maryland)

sophisticated equipment. Yet Waller's findings have withstood the test of time.

Waller's background is most interesting. He was born on a farm in Kent. His father, a strict vegetarian, moved the family to Nice, where Augustus remained until he was 14. After his father died, he was sent back to England to live with a Dr. William Lambe, also a vegetarian. Augustus went to medical school in Paris, graduating in 1840. Here he must have become interested in histology and familiar with the work

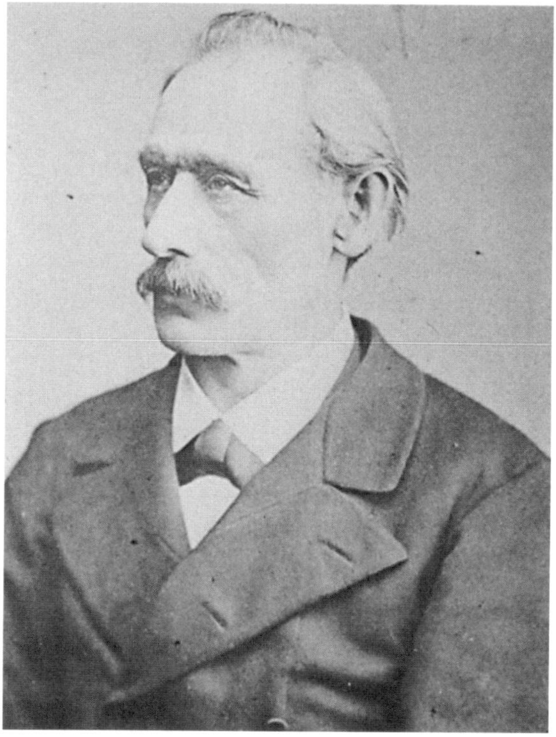

Carl von Langer. (From Nader, J. [ed.]: Medicinal-Kalender. vol. 36. part 1. Vienna, Carl Fromme, 1881. Courtesy of the Library of the College of Physicians of Philadelphia)

being done with good microscopes. Two years after graduation, he started a practice in Kensington, apparently doing well. He also set up his own laboratory and published two papers of classical experimentation. The first paper was a rediscovery of the diapedesis of white blood corpuscles through capillary walls. The second paper was the classic on degeneration and regeneration of the nerve, in 1850.

About 1852, after 10 years of practice, he moved to Bonn, Germany, where he and Julius L. Budge (1811–1888) demonstrated the ciliospinal center in the spinal cord and showed the vasoconstrictor action of the cervical sympathetic nerves. This work, complementing that of Claude Bernard and Brown-Séquard, was the signal for opening a new field of knowledge of the sympathetic nervous system. Waller and Budge shared a prize from the Paris Academy of Sciences for their work, and 4 years later, Waller, by himself, was the recipient of the same prize. He was also honored by the Royal Society of London.

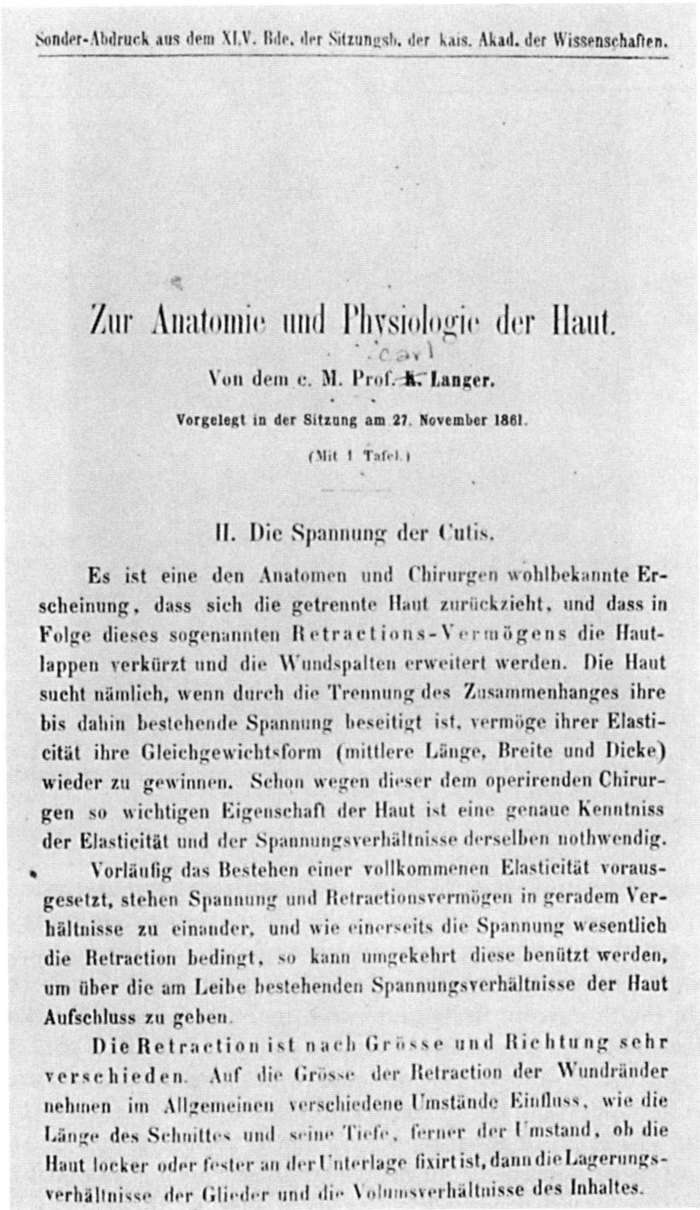

Sonder-Abdruck aus dem XLV. Bde. der Sitzungsb. der kais. Akad. der Wissenschaften.

Zur Anatomie und Physiologie der Haut.

Von dem c. M. Prof. K. Langer.

Vorgelegt in der Sitzung am 27. November 1861.

(Mit 1 Tafel.)

II. Die Spannung der Cutis.

Es ist eine den Anatomen und Chirurgen wohlbekannte Erscheinung, dass sich die getrennte Haut zurückzieht, und dass in Folge dieses sogenannten Retractions-Vermögens die Hautlappen verkürzt und die Wundspalten erweitert werden. Die Haut sucht nämlich, wenn durch die Trennung des Zusammenhanges ihre bis dahin bestehende Spannung beseitigt ist, vermöge ihrer Elasticität ihre Gleichgewichtsform (mittlere Länge, Breite und Dicke) wieder zu gewinnen. Schon wegen dieser dem operirenden Chirurgen so wichtigen Eigenschaft der Haut ist eine genaue Kenntniss der Elasticität und der Spannungsverhältnisse derselben nothwendig.

Vorläufig das Bestehen einer vollkommenen Elasticität vorausgesetzt, stehen Spannung und Retractionsvermögen in geradem Verhältnisse zu einander, und wie einerseits die Spannung wesentlich die Retraction bedingt, so kann umgekehrt diese benützt werden, um über die am Leibe bestehenden Spannungsverhältnisse der Haut Aufschluss zu geben.

Die Retraction ist nach Grösse und Richtung sehr verschieden. Auf die Grösse der Retraction der Wundränder nehmen im Allgemeinen verschiedene Umstände Einfluss, wie die Länge des Schnittes und seine Tiefe, ferner der Umstand, ob die Haut locker oder fester an der Unterlage fixirt ist, dann die Lagerungsverhältnisse der Glieder und die Volumsverhältnisse des Inhaltes.

Carl von Langer: Zur Anatomie und Physiologie der Haut. II. Die Spannung der Cutis. Sitzungsb. kais. Akad. Wiss., *45*:171–194, 1861. (Courtesy of the Library of the New York Academy of Medicine)

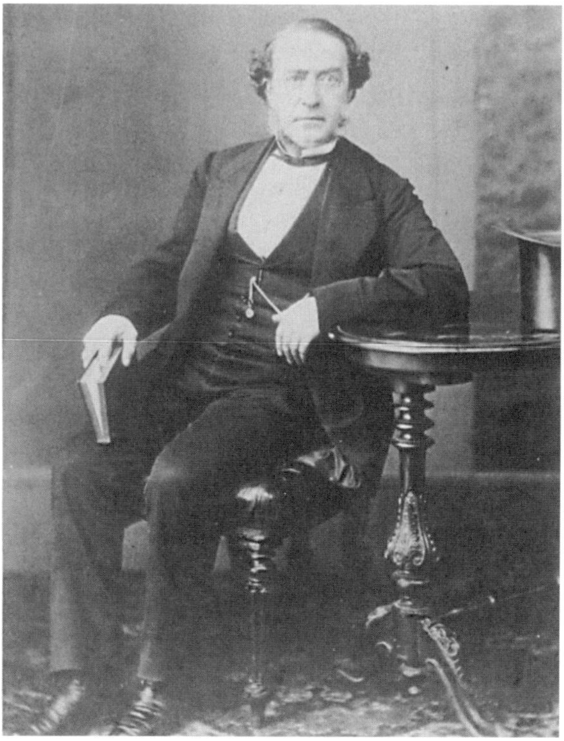

Alfred Baring Garrod. (Courtesy of the Library of the New York Academy of Medicine)

He spent 4 fruitful years in Bonn and then went to Flouren's laboratory in Paris (see Paget), but here Waller developed a low-grade febrile disease, which caused him to return to England. In 1858 he was made professor of physiology in Birmingham; but again, his illness forced him to resign. He then went to Belgium and finally to Geneva, Switzerland, hoping for relief. He died there of angina pectoris in 1870. A son, Augustus, became a well-known physiologist in England, and when someone spoke of his father and the monumental work that he had done, he said, "I am the Wallerian degeneration."

Most of us remember, from our introduction to the study of human anatomy, the drawing showing Langer's lines in the skin. **Carl von Langer** (1819–1887) authored a well-known textbook of systematic and topographic anatomy, as well as a work on the anatomy of the joints.

He was born in Vienna, but took part of his medical training in Prague, returning to Vienna to become prosector of anatomy. When qualified, he was professor of zoology at the University of Pest, but returned to Vienna

ON AN

UNUSUAL FORM OF NODULE UPON THE JOINTS OF THE FINGERS.

BY

ARCHIBALD E. GARROD, M.D.

Nodular excrescences of various kinds are met with in the neighbourhood of the finger-joints. In children and young adults subcutaneous rheumatic nodules not infrequently occur in such situations, and in older patients the finger-joints are common seats of urate of sodium deposits and of the osteophytes of rheumatoid arthritis. Moreover, the hands of those engaged in manual labour may exhibit thickenings of the skin which constitute distinct excrescences.

In the course of the last few years I have met with three cases characterised by the presence upon the finger-joints of nodules or cushions which did not appear to conform to any of the recognised types, and as all the cases seemed to be examples of the same morbid condition, and presented features of some interest, I venture to record them here, although my observations upon them have been purely clinical, and I have no knowledge of their morbid anatomy.

CASE I.—The first case was that of a young man, aged 20, whose occupation involved much writing. Although he was a sufferer from dyspepsia, he enjoyed fairly good health, and exhibited no sign of organic disease of any viscus.

The patient came of a gouty family, his paternal grandfather having been a martyr to that disease, and his father having Dupuytren's contracture of the fingers. His mother was said to be somewhat rheumatic.

On looking at his hands, one was at once struck by their peculiar appearance; nodules of about the size of half a hazel-

Archibald Edward Garrod: On an unusual form of nodule upon the joints of the fingers. St. Bartholomew's Hosp. Rep., *29*:157–161, 1893. (Courtesy of the National Library of Medicine, Bethesda, Maryland)

and took the chair of anatomy, first at the Joseph Academy, then at the University of Vienna. He died there in 1887. A memorial was placed in the arcade of the University of Vienna in 1903, and the presentation made by Toldt, another famous name in anatomy.

Langer's lines are of interest to surgeons in the study of the placement and direction of incisions in the skin, but they should not be confused with the flexion creases and other lines of tension in the skin. Darrel Shaw, in an article in *Plastic and Reconstructive Surgery*, discussed these and the lines of Langer.

In the eighteenth century, Heberden was the master clinician, with classic descriptions of disease states—without a stethoscope, thermometer, microscope, or laboratory aids. In the nineteenth century, **Alfred Baring Garrod** (1819–1907) took his place. He was the one to separate

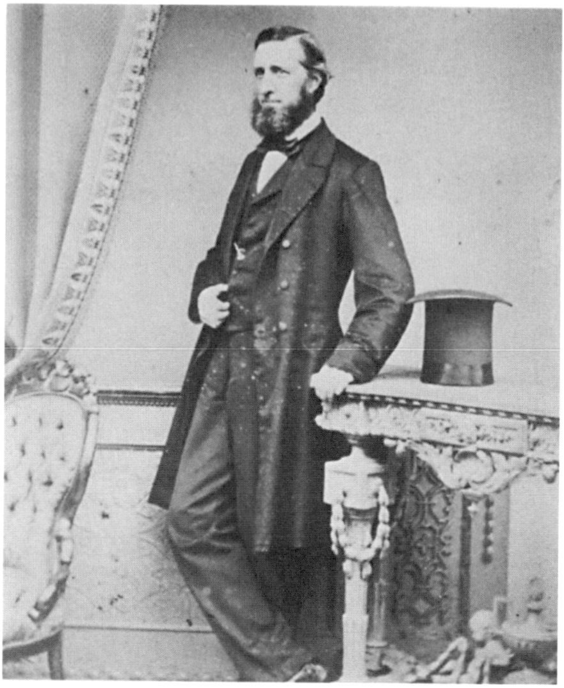

Alfred Poland. (Courtesy of The Wills Library and the Department of Medical Photography, Guy's Hospital Medical School, London)

gout from other rheumatic disorders by identifying the uric acid crystals in the serum and developing what he called the thread test. He recognized the use of colchicum, even saying its effect would be of diagnostic value. His textbook went through thirteen editions. A son, **Archibald Edward Garrod** described the nodules on the dorsum of the middle joints that often appear in patients with Dupuytren's disease. He wrote the still authoritative text, *Inborn Errors of Metabolism.* In 1920 he succeeded Sir William Osler as regius professor of medicine at Oxford.

In 1843, "after an unusually satisfactory examination," 23-year-old **Alfred Poland** (1820–1872) was made a member of the Royal College of Surgeons. Poland, born in Blackheath, was the son of Sir William Poland. We remember Poland for his description of the brachy-syndactyly associated with absence of the pectoral muscle, which he noted in a cadaver while he was a demonstrator in anatomy at Guy's. He reported this in 1841. Completing his surgical studies under Charles Aston Key, he went on to become an excellent surgeon, at first showing an interest in eye surgery; however, when he later was appointed full surgeon, he devoted more time to general surgery. He won three unusual prizes: one for an

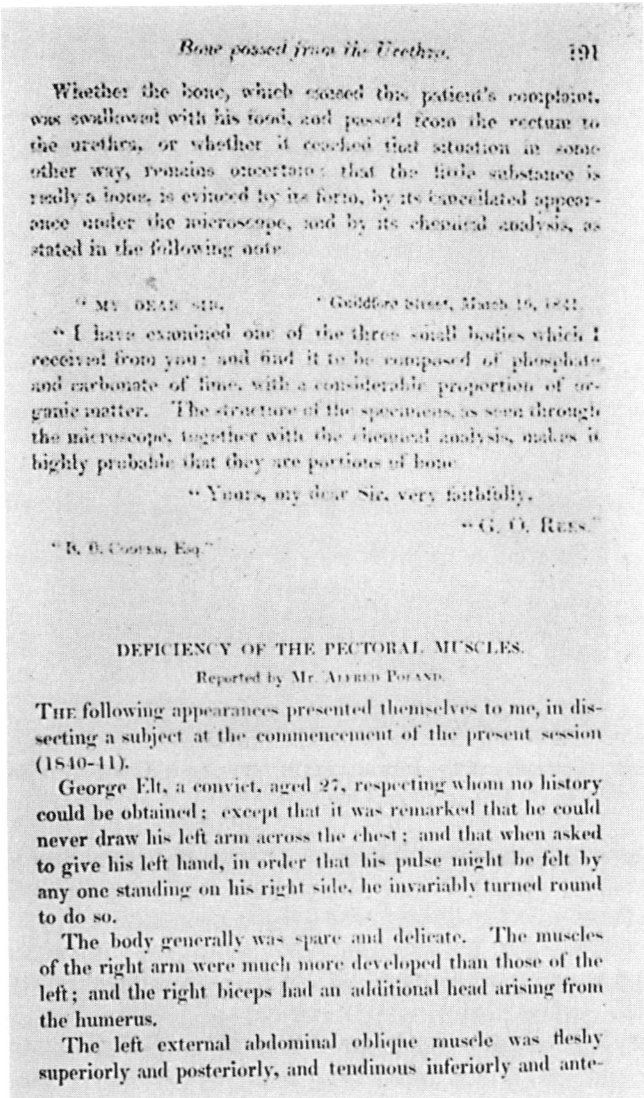

Bone passed from the Urethra. 191

Whether the bone, which caused this patient's complaint, was swallowed with his food, and passed from the rectum to the urethra, or whether it reached that situation in some other way, remains uncertain: that the little substance is really a bone, is evinced by its form, by its cancellated appearance under the microscope, and by its chemical analysis, as stated in the following note.

"My dear Sir, "Guildford Street, March 16, 1841.

"I have examined one of the three small bodies which I received from you; and find it to be composed of phosphate and carbonate of lime, with a considerable proportion of organic matter. The structure of the specimens, as seen through the microscope, together with the chemical analysis, makes it highly probable that they are portions of bone.

"Yours, my dear Sir, very faithfully,

"G. O. Rees."

"B. B. Cooper, Esq."

DEFICIENCY OF THE PECTORAL MUSCLES.

Reported by Mr. Alfred Poland.

The following appearances presented themselves to me, in dissecting a subject at the commencement of the present session (1840-41).

George Elt, a convict, aged 27, respecting whom no history could be obtained; except that it was remarked that he could never draw his left arm across the chest; and that when asked to give his left hand, in order that his pulse might be felt by any one standing on his right side, he invariably turned round to do so.

The body generally was spare and delicate. The muscles of the right arm were much more developed than those of the left; and the right biceps had an additional head arising from the humerus.

The left external abdominal oblique muscle was fleshy superiorly and posteriorly, and tendinous inferiorly and ante-

Alfred Poland: Deficiency of the pectoral muscles. Guy's Hosp. Rep., 6:191–193, 1841. (Courtesy of the Library of the New York Academy of Medicine)

anatomical study of the nerves of the orbit; another, the Fothergill Medal, for a study of injuries and wounds of the abdomen; and the Jacksonian Prize for a dissertation on gunshot wounds and their treatment. He was an excellent lecturer, his style being described as clear and brief, and his manner was that of a man with a retiring disposition and modest de-

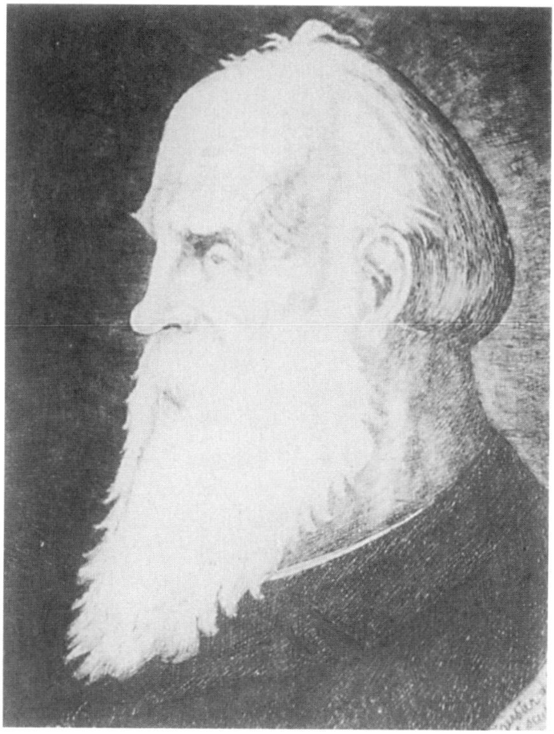

Karl Thiersch. (Courtesy of the Library of the New York Academy of Medicine)

meanor. He edited the Guy's Hospital reports and was a frequent contributor.

He developed a severe illness, said to have been induced by a purulent infection contracted in the hospital work, which cut short his activities and forced him to cancel his lectures and retire from the city. After some improvement in his health, which was only temporary, he was embittered by severe domestic trials and died in 1872.

Poland's time in London was during a stirring period. His report of the brachy-syndactyly was done in 1841, the year of Astley Cooper's death. Charles Bell had returned to Edinburgh, Duchenne was just beginning his work in Paris, and Paget was still at St. Bart's, not yet an appointed surgeon. Little was in London, having introduced the subcutaneous tenotomy procedure for clubfoot, and had just recently founded the Royal Orthopaedic Hospital. Waller had just graduated from the University of Paris. It was a period of many great men, and Alfred Poland could have been one of them, had he survived the vicissitudes of illness and marriage.

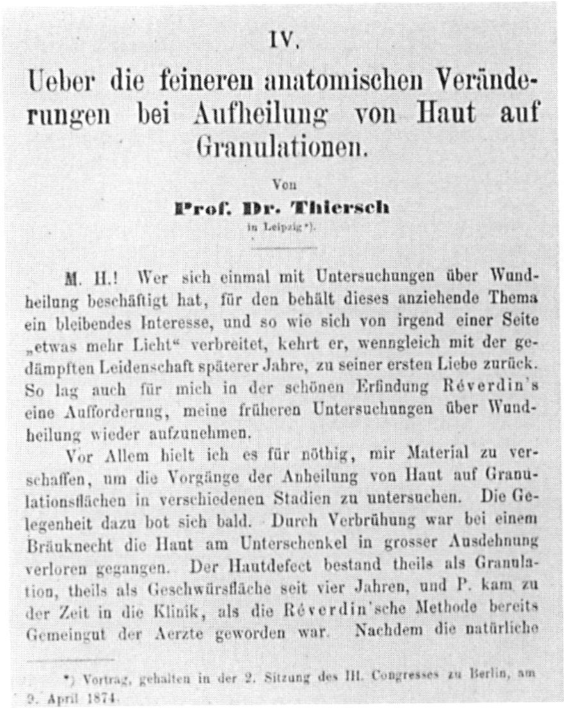

IV.

Ueber die feineren anatomischen Veränderungen bei Aufheilung von Haut auf Granulationen.

Von

Prof. Dr. Thiersch

in Leipzig *).

M. H.! Wer sich einmal mit Untersuchungen über Wundheilung beschäftigt hat, für den behält dieses anziehende Thema ein bleibendes Interesse, und so wie sich von irgend einer Seite „etwas mehr Licht“ verbreitet, kehrt er, wenngleich mit der gedämpften Leidenschaft späterer Jahre, zu seiner ersten Liebe zurück. So lag auch für mich in der schönen Erfindung Réverdin's eine Aufforderung, meine früheren Untersuchungen über Wundheilung wieder aufzunehmen.

Vor Allem hielt ich es für nöthig, mir Material zu verschaffen, um die Vorgänge der Anheilung von Haut auf Granulationsflächen in verschiedenen Stadien zu untersuchen. Die Gelegenheit dazu bot sich bald. Durch Verbrühung war bei einem Bräuknecht die Haut am Unterschenkel in grosser Ausdehnung verloren gegangen. Der Hautdefect bestand theils als Granulation, theils als Geschwürsfläche seit vier Jahren, und P. kam zu der Zeit in die Klinik, als die Réverdin'sche Methode bereits Gemeingut der Aerzte geworden war. Nachdem die natürliche

*) Vortrag, gehalten in der 2. Sitzung des III. Congresses zu Berlin, am 9. April 1874.

Karl Thiersch: Ueber die feineren anatomischen Veränderungen bei Aufheilung von Haut auf Granulationen. Verh. Dtsch. Ges. Chir. (Berlin), 3:69–75, 1874. (Courtesy of the Library of the College of Physicians of Philadelphia)

In Germany, one of Stromeyer's pupils was developing a reputation as a surgeon, anatomist, and investigator. **Karl Thiersch** (1822–1895) is remembered primarily for his studies on transplantation of skin, published in 1874, although Reverdin had done the same in 1869 and Ollier in 1872. Even as early as 1823, Christian Bünger, working with Carl F. von Graefe, had reconstructed a nose by using skin from the upper thigh, with partial success. Jonathan Mason Warren in Boston had transplanted skin from arm to nose, as did Pancoast, who reconstructed an ear with a free graft. Jerome P. Webster and Martha Gnudi, in their study, *The Life and Times of Gaspare Tagliacozzi*, record the works of these various surgeons, none of whom gave credit to one Giuseppe Baronio, who in 1804 successfully transplanted full-thickness skin from one area to another on sheep.

But Thiersch was probably thinking also of another problem, that is, the growth of epithelial cells. In fact, in 1865 he had published a monograph on epithelial cancer, presenting evidence of growth of these epithelial cells from other epithelial cells and refuting the idea of Koch that all tumors arose from the mesenchyme.

Thiersch's 1874 work was a study of the transplantation of skin, without any visible subcutaneous tissue. He was able to show the histological development of blood vessels as early as 18 hours after the graft. He did this by using clinical material—patients who required amputation of a leg for various reasons—and transplanting the skin at various times before the limb was removed.

Thiersch was born in Munich, where his father was professor of classics in the university and where Stromeyer for a time was professor of surgery. Thiersch studied in Berlin, Vienna, and Paris and graduated in 1848 from Munich. He then served as a prosector in anatomy. In 1850 he served in the Schleswig-Holstein war with Denmark, under Stromeyer, who was surgeon general of the Hanoverian army. Later they both were in the Franco-Prussian war of 1870, where Thiersch was a consultant, and Volkmann served under Thiersch.

From 1854 to 1867 Thiersch was professor at Erlangen. He then went to Leipzig, where he remained for 28 years. It was apparently during the 1870 war that he became impressed with Lister's idea of antisepsis and was one of Europe's first surgeons to introduce this system in his clinic. He was also instrumental in the design of the new hospital in Leipzig, introducing barracks or pavilions as a means of reducing the spread of infection.

He was described as being a careful and accurate observer, especially competent in plastic surgery of the head and neck, and with particular concern for children. He spoke of himself as being an anatomist who had strayed into surgery.

Another name connected with a type of skin graft is that of **John Reissberg Wolfe** (1824–1904), credited with development of the free full-thickness skin graft. He was an eye surgeon. In 1875, for repair of a lower eyelid that was scarred from a blast injury, he excised the scar, sutured the lids together, and then fitted into the defect, like a watch glass, a free graft 2 inches long and 1 inch wide, taken from the forearm. On one-third of the graft he left the areolar tissue, but in the other portion he removed all until a "white" surface remained. According to the report, the graft was successful in all areas, although the removal of all subcutaneous tissue is today the preferred method of preparing the full-thickness skin graft. A similar type of graft had been reported by Lawson in 1870, in an operation for ectropion, and also by Le Fort in 1872. Finally, in 1893 Fedor Krause reported his technique and popularized the use of what today we call the full-thickness, or Wolfe-Krause, graft. Thiersch's original grafts were, for all practical purposes, full-thickness skin; later, in 1886 his perfected method was the same as that of Ollier's report of 1872. Both transplanted large films of epidermis with a thin layer of dermis, or what we would today call split-skin grafts. Reverdin had

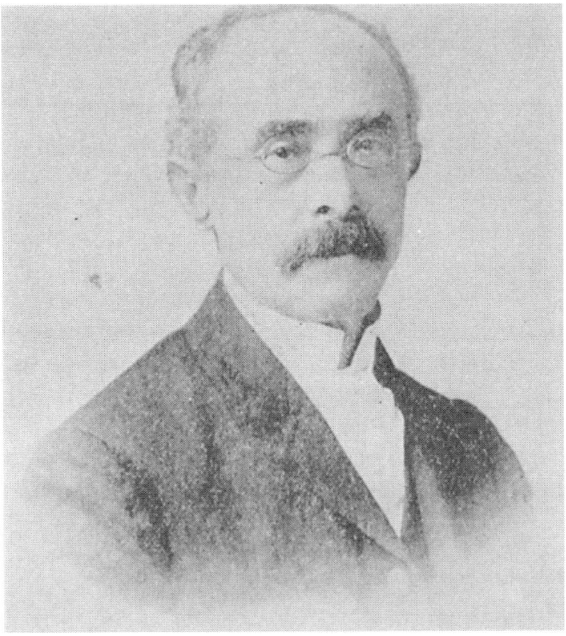

John Reissberg Wolfe. (Courtesy of the Library of the New York Academy of Medicine)

called his grafts "epidermal," but later admitted taking part of the corium.

J. R. Wolfe was probably a most interesting man, and it is unfortunate that we do not have his own story of his life. He was born in Breslau of Hungarian-Jewish ancestry and in 1848 came to Glasgow to become the tutor in Hebrew for the Free Church of Scotland. In 1853 he published the *Practical Hebrew Grammar.* He was graduated in medicine from the University of Glasgow in 1856, and, for some reason, practiced in Salonika for more than 2 years. He studied ophthalmology in Paris under Desmarres and then served a term in Garibaldi's army. He then returned to Scotland, but practiced in Aberdeen for 5 years before going to Glasgow, where he was in private practice and worked at what later became the Royal Eye Infirmary. A massive textbook of 450 pages, *Diseases and Injuries of the Eye,* was published in 1880, just 5 years after the reported full-thickness graft. In 1889 he became professor at St. Mungo's, the forerunner of the eye department of the University of Glasgow. He subsequently practiced for several years in Melbourne, Australia. He retired and returned to Glasgow, where he died in 1904. He had an extraordinary life, filled with many experiences in the most varied parts of the world. He had two sons, who both graduated in medicine.

A NEW METHOD OF PERFORMING PLASTIC OPERATIONS.

By J. R. WOLFE, M.D., F.R.C.S.Ed.,
Surgeon to the Glasgow Ophthalmic Institution; Lecturer on Ophthalmic Surgery in Anderson's University.

It is now nearly three hundred years since Tagliacozzi published his great work on *Plastic Operations;* and, notwithstanding the admiration which the work of the Bologna professor had elicited, it is remarkable how comparatively little has since been done for the cultivation of plastic surgery. The reasons are obvious. The fact is that, in operations on the nose, eyelids, and face—the most interesting regions for improving deformities—Tagliacozzi's method of taking flaps from the arm has been generally abandoned, on account of the extreme discomfort which it involves; and the practice of taking flaps from the forehead or face having been the only one in vogue, the procedure came to be considered more serious. In addition, when we take into account the elements of failure, from shrinking of the flap, from erysipelas or gangrene, it is not to be wondered at that surgeons are generally chary of resorting to the expedient, except in great emergencies. It amounts to this: we are to cut skin off the face to repair the face; and, in doing so, we run great risk of failure. To render plastic operations on the face more acceptable, and to bring them within a wider scope of utility, the following conditions must be fulfilled. 1. We must take a flap from the arm, or from any other part but the face. 2. We must seek to eliminate the elements of failure. I propose, in this short communication, to indicate the means of fulfilling both these conditions.

First, Tagliacozzi laid down the rule, which has ever since been considered as the primary law, and *sine quâ non* to the success of the operation, that the flap must retain its connection to the adjacent living structure by a pedicle which is to be severed only after complete union and cicatrisation of the raw surfaces. This pedicle has, in my opinion, been a source of great embarrassment to surgeons, and tended rather to retard the progress of plastic surgery. From my observations on transplantation of structures from the lower animals and on skin-grafting, as well as on plastic operations, I have long held it demonstrated, that in most cases the pedicle is not essential, if indeed it do contribute anything, to the vitality of flap. This being once established, we are henceforward free to choose our bit of skin from any part of the body we may find suitable.

My next endeavour has been to eliminate the elements of failure. The principal cause of failure I find to be in the subcutaneous structures. If we wish a skin-flap to adhere to a new surface by first intention or agglutination, we must be sure that it is cleared of all areolar tissue, and properly fixed in its new place. The following case will illustrate the points referred to.

Formation of the Lower Eyelid with Skin from the Forearm.—P. C., aged 25, a quarrier, was admitted into the Glasgow Ophthalmic Institution, with his face, eyes, and eyelids injured by an explosion of powder. I showed the man recently to the Edinburgh meeting of the Association, as an instance of conjunctival transplantation from the rabbit.* The right upper eyelid, which was strongly everted, I partially succeeded in correcting by skin-granting. The lower right eyelid being completely everted, its integument totally destroyed, and the skin of the face consisting of discoloured cicatrices not by any means suitable for plastic operations, I formed a new lower eyelid in the following manner. The edges of the upper and lower eyelids having been vivified, I introduced three ligatures into the border of the lower eyelid, which I entrusted to my assistant. By means of these ligatures, he used traction, whilst I dissected the whole of the cicatricial tissue, and thus liberated the subjacent structure. The ligatures were then introduced into the upper eyelid, and the edges of the upper and lower eyelids were thus united. I then elevated the edges of the wound, preparing them to receive the

* This patient had to undergo several operations before his eyes were rendered serviceable and his face presentable. Left eye: 1. Artificial pupil; 2. Conjunctival transplantation from rabbit. Right eye: 1. Paracentesis for onyx and hypopion; 2. Skin-grafting on upper eyelid; 3. Plastic operation on lower eyelid. All these operations were done without chloroform.

John Reissberg Wolfe: A new method of performing plastic operations. Br. Med. J., 2:360–361, 1875. (Courtesy of the Library of the College of Physicians of Philadelphia)

The problem of transplanting skin had interested many surgeons, and the names of some of these are commonly used today. Most of these have dealt with the ways of grafting free skin. The pedicle method was already known and dated back into ancient history, but here, over the span of a few years, we see free grafts of everything from epidermis to full-thickness skin. It will be a long time before any new developments take place, and then not until Filatov and Gillies, independently, "tube" the pedicle.

J. R. Wolfe of the skin graft should not be confused with Julius Wolff (1836–1902) of West Prussia, the originator of the law of bone growth. This Wolff began to study the problem at the suggestion of professor Langenbeck, after Ollier had published his original work. Wolff's law finally evolved and was defined in typical Teutonic fashion as, change in structure and form is followed by changes in the architecture and secondary alterations in external conformation in accordance with mathematical laws. It was Keith who said that Wolff's law represents a stage upon which the actors, that is, the osteoblasts, never appear. John B. Murphy, Chicago's famous surgeon, said it more succinctly, "The amount of growth in a bone depends upon the need for it."

Surgery of the hand demands a clear view of the intricate parts, and to operate in a bloody field compromises our efforts and may lead to disaster. Our modern pneumatic tourniquets are so efficient that it is difficult to imagine what it must have been like before. Restricting the blood flow in an extremity by some means has surely been done since ancient times. We know that Jean-Louis Petit (1674–1750) used a screw tourniquet of his own design, and others must have had similar ideas. But when conservative surgery of the extremities became the accepted treatment, a bloodless field became essential.

Johann Friedrich August von Esmarch (1823–1908) developed the use of an elastic bandage, made of woven rubber, to exsanguinate the extremity. Several turns of rubber tubing were then applied proximally, the two ends of which were locked together with a hook and chain. He used this in operations such as bony resections for osteomyelitis, and he carefully pointed out that in such cases, where infection is present, one should not wrap the whole limb with the rubber bandage but instead simply elevate the extremity before applying the encircling tourniquet.

Esmarch was born in Tonning in Schleswig-Holstein, which was to be the site of friction between Germany and Denmark soon after. He studied in the local schools and took his medical training at Kiel and Göttingen, first under Langenbeck and then under Stromeyer, whom he later succeeded as professor. He married Stromeyer's daughter. He was active in the insurrection against Denmark, taking part in the war of 1848–50 along with Stromeyer, who was surgeon general of the Hanover forces. It

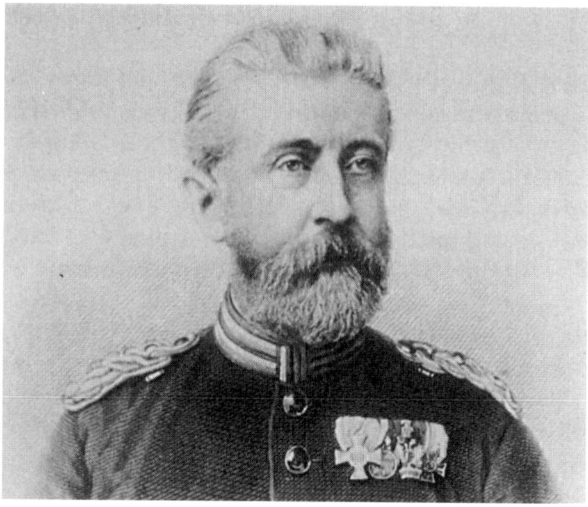

Johann Friedrich August von Esmarch. (Courtesy of the Library of the New York Academy of Medicine)

58.

(Chirurgie No. 19.)

Ueber künstliche Blutleere bei Operationen.

Von

Prof. F. Esmarch

in Kiel.

Meine Herren! Sie Alle sind gestern Zeugen gewesen einer schwierigen und langdauernden Operation, bei welcher die Patientin sehr viel Blut verlor, trotz aller Vorsicht, die dabei angewendet wurde.

Es handelte sich um die Exstirpation einer kindskopfgrossen Geschwulst, eines blutreichen Markschwammes, welcher die ganze obere Halsgegend rechterseits einnahm. Es fand sich, dass die Neubildung nicht nur einen Theil der Parotis, sondern auch die benachbarten Muskeln, den Kopfnicker, den Mylohyoideus und den hintern Bauch des Digastricus derartig ergriffen hatte, dass ich mich genöthigt sah, beträchtliche Stücke von allen diesen Theilen mitwegzunehmen, sodass am Schlusse der Operation die Vena jugularis interna und die Carotis in grosser Ausdehnung in der Wunde freilagen.

Was die Operation vor Allem schwierig machte, war die ausserordentlich starke Blutung. Sie erinnern sich, dass fast bei jedem Schnitte, obwohl ich dieselben aus Vorsicht sehr klein machte, eine oder mehrere Arterien spritzten oder Venen ihr dunkles Blut über das Operationsfeld ergossen. Sie sahen, wie ich den Blutverlust dadurch möglichst zu verringern suchte, dass ich nach jedem Schnitte die blutenden Gefässe mit Schieberpincetten fasste und diese hängen liess, während ich weiter operirte. Mehr als ein Mal hingen sämmtliche 21 Pincetten, welche ich bei grossen Operationen immer zur Hand habe, in der Wunde, und sah ich mich genöthigt, erst die gefassten Gefässe zu unterbinden, ehe ich weiter in die Tiefe dringen konnte. Als

Klin. Vorträge, 58. (Chir. 19.) 31

Johann Friedrich August von Esmarch: Ueber künstliche Blutleere bei Operationen. Samml. Klin. Vortr., *58* (Chir. 19):373–384, 1873. (Courtesy of the Library of the College of Physicians of Philadelphia)

was in this war that conservative surgery of injuries by resection rather than by radical amputation was adopted, and he published an account of his experiences with resection of parts damaged by bullet wounds. His surgical life became intimately connected with war and with care of the wounded. He devised a first-aid packet for each soldier to carry and promoted better and earlier care of the wounded. He was one of the instigators of the pavilion system of hospital construction and, as Thiersch was doing, introduced the Lister methods on his service.

During the Franco-Prussian war of 1870, he served as chief of a large hospital and later carried over his ideas of first-aid care to civilian casualties. Using the plan of the St. John Society in England, he formed a Samaritan association, with branches in each village. He wrote a *Textbook for Samaritans*, and another, *Early Aid in Injuries and Accidents*, was translated into English and published in Philadelphia in 1883.

His second wife was a princess of Schleswig-Holstein and an aunt of the German empress. He was unchanged by such titled relatives and continued his work and teaching, being highly respected by surgeons of all countries. He was a worthy successor to his chief, Stromeyer, and a credit to his first professor, Langenbeck.

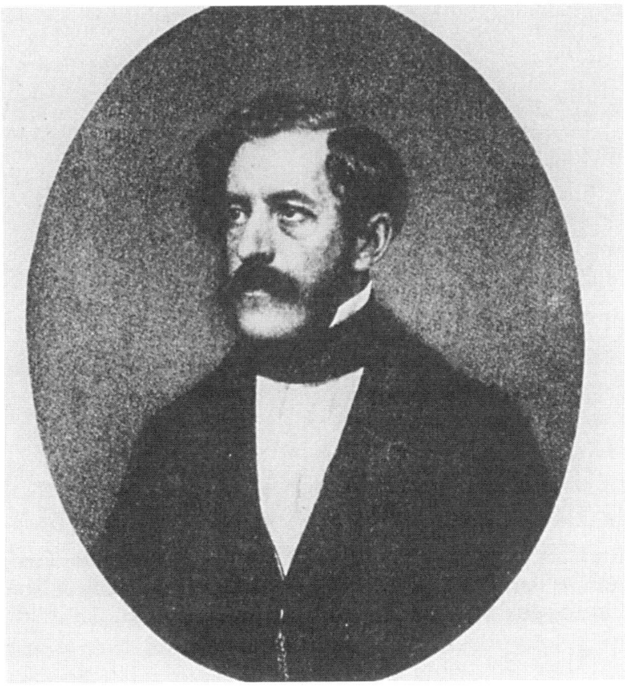

Bernhard Rudolf Konrad von Langenbeck. (From Garrison, F. H.: An Introduction to the History of Medicine. ed. 4. Philadelphia, W. B. Saunders, 1929)

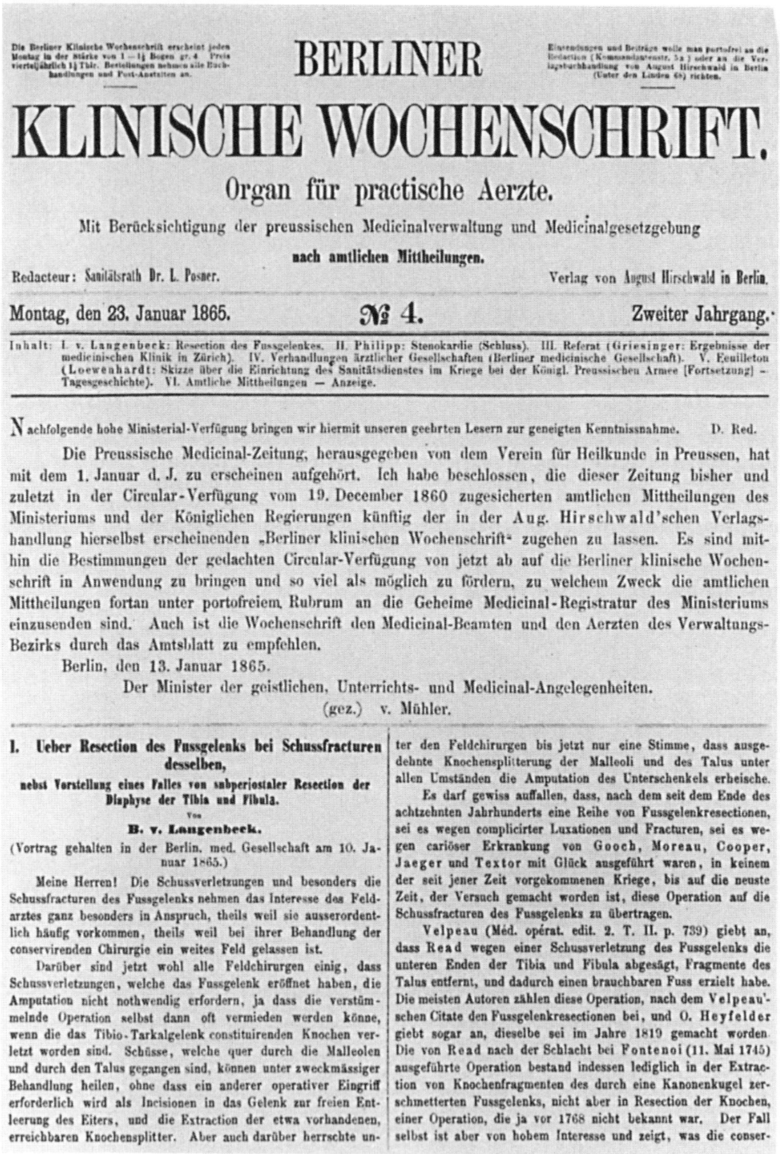

Die Berliner Klinische Wochenschrift erscheint jeden Montag in der Stärke von 1–1½ Bogen gr. 4. Preis vierteljährlich 1⅓ Thlr. Bestellungen nehmen alle Buchhandlungen und Post-Anstalten an.

BERLINER

Einsendungen und Beiträge wolle man portofrei an die Redaction (Kommandantenstr. 5a) oder an die Verlagsbuchhandlung von August Hirschwald in Berlin (Unter den Linden 68) richten.

KLINISCHE WOCHENSCHRIFT.

Organ für practische Aerzte.

Mit Berücksichtigung der preussischen Medicinalverwaltung und Medicinalgesetzgebung

nach amtlichen Mittheilungen.

Redacteur: Sanitätsrath Dr. L. Posner. Verlag von August Hirschwald in Berlin.

Montag, den 23. Januar 1865. № 4. Zweiter Jahrgang.

Inhalt: I. v. Langenbeck: Resection des Fussgelenkes. II. Philipp: Stenokardie (Schluss). III. Referat (Griesinger: Ergebnisse der medicinischen Klinik in Zürich). IV. Verhandlungen ärztlicher Gesellschaften (Berliner medicinische Gesellschaft). V. Feuilleton (Loewenhardt: Skizze über die Einrichtung des Sanitätsdienstes im Kriege bei der Königl. Preussischen Armee [Fortsetzung] – Tagesgeschichte). VI. Amtliche Mittheilungen — Anzeige.

Nachfolgende hohe Ministerial-Verfügung bringen wir hiermit unseren geehrten Lesern zur geneigten Kenntnissnahme. D. Red.

Die Preussische Medicinal-Zeitung, herausgegeben von dem Verein für Heilkunde in Preussen, hat mit dem 1. Januar d. J. zu erscheinen aufgehört. Ich habe beschlossen, die dieser Zeitung bisher und zuletzt in der Circular-Verfügung vom 19. December 1860 zugesicherten amtlichen Mittheilungen des Ministeriums und der Königlichen Regierungen künftig der in der Aug. Hirschwald'schen Verlagshandlung hierselbst erscheinenden „Berliner klinischen Wochenschrift" zugehen zu lassen. Es sind mithin die Bestimmungen der gedachten Circular-Verfügung von jetzt ab auf die Berliner klinische Wochenschrift in Anwendung zu bringen und so viel als möglich zu fördern, zu welchem Zweck die amtlichen Mittheilungen fortan unter portofreiem Rubrum an die Geheime Medicinal-Registratur des Ministeriums einzusenden sind. Auch ist die Wochenschrift den Medicinal-Beamten und den Aerzten des Verwaltungs-Bezirks durch das Amtsblatt zu empfehlen.

Berlin, den 13. Januar 1865.

Der Minister der geistlichen, Unterrichts- und Medicinal-Angelegenheiten.

(gez.) v. Mühler.

I. Ueber Resection des Fussgelenks bei Schussfracturen desselben,

nebst Vorstellung eines Falles von subperiostaler Resection der Diaphyse der Tibia und Fibula.

Von

B. v. Langenbeck.

(Vortrag gehalten in der Berlin. med. Gesellschaft am 10. Januar 1865.)

Meine Herren! Die Schussverletzungen und besonders die Schussfracturen des Fussgelenks nehmen das Interesse des Feldarztes ganz besonders in Anspruch, theils weil sie ausserordentlich häufig vorkommen, theils weil bei ihrer Behandlung der conservirenden Chirurgie ein weites Feld gelassen ist.

Darüber sind jetzt wohl alle Feldchirurgen einig, dass Schussverletzungen, welche das Fussgelenk eröffnet haben, die Amputation nicht nothwendig erfordern, ja dass die verstümmelnde Operation selbst dann oft vermieden werden könne, wenn die das Tibio-Tarkalgelenk constituirenden Knochen verletzt worden sind. Schüsse, welche quer durch die Malleolen und durch den Talus gegangen sind, können unter zweckmässiger Behandlung heilen, ohne dass ein anderer operativer Eingriff erforderlich wird als Incisionen in das Gelenk zur freien Entleerung des Eiters, und die Extraction der etwa vorhandenen, erreichbaren Knochensplitter. Aber auch darüber herrschte unter den Feldchirurgen bis jetzt nur eine Stimme, dass ausgedehnte Knochensplitterung der Malleoli und des Talus unter allen Umständen die Amputation des Unterschenkels erheische.

Es darf gewiss auffallen, dass, nach dem seit dem Ende des achtzehnten Jahrhunderts eine Reihe von Fussgelenkresectionen, sei es wegen complicirter Luxationen und Fracturen, sei es wegen cariöser Erkrankung von Gooch, Moreau, Cooper, Jaeger und Textor mit Glück ausgeführt waren, in keinem der seit jener Zeit vorgekommenen Kriege, bis auf die neuste Zeit, der Versuch gemacht worden ist, diese Operation auf die Schussfracturen des Fussgelenks zu übertragen.

Velpeau (Méd. opérat. edit. 2. T. II. p. 739) giebt an, dass Read wegen einer Schussverletzung des Fussgelenks die unteren Enden der Tibia und Fibula abgesägt, Fragmente des Talus entfernt, und dadurch einen brauchbaren Fuss erzielt habe. Die meisten Autoren zählen diese Operation, nach dem Velpeau'schen Citate den Fussgelenkresectionen bei, und O. Heyfelder giebt sogar an, dieselbe sei im Jahre 1819 gemacht worden. Die von Read nach der Schlacht bei Fontenoi (11. Mai 1745) ausgeführte Operation bestand indessen lediglich in der Extraction von Knochenfragmenten des durch eine Kanonenkugel zerschmetterten Fussgelenks, nicht aber in Resection der Knochen, einer Operation, die ja vor 1768 nicht bekannt war. Der Fall selbst ist aber von hohem Interesse und zeigt, was die conser-

Bernhard Rudolf Konrad von Langenbeck: Ueber Resection des Fussgelenks bei Schussfracturen. Berl. Klin. Wochenschr., *2*, 1865. (Courtesy of The Francis A. Countway Library of Medicine, Boston, Massachusetts)

It is fitting that mention be made of the surgical progenitor of a remarkable group of German surgeons. **Bernhard Rudolf Konrad von Langenbeck** (1810–1887) was born in Horneburg and was a nephew of a

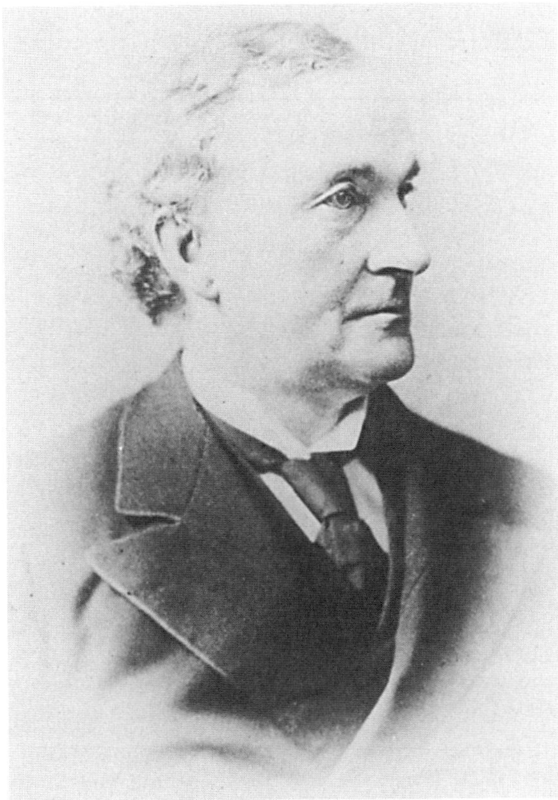

Henry Austin Martin. (Courtesy of The Francis A. Countway Library of Medicine, Boston, Massachusetts)

surgeon, Konrad J. M. Langenbeck. He graduated in 1835, traveled to France and England, and became privatdocent at Göttingen and then professor at Kiel until 1847, when he took the chair at Berlin. He trained Esmarch, Thiersch, and Trendelenburg and was chief over Billroth, who later made the Allgemeine Krankenhaus in Vienna world famous. Billroth, in turn, trained many surgeons whose names are eponyms in general surgery. One was Emil Theodor Kocher, who, in turn, trained de Quervain. Langenbeck was a great teacher, and his influence on surgery was a big factor in the rise of German surgery. I am sure that his surgical "sons" and "grandsons" would agree with me in saying that he was certainly one of those giants upon whose shoulders they stood to see further.

For many years the Esmarch tourniquet was used, and then it was found that the woven rubber bandage could be left in place proximally

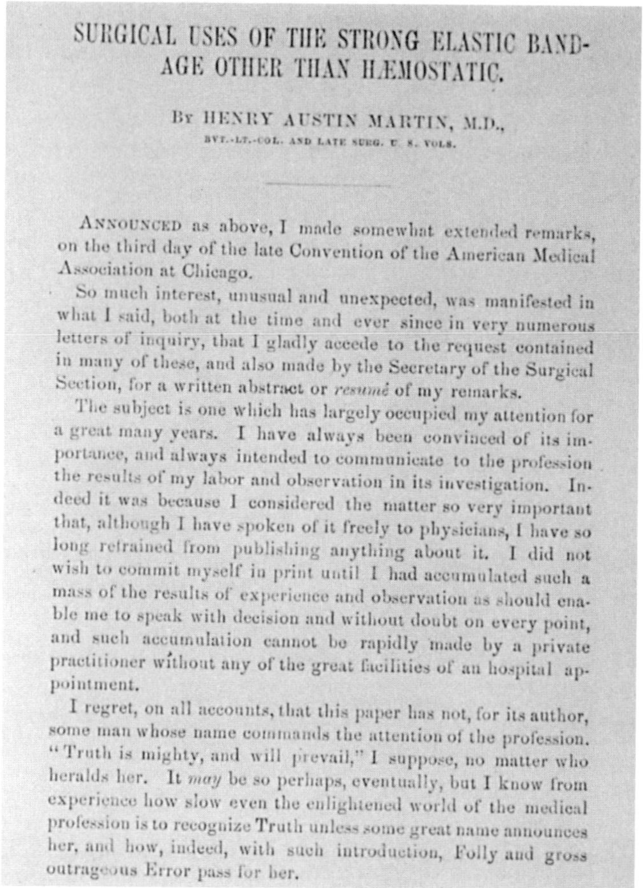

SURGICAL USES OF THE STRONG ELASTIC BANDAGE OTHER THAN HÆMOSTATIC.

By HENRY AUSTIN MARTIN, M.D.,

BVT.-LT.-COL. AND LATE SURG. U. S. VOLS.

ANNOUNCED as above, I made somewhat extended remarks, on the third day of the late Convention of the American Medical Association at Chicago.

So much interest, unusual and unexpected, was manifested in what I said, both at the time and ever since in very numerous letters of inquiry, that I gladly accede to the request contained in many of these, and also made by the Secretary of the Surgical Section, for a written abstract or *resumé* of my remarks.

The subject is one which has largely occupied my attention for a great many years. I have always been convinced of its importance, and always intended to communicate to the profession the results of my labor and observation in its investigation. Indeed it was because I considered the matter so very important that, although I have spoken of it freely to physicians, I have so long refrained from publishing anything about it. I did not wish to commit myself in print until I had accumulated such a mass of the results of experience and observation as should enable me to speak with decision and without doubt on every point, and such accumulation cannot be rapidly made by a private practitioner without any of the great facilities of an hospital appointment.

I regret, on all accounts, that this paper has not, for its author, some man whose name commands the attention of the profession. "Truth is mighty, and will prevail," I suppose, no matter who heralds her. It *may* be so perhaps, eventually, but I know from experience how slow even the enlightened world of the medical profession is to recognize Truth unless some great name announces her, and how, indeed, with such introduction, Folly and gross outrageous Error pass for her.

Henry Austin Martin: Surgical uses of the strong elastic bandage other than haemostatic. Trans. Am. Med. Assoc., *28*:589–610, 1877. (Courtesy of the Library of the College of Physicians of Philadelphia)

and the distal part removed. This avoided the use of the cumbersome rubber tubing, with its hook and chain. But in 1877, a Boston surgeon used a thin rubber bandage for compression, just as today we use an elastic bandage, and this took the place of the heavy, unwieldly Esmarch bandage.

Henry Austin Martin (1824–1884) used this thin rubber bandage—now known by his name—in treating indolent ulcers, but never as a means of exsanguinating the part. In fact, he said that it could not arrest the circulation.

Martin was born in London, the descendant of a distinguished family of Huguenots who had emigrated to Ireland in the 1600s. Coming to America as a boy, he graduated from Harvard Medical School in 1845 and practiced in Roxbury, a suburb of Boston. He was a surgeon, active in the Civil War for Hancock's corps. References have been made to his performing a ligation of the femoral artery and a primary resection of the upper end of the femur, and to his development of an extension apparatus used after excision of the humerus. He wrote on the treatment of fistula-in-ano and a method of tracheotomy without a cannula. At an international medical congress, he said that he had successfully used his elastic rubber bandage in the treatment, after aspiration, of more than 140 knee joint effusions, requiring more than 400 needle punctures. He emphasized that these were all done without any antiseptic precautions except for cleanliness of the needles.

Martin's name should not be recalled, however, for a glorified elastic bandage, but rather for his work on smallpox vaccination. He was so impressed by Jenner's work that he became engrossed in the study of vaccination and of means of improving the results. He collected all writings on the subject and was said to have had the most complete library on the subject except for that in the British Museum.

At that time, vaccine was propagated from arm to arm. The "humanized" virus was stored by saving the crusts. Martin believed that these methods were too slow, that the incidence of the disease was increasing, and that the vaccine was becoming weaker or attenuated. When two articles appeared in the French literature about propagating the virus in animals, he was so impressed that he sent an agent to Paris to bring back this new viral strain, which had been grown from a case of spontaneous cowpox in France. He vaccinated his own herd of fifty cows and successfully maintained the virus. After 3 years of comparing this fresh virus, propagated on animals, with that of the "humanized" type, he was convinced not only that it was more efficacious but that it reduced the chance of transmitting other diseases. A bitter controversy resulted; but the idea gradually caught on, and the procedure spread and became universally adopted.

Martin was an intense man, with a wide knowledge of the classics as well as the medical literature, and he was described as being a fine speaker. He was generous in referring to the works of others, if merited, but was scathing in his criticism of what he considered to be wrong. Proud, imperious, and brooking no personal affront, he could be forcible and argumentative, often denunciatory. These are terms that were used by one of his biographers.

Reading his paper on the elastic bandage—which he wrote for the surgical section of the American Medical Association—one gets the feeling that he was somewhat pompous and condescending. He used more than 300 words to introduce the subject, a form of presentation that would scarcely pass the desk of any modern editor.

When he was nearly 60 years of age, he developed diabetes and failed rapidly, dying within a year. He had two sons, both of whom became physicians. Some of his admirers thought that he, rather than Waterhouse, should have been called the Jenner of America.

THE MID-NINETEENTH CENTURY

Wars have usually resulted in great progress in surgery. The Civil War in the United States saw the development of pavilion-type hospitals, an idea carried on in Germany by Esmarch and Thiersch, and a system of evacuation of the wounded by the then surgeon general, Letterman. A work on nerve injuries was the direct result of the efforts of a most unusual man.

Silas Weir Mitchell (1829–1914)—brilliant and versatile, a novelist and a poet, neurologist and investigator of drug actions—is noted for his descriptions of ascending neuritis, causalgia, and erythromelalgia, the last being the only state known specifically by his name. His book, published in 1872, *Injuries of Nerves and Their Consequences*, should be required reading of all surgeons interested in peripheral nerves.

Mitchell was born in Philadelphia of a father who was a distinguished physician, and he was the seventh physician in three generations of the family. A fundamentalist upbringing, with compulsory church and Sunday school, strict observance of the Sabbath, and abhorrence of card playing as an evil pastime, did not deter his mischievousness, which was said to have led to a poor record in school, making a general nuisance of himself, and a penchant for pinching the melons and peaches of the nearby farmer's orchards. He was only 15 when he entered the university, and his father was so perturbed that he thought it inadvisable for him to try to study medicine. Mitchell settled down, however, and by the time he was graduated in 1850, he was the leader in his class.

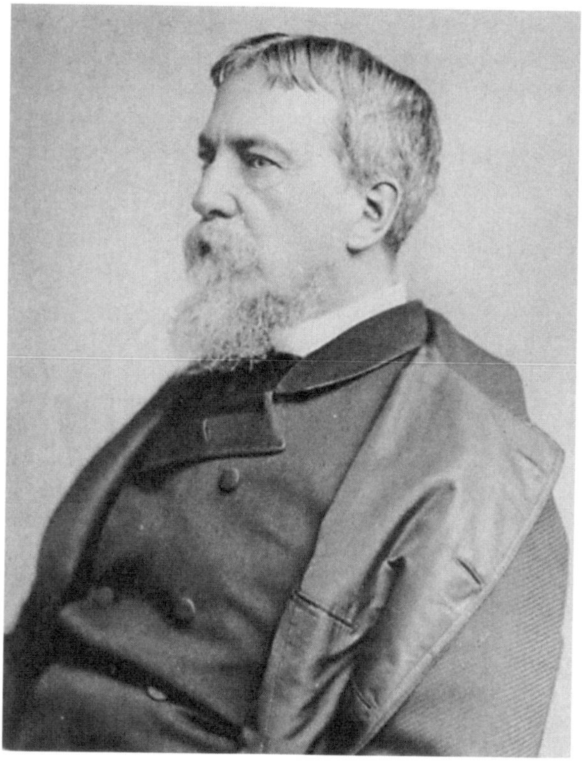

Silas Weir Mitchell. (Courtesy of the Library of the New York Academy of Medicine)

Mitchell spent a year of study in Paris; his interest seemed to be in physiology, and here he was most impressed by Claude Bernard. Returning to Philadelphia, he began a study of the effect of snake venom, a subject that was to interest him for many years, and also investigated the action of drugs. One of his co-workers, Hammond, later became the surgeon general, and when the Civil War broke out, Mitchell was placed in charge of a hospital for nervous diseases. Here he, Morehouse, and W. W. Keen, who was the surgeon, began the compilation of records of wounded men, which provided the material for the volume, *Gunshot Wounds and Other Injuries of the Nerves.* Published in 1864, this book contained the first description of the condition called causalgia, and all of their material was later used for the classic of 1872. Mitchell knew that the opportunity to study such a large and varied number of these problems was unique, and he made the most of it, with detailed histories, findings on examination, and follow-up reports. When an opportunity such as

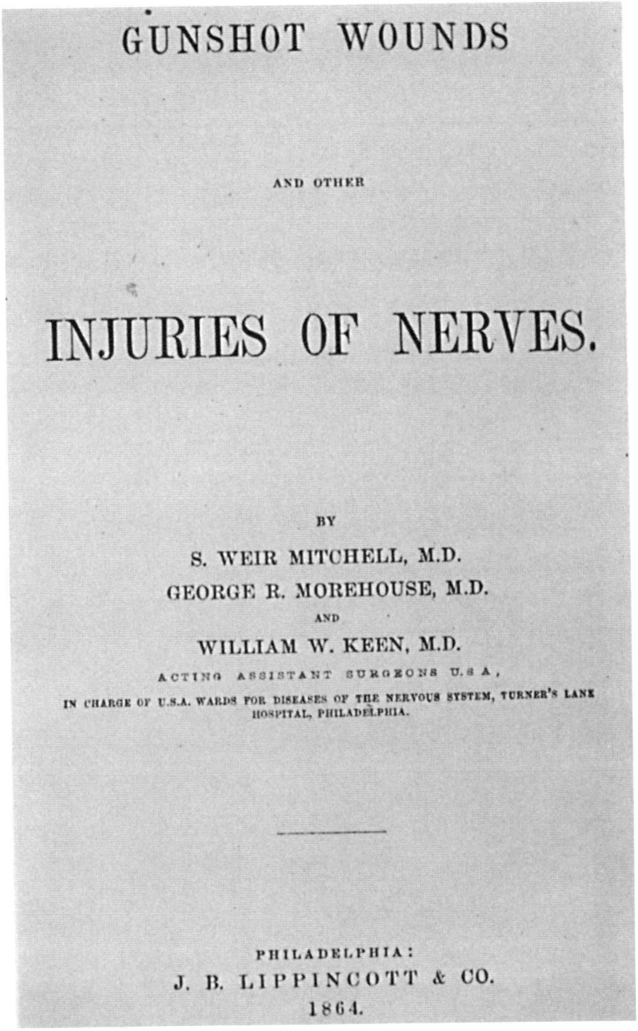

GUNSHOT WOUNDS

AND OTHER

INJURIES OF NERVES.

BY

S. WEIR MITCHELL, M.D.
GEORGE R. MOREHOUSE, M.D.
AND
WILLIAM W. KEEN, M.D.

ACTING ASSISTANT SURGEONS U.S.A.,
IN CHARGE OF U.S.A. WARDS FOR DISEASES OF THE NERVOUS SYSTEM, TURNER'S LANE HOSPITAL, PHILADELPHIA.

PHILADELPHIA:
J. B. LIPPINCOTT & CO.
1864.

Silas Weir Mitchell, George R. Morehouse, and William W. Keen: Gunshot Wounds and Other Injuries of Nerves. Philadelphia, J. B. Lippincott, 1864. (Courtesy of the Library of the College of Physicians of Philadelphia)

this comes, one must be prepared. He was ready in 1861, as was Tinel, who also used the same kind of opportunity to study nerve wounds in World War I. Sir Herbert Seddon and his Oxford group did the same for nerve wounds in World War II.

Mitchell's contributions to neurology can be grouped thusly—clinical observations of great detail of injury and disease; experimental investiga-

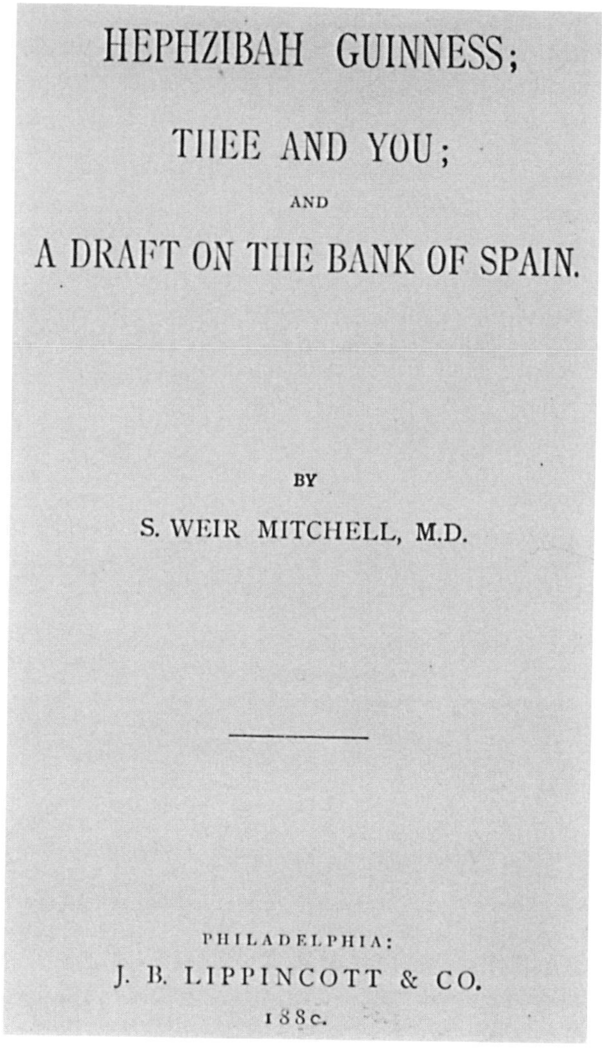

HEPHZIBAH GUINNESS;

THEE AND YOU;

AND

A DRAFT ON THE BANK OF SPAIN.

BY

S. WEIR MITCHELL, M.D.

PHILADELPHIA:

J. B. LIPPINCOTT & CO.

1880.

Silas Weir Mitchell: Hephzibah Guinness; Thee and You; and A Draft on the Bank of Spain. Philadelphia, J. B. Lippincott, 1880. (Courtesy of the Library of the College of Physicians of Philadelphia)

tion of the function of the cerebellum; descriptions of new clinical entities, and also the therapy of such disease, including the use of drugs. In addition to the studies of snake venom, he investigated the effects of morphine and atropine and the use of amyl nitrate to abort epileptic attacks. He used splints for local rest of affected parts, and he used ice and local sprays to alleviate spasm. He also used massage and faradic current. (Did Mitchell meet Duchenne while on his tour of Paris?)

He was one of those people with imagination. One idea or a way to investigate some problem led to another and another. Keen, who worked with him, said that to spend an hour with Mitchell caused such a turmoil in his mind that he could not sleep. Another described him as being "yeasty." He must have been a most interesting man. Such a wealth of knowledge of his own field, with obviously wide interests in other arts, along with his literary background, would make him a good conversationalist. He is reported to have said that a man is successful if he is at the top of his profession, has written a successful novel, and has killed a king salmon. That is quite a series of achievements, and he did all three and more.

Mitchell was turned down for the chair of physiology by both the University of Pennsylvania and Jefferson Medical College. He organized the Infirmary for Nervous Diseases and developed a faithful following of students and patients. Apparently, he became more and more interested in psychiatric disorders as he grew older. His treatment of mental disease was not accepted at first. He is considered to be one of the earliest psychoanalysts.

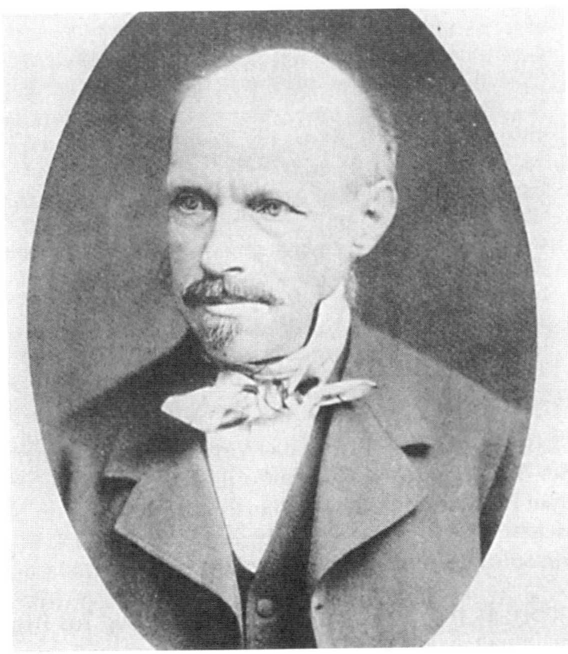

Georg Meissner. (From Beilage Munch. Med. Wochenschr., 52[2]:164, 1905. Courtesy of the Library of the New York Academy of Medicine)

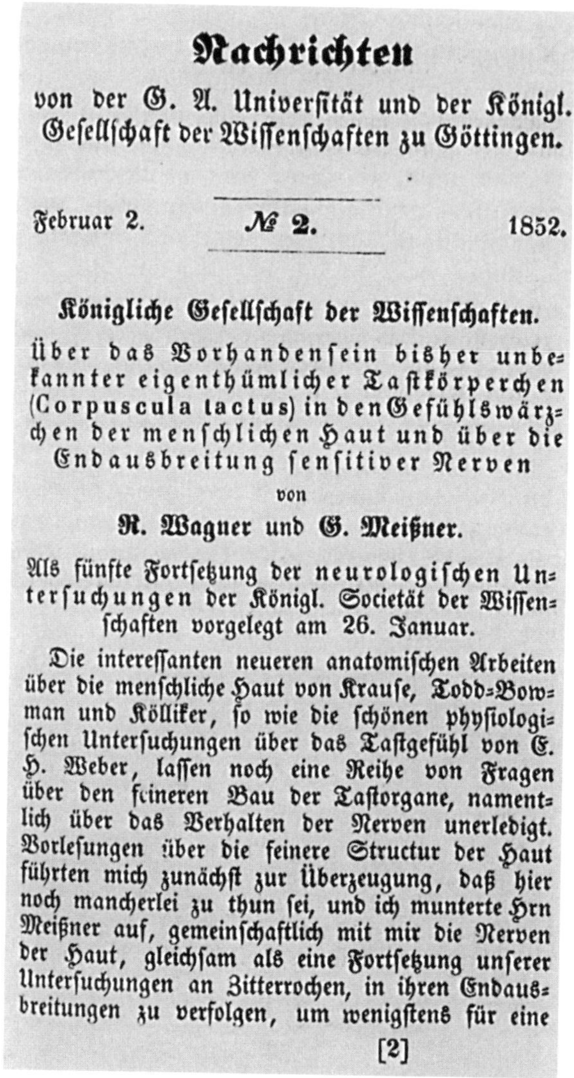

Nachrichten

von der G. A. Universität und der Königl. Gesellschaft der Wissenschaften zu Göttingen.

Februar 2. **№ 2.** 1852.

Königliche Gesellschaft der Wissenschaften.

Über das Vorhandensein bisher unbekannter eigenthümlicher Tastkörperchen (Corpuscula tactus) in den Gefühlswärzchen der menschlichen Haut und über die Endausbreitung sensitiver Nerven

von

R. Wagner und G. Meißner.

Als fünfte Fortsetzung der neurologischen Untersuchungen der Königl. Societät der Wissenschaften vorgelegt am 26. Januar.

Die interessanten neueren anatomischen Arbeiten über die menschliche Haut von Krause, Todd-Bowman und Kölliker, so wie die schönen physiologischen Untersuchungen über das Tastgefühl von E. H. Weber, lassen noch eine Reihe von Fragen über den feineren Bau der Tastorgane, namentlich über das Verhalten der Nerven unerledigt. Vorlesungen über die feinere Structur der Haut führten mich zunächst zur Überzeugung, daß hier noch mancherlei zu thun sei, und ich munterte Hrn Meißner auf, gemeinschaftlich mit mir die Nerven der Haut, gleichsam als eine Fortsetzung unserer Untersuchungen an Zitterrochen, in ihren Endausbreitungen zu verfolgen, um wenigstens für eine

[2]

R. Wagner and Georg Meissner: Über das Vorhandensein bisher unbekannter eigenthümlicher Tastkörperchen (Corpuscula tactus) in den Gefühlswärzchen der menschlichen Haut und über die Endausbreitung sensitiver Nerven. Nach. Königl. Gesellschaft Wissenschaften (Göttingen), 2:17–32, 1852. (Courtesy of the American Philosophical Society, Philadelphia, Pennsylvania)

More and more as the years went on he increased his literary output, writing poems, short stories, and novels. *Westways* was a novel about his impressions of Gettysburg just after the battle. Some of his books showed his interest in psychic disturbances.

He died at age 85 after an attack of influenza, still sufficiently mentally alert at the beginning of these last days to read the proof of one of his poems, but finally he became delirious with fantasies of being a surgeon at the Battle of Gettysburg.

He was a giant in medicine, especially in the fields of neurology and the injuries and diseases of the peripheral nerves, but he was a man who was prepared when the opportunity came, with an inquisitive mind and an ability to express himself. Wars are the proving grounds of surgeons, but the field of surgery of peripheral nerves owes its existence to men such as Silas Weir Mitchell.

Early in the 1800s, the laboratory of Johannes Müller, in Berlin, was one of the most renowned anatomy schools in Europe. Schwann was there when Little came to study for his medical degree, and Henle and Remak were also there.

Georg Meissner (1829–1905) was a student there later, and early in his studies described the skin corpuscle that is named after him. A little later, when he was at Basle, he described the Meissner plexus of the intestine. He went from Müller's laboratory directly to the professorship of anatomy and physiology at Basle, at the age of 26.

Meissner was born in Hanover and, as so many others, took his medical training in various places, first at Berlin and then Munich, before taking his degree at Göttingen, where Langenbeck was professor. After a 3-year term at Basle, he moved to Freiburg. He finally settled at Göttingen as chief. He was apparently a brilliant student, and he became a professor at the age of 26.

He was an experimental physiologist, and he made valuable contributions to the study of digestive processes and made physiochemical studies of hippuric acid.

His difficult personality caused him to have few friends, and, though respected by students and colleagues, he was severely criticized for some of his work.

With Henle he edited the *Fortschritte der Anatomie und Physiologie* until 1872, when his scientific contributions stopped. He lived more than 30 years more and died of a stroke at age 76. He is said to have burned many of his notes and papers. He was 43 years of age when he stopped publishing, and what he might have contributed after that was deliberately destroyed.

Richard von Volkmann (1830–1889) is one of the best known of the German surgeons of the mid-nineteenth century; we frequently use his name in describing an ischemic contracture of the muscles of the forearm. His description of this ischemic contracture, published in 1881, was really one of his minor contributions. In it he said that, for many years, he had called attention to a form of paralysis and contracture following the

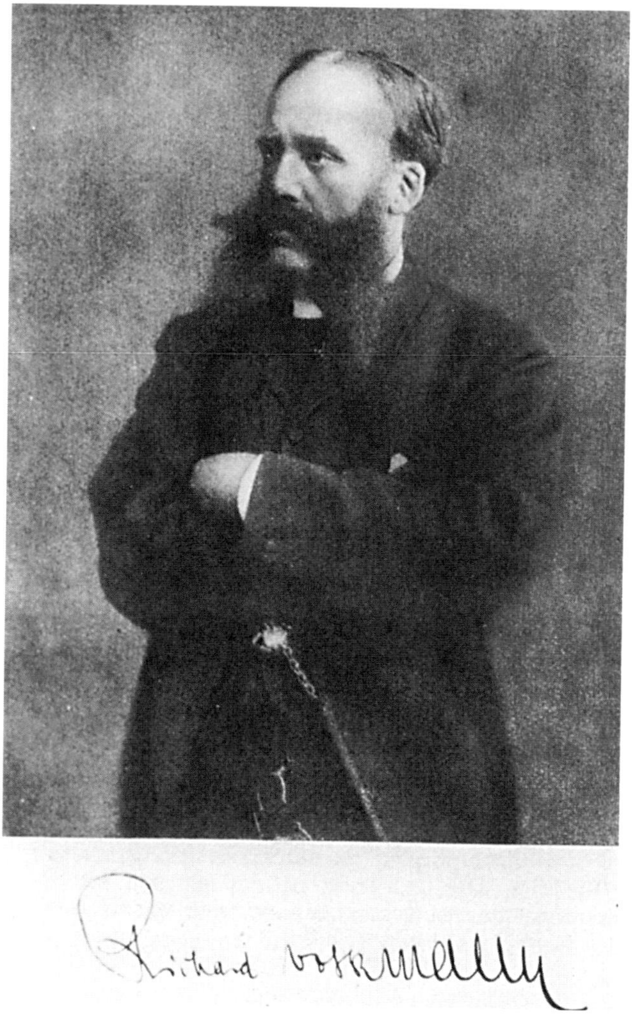

Richard von Volkmann. (From Trendelenburg, F.: Die Ersten 25 Jahre der Deutschen Gesellschaft für Chirurgie; ein Beitrag zur Geschichte der Chirurgie. Berlin, Verlag von Julius Springer, 1923. Courtesy of the Library of the College of Physicians of Philadelphia)

use of a tight bandage, which was not due to the effect on nerves but was of muscular origin, caused by a lack of oxygen. He believed that this was due to arterial blockage and that the *concurrent venous stasis* seemed to hasten the paralysis. The point of this short paper was to bring out the difference between these contractures of rapid development and those

Centralblatt

für

CHIRURGIE

herausgegeben

von

F. König, in Göttingen. **E. Richter,** in Breslau. **R. Volkmann,** in Halle a/S.

Achter Jahrgang.

Wöchentlich eine Nummer. Preis des Jahrgangs 20 Mark, bei halbjähriger Pränumeration. Zu beziehen durch alle Buchhandlungen und Postanstalten.

Nº. 51. Sonnabend, den 24. December. **1881.**

Inhalt: Volkmann, Die ischaemischen Muskellähmungen und Kontrakturen. — **Wittelshöfer,** Ein Instrument zur Operation der Phimose. (Original-Mittheilungen).
Macewen, Chromgut. — **Albert,** Fehlen der Hirnpulsation. — **Maier,** Ganglien der harnabführenden Wege. — **Winckel,** Pathologie der weiblichen Sexualorgane. — **Shaffer,** Gelenkneurosen. — **Ollier,** Hüftgelenkresektion. — **Tillaux,** Lisfranc'sche Amputation.
Del Greco, Galvanokaustische Schere. — **Paquet,** Oberkiefergeschwulst. — **Radulowitsch,** Kanüle in der Luftröhre. — **Mangiagalli,** Peritonealplastik.

Die ischaemischen Muskellähmungen und -Kontrakturen.

Von

Richard Volkmann.

Bereits vor einer längeren Reihe von Jahren habe ich darauf aufmerksam gemacht, dass die nach zu fest angelegten Verbänden zuweilen eintretenden Lähmungen und Kontrakturen der Glieder nicht, wie man bis dahin angenommen, auf Lähmungen der Nerven durch den Druck beruhen, sondern durch einen raschen und massenhaften Zerfall der kontraktilen Substanz und die auf ihn folgenden reaktiven und regenerativen Vorgänge entstünden. Die Lähmung und Kontraktur sei als eine rein myogene aufzufassen[1].

Eine Reihe seitdem gemachter neuer Erfahrungen hat die Richtigkeit dieser Behauptung lediglich bestätigt, uns zugleich aber auch bestimmtere Anschauungen über den Charakter der hier in Frage kommenden Vorgänge und Processe gewinnen lassen. Ich möchte daher meine gegenwärtigen Anschauungen in folgende Sätze zusammenfassen:

[1] Volkmann, Krankheiten der Bewegungsorgane p. 846 und Beiträge zur Chirurgie, Leipzig 1875. p. 219. Kraske, Centralbl. f. Chirurgie 1879. No. 12.

51

Richard von Volkmann: Die ischaemischen Muskellähmungen und -Kontrakturen. Centralblatt Chir., *8*:801–803, 1881. (Courtesy of the Library of the College of Physicians of Philadelphia)

which developed late, after nerve paralyses. The fact that he mentioned the venous stasis implies that he believed the arterial block alone was not the sole cause, for this—such as from emboli—results in gangrene of distal parts, something that does not occur with Volkmann's ischemic paralysis.

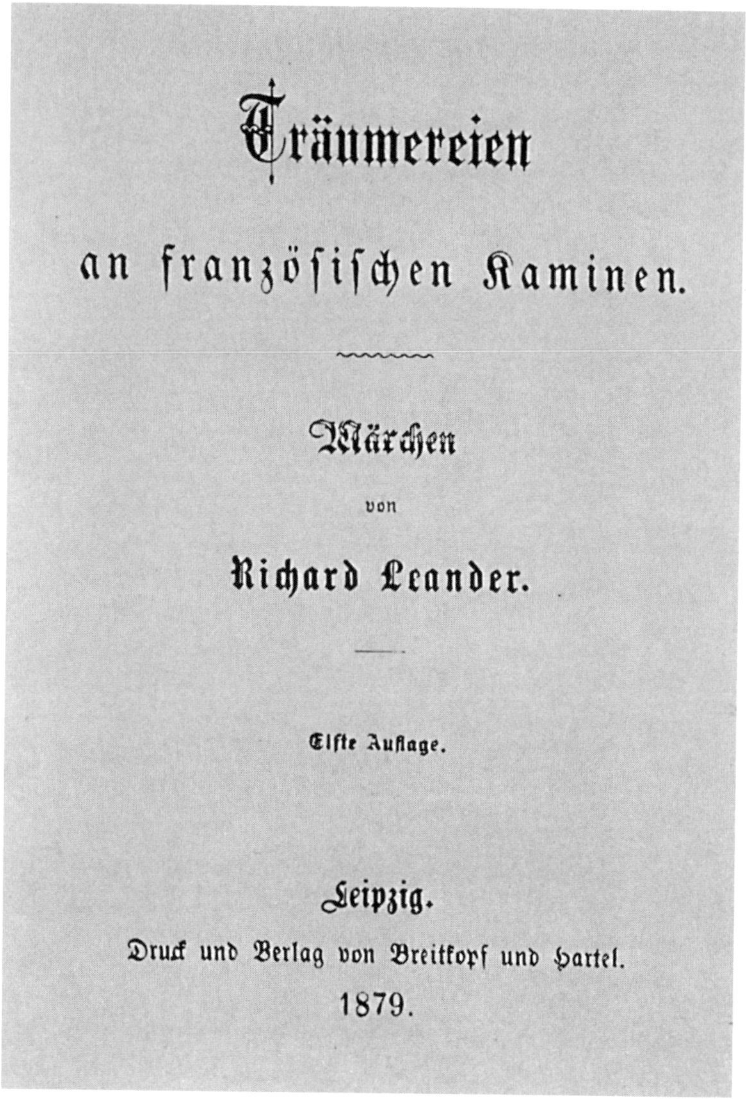
Träumereien

an französischen Kaminen.

Märchen

von

Richard Leander.

Elfte Auflage.

Leipzig.

Druck und Verlag von Breitkopf und Härtel.

1879.

Richard Leander (Richard von Volkmann): Träumereien an französischen Kaminen. Leipzig, Breitkopf und Härtel, 1879. (Courtesy of the General Research and Humanities Division, The New York Public Library; Astor, Lenox and Tilden Foundations)

Volkmann's fame, however, should rest on other things. He was the champion of Listerism in Germany. Both he and Thiersch served in the German army during the Franco-Prussian War of 1870, and it was this experience that led them to use Lister's ideas in their clinics. Volkmann had tried to carry out this system in the field hospitals. One of his papers concerning osteotomy had a foreword written by Lister.

Volkmann's father was professor of physiology at Halle for many years, and Richard grew up there, although he was born in Leipzig. As was the custom, he did his medical studies in various schools. He took his degree at the University of Berlin. His doctoral dissertation was said to have been given in fluent Latin. Two years later he was named privatdocent at Halle. From this he went to the professorship and spent his entire professional life there. Years later, when Langenbeck, the famous teacher of so many surgeons, retired at Berlin, Volkmann was offered the chair, but declined it. The attraction of Halle must have been very strong for Volkmann, for this chair was probably the highest honor a surgeon could receive. Few men would have been able to turn down such an offer. Billroth did also, but he was in Vienna, itself a city of world renown, and his clinic at Allgemeine Krankenhaus was one of the best. Billroth had a more compelling reason, though, for he was intensely interested in music. Vienna was famous for its musical contributions, and Billroth's personal friend Brahms refused to leave.

The war with France in 1870 saw Volkmann with headquarters of the Fourth Army Corps, and, during the Siege of Paris, stationed at Soisy. Here he wrote, in simple language, stories for his children. These were fairy tales and fantasies later published as *Reveries at French Firesides (Träumereien an französischen Kaminen)* under the pen name, Richard Leander. There were fourteen editions in 19 years, and even as late as 1908, an American edition was used as reading matter and was recommended for the early study of the German language.

His work included a description of the development of cancer among paraffin workers, probably the first report of excision of the rectum for cancer, and a paper that dermatologists consider a classic in their field. He founded a surgical journal, and many of his writings were published in England.

Richard von Volkmann has always been one of my favorites. He was a scholar, a surgeon, and a gentleman. We do well to honor his name, even if the contribution for which we do so, in our special field, was a relatively minor one. But this has happened often: Heberden's nodes, for example, were just a passing observation of a clinical finding, as was Madelung's description of the wrist deformity. Clinical observations have given us many eponyms, and even today, with all of our sophisticated diagnostic equipment and other aids, simple observation and recording of abnormal states may yet give rise to others. Is this not a good reason to insist on careful, detailed reports of the physical examination of patients? The art of surgery consists of this ability to seek out and find the abnormal and the unusual, and never to be satisfied with the obvious.

An astute examiner is not the automaton carrying out a prescribed ritual, but a thinking observer. He knows the normal, and, therefore, anything abnormal, anything out of place, stands out in bold relief. I can recall a trip into the mountains with an old experienced guide who was sitting at the bottom of a hillside looking for the mule deer, a species native to that area. He scanned the hillside—which was as familiar to him as his own front yard—and then suddenly pointed out a group of animals slowly making their way across the saddle into another valley. They were noted because there was something different, something "wrong" in the view. Only with good binoculars could we be sure that these were the objects of our search, but he had picked out the abnormality of the scene, the unordinary aspect. Such is the training we must develop in our examination of patients, this ability to note the minor deviations from the average, and then once noting them, to follow through: to ask why is this present, what does it mean?

These men whose names we recall were patient and thorough in their observations. To read their reports, such as the classic description of Raynaud's disease, should be a stimulus to better clinical reports. These men used their senses to observe and then recorded their findings clearly, accurately, and, in most instances, with a good style.

Wars have always provided the opportunity for testing surgical judgments and verifying some procedures. Allbutt wrote, "How fertile the blood of warriors in training surgeons." But it was not until after the Civil War in the United States and the Franco-Prussian War of 1870, that conservative surgery of the extremities became a general practice. Amputation was the rule, and although better primary care and evacuation were practiced and "hospital" gangrene was lessened by the pavilion type of construction, the principles of Listerism could not be carried out in the field. Both Thiersch and Volkmann were successful only after they returned and established the proper control in their clinics.

There was a man, however, on the other side, in France, who was making a remarkable record in the treatment of wounds by resection. **Louis Xavier Edouard Léopold Ollier** (1830–1900), well remembered today for a type of skin graft as well as for his description of dyschondroplasia, lived during these years of rapid advances in medicine and surgery. The microscope had come into clinical use, and antisepsis was being developed. Also, Ollier saw the discovery of Röntgen's rays during his time.

In surgery of the upper extremity, we use Ollier's name for the modern skin graft (usually combining it with that of Thiersch), implying a split graft—as opposed to a full-thickness graft, called the Wolfe-Krause graft. This work in the skin transplantation, however, was done later in his surgical life. He first took up the study of bone regeneration. The disease dyschondroplasia was described only 3 years before he died.

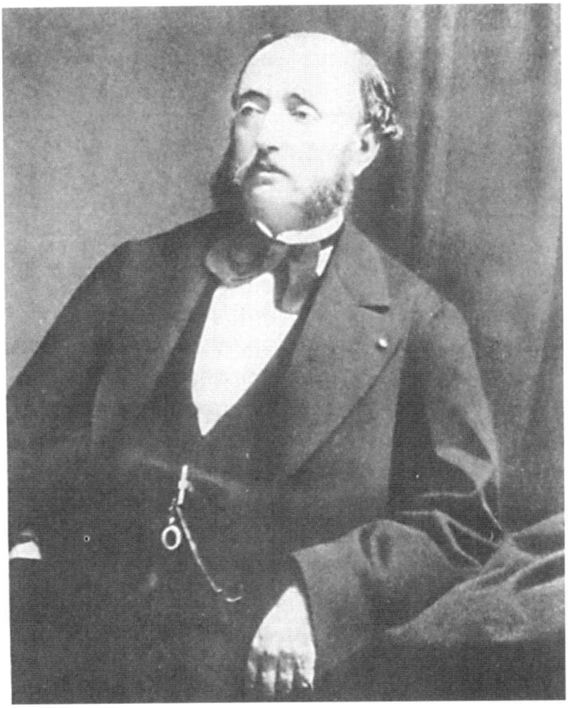

Louis Xavier Edouard Léopold Ollier. (From Médecins Célèbres. Geneva, Lucien Mazenod, 1947. Courtesy of the New York Academy of Medicine)

Ollier was born in Vans in the district of Ardèche, studied natural sciences at Montpellier, and became an assistant in botany. To gain clinical experience in medicine he went to Lyon to intern and finally completed his medical training and took his degree at Montpellier in 1856.

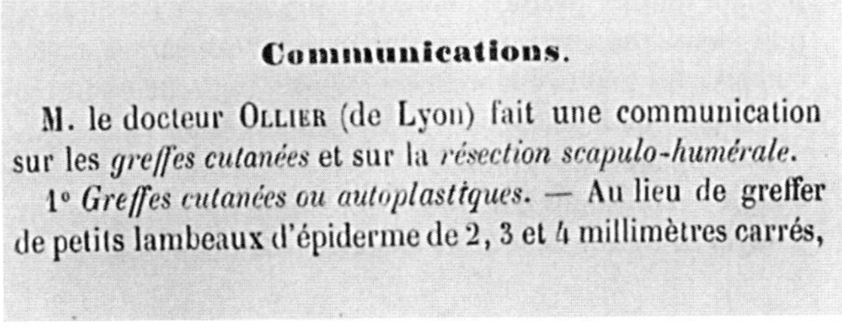

Communications.

M. le docteur OLLIER (de Lyon) fait une communication sur les *greffes cutanées* et sur la *résection scapulo-humérale.*

1° *Greffes cutanées ou autoplastiques.* — Au lieu de greffer de petits lambeaux d'épiderme de 2, 3 et 4 millimètres carrés,

Louis Xavier Edouard Léopold Ollier: Greffes cutanées ou autoplastiques. Bull. Acad. Med. (Paris), *1* (2):243–246, 1872. (Courtesy of the Library of the College of Physicians of Philadelphia)

The next year we find him in Paris, in the laboratory of Chauveau, where he transplanted tibial periosteum to the neck of a rabbit. New bone developed. Using this principle of subperiosteal resection, he excised bones and joints and published his results 10 years later. The Franco-Prussian War provided him with ample opportunity to test his operation. The results were very good, and he received one of France's highest honors for his work.

He became intensely interested in the problems of bone growth, and he later showed that the deep layer of the periosteum had the potential growth ability. This resulted in a conflict with Macewen, who, being unable to duplicate Ollier's work, became convinced that the periosteum was only a limiting membrane. Macewen used tibial bone without periosteum, and this type of graft, combined with the internal fixation or splint developed by Lane, became the basis for the modern operation of bone grafting. Macewen was wrong, as Leo Mayer showed with experiments done while he was in Munich with Lange. Macewen's grafts were only a framework for new bone growth. Today, the osteoperiosteal graft provides the stability and the growth potential.

Ollier was the first to excise an epiphysis to stop bone growth and correct deformity, after he had studied the relation of growth to epiphyseal activity. Keith tells the interesting story of the study of bone growth, illustrating so well how an inquisitive mind reacts to a new experience. Just as Schwann, after a dinner conversation with Schleiden, began to realize the full potential of the studies they both were making on cells, so it was that a young surgeon of Guy's Hospital, J. B. Belchier (1706–1785), had dinner with his friend, a calico printer. The main course was a leg of pork, and when Belchier noted the red color of the bone, his curiosity was aroused. Questions led to the finding that the printer had fed his pigs a bran mixture that had been soaked with the strong purple dye used in the printing of the fabric. This madder came from the root of the plant *Rubia tinctorum*. Duhamel (1700–1782), a French squire, not a physician, took up the idea, fed the madder in alternate diets, and found the "rings of growth." He concluded that periosteum was the mother of bone and that growth took place only at the ends of the bone. At this time, Albrecht von Haller, who was the first professor at Göttingen, was teaching that periosteum did not form bone, that all bone growth came from the blood vessels. John Hunter agreed with him, although he believed that there was absorption as well as deposition of bone. Much later, Goodsir would show—using a microscope that had been improved by Lister's father—the distinction between osteoblasts and osteoclasts.

Ollier, of course, knew of Duhamel's work and firmly believed in the generative powers of the periosteum. His operation of subperiosteal resection allowed new bone to develop. Although he was not the first—others having done similar procedures for osteomyelitis—his work of

1891, *Treating Bony Resections*, is a valuable contribution. His work on skin grafting was published in 1872, antedating Thiersch's final report of 1886, in which no mention was made of Ollier's work.

Ollier was most particular concerning follow-up reports on his patients. He said that, "It is in the verification and criticism of old results that is to be found true consecration of operative methods, which are intended to be used for the purposes of conservative surgery." Yet many years would elapse before the founding of "follow-up clinics" to study the results of operative procedures, such as the one of Codman at the Massachusetts General Hospital.

Ollier has earned the respect of surgeons, and we honor his name in recalling the procedures he developed and the diseases he described.

Most of the men whose names we have used and whose lives we have discussed, other than anatomists or physiologists, were surgeons in a most general sense. The development of surgical specialties is more recent, but there was a man whose interest in the problems of the urinary tract came at the same time as the development of the cystoscope and who became famous for his teaching and experience in this surgical field. We use his name, however, to recall one of his earliest works in anatomy.

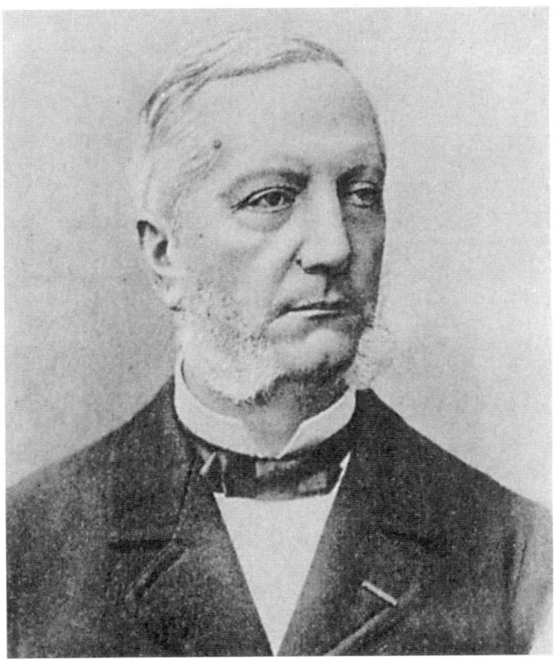

Felix Jean Casimir Guyon. (From Ferrannini [ed.]: Eleventh congrée internationale de medecin, Rome. Numero Souvenir. Les grande medécines contemporains. Ital. Med.-Chir. [Naples], *1*, 1893–1894. Courtesy of the Library of the New York Academy of Medicine)

NOTE SUR UNE DISPOSITION ANATOMIQUE PROPRE A LA FACE ANTÉRIEURE DE LA RÉGION DU POIGNET ET NON ENCORE DÉCRITE, par le docteur F. GUYON.

Il existe à la face antérieure du poignet, immédiatement en dedans du pisiforme, à la racine de la région de l'hypothénar, une petite loge intra-aponévrotique contenant un peloton graisseux facile à déplacer par la pression, et venant alors faire une saillie remarquable au-dessus du pli cutané transversal qui marque les limites de la main et de l'avant-bras.

C'est la facilité avec laquelle on peut mettre cette disposition en évidence chez tous les sujets qui m'a amené à faire des dissections que j'ai montrées cet hiver à M. Malgaigne, et que j'ai depuis soumises au jugement de la Société.

Ce qu'il y a de curieux dans le fait que je signale, c'est que chez certains individus, chez moi-même, par exemple, le peloton graisseux déplacé par la pression est assez volumineux pour que je me sois demandé tout d'abord s'il ne s'agissait pas d'un état anormal de la synoviale des tendons. Voici, en effet, ce que l'on observe : en pressant sur la racine de l'hypothénar, on voit immédiatement se dessiner et faire saillie dans le point indiqué deux ou trois petits lobules simulant très bien à travers la peau le fond d'un cul-de-sac distendu, et disparaissant, semble-t-il, sous le ligament antérieur du carpe dès que l'on suspend la pression.

En y réfléchissant, on peut, il est vrai, rejeter l'idée d'une petite hydropisie de la synoviale, et je dois dire que mon ami et

Felix Jean Casimir Guyon: Note sur une disposition anatomique a la face antérieure de la région du poignet et non encore décrite. Bull. Soc. Anat., *36*:184–186, 1861. (Courtesy of the Library of the College of Physicians of Philadelphia)

He was **Felix Jean Casimir Guyon** (1831–1920), who was born at Ile-Bourbon, went to school at Nantes, and was graduated in Paris in 1858. His interest at this time was in anatomy. He followed the same pattern as Denonvilliers, who 2 years before had published his work on plastic surgery, but whose original interest had been in anatomy, and who had actually succeeded Breschet in the chair of anatomy. Guyon, in the same fashion, became professor of surgical pathology. He was secretary of the Société d'Chirurgie in 1874, when a memorial was held in honor of Denonvilliers. A short description of the "Loge de Guyon" on the anterior aspect of the wrist was written in his early years.* Later, he concentrated on the urinary tract, its anatomy and its diseases.

*For a recent study, see Grantham, S. A.: Ulnar nerve compression in the loge de Guyon. JAMA, *197*:509–510, 1966.

Guyon was an excellent surgeon, especially noted for the success of his lithotomies and for operations on the prostate gland. He was chief of service at Necker Hospital in Paris and drew students and surgeons from many countries. Respected for his personal qualities as well as for his organizational ability, he was instrumental in founding the International Urological Society and was its president. When in 1914 the Congress of the Society was to be held in Berlin, Guyon declined the honor of being honorary president, but his German confreres, despite the feeling at the onset of World War I, made him an honorary member. He retired in 1907, and he died in 1920, having lived through most of the nineteenth century and having been a part of the tremendous changes in surgery in that period.

In 1869 **Johann Friedrich Horner** (1831–1886) described a special form of ptosis, now known as Horner's syndrome. Changes in the eye had been noted by Petit as early as 1727, when he was severing intercostal

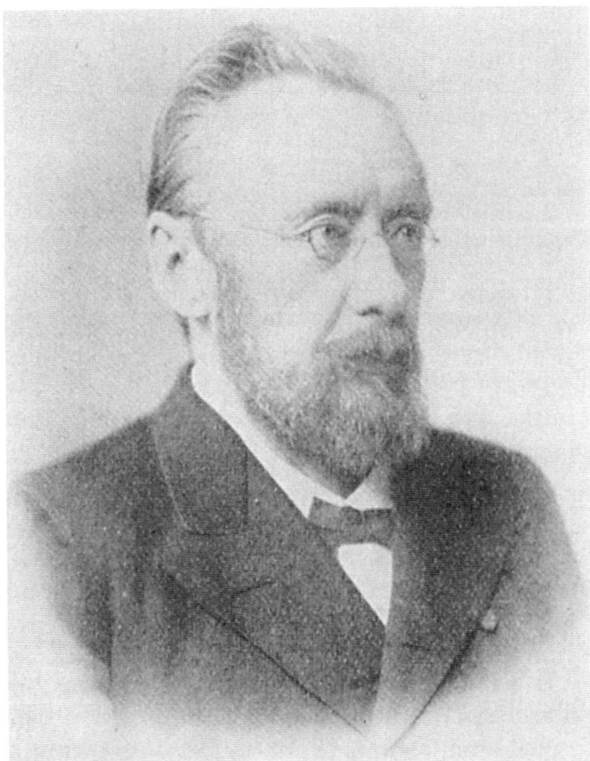

Johann Friedrich Horner. (From Schweiz. Med. Wochenschr., *14*:343, 1933. Courtesy of the Library of the New York Academy of Medicine)

Ueber eine Form von Ptosis.

Von

F. Horner.

Wohl manchem meiner Collegen sind Fälle von Ptosis incompleta vorgekommen, die bei erwachsenen Individuen langsam entstanden waren, jeder begleitenden Lähmungserscheinung im Oculomotoriusgebiet entbehrten und die auffallende Erscheinung einer Myosis der gleichseitigen Pupille darboten. Mir war dieses Bild kein neuer Symptomencomplex, als sich mir Ende November vorigen Jahres eine 40jährige Frau mit demselben vorstellte; ja wenige Wochen später sah ich ihn wieder, und abermals bei einer Frau fast gleichen Alters; aber nie war es mir möglich gewesen, für die Auffassung dieser Ptosisform so anregende Beobachtungen zu sammeln, wie in jenem ersterwähnten Fall. Es sei mir erlaubt, hier über diese Kranke Bericht zu erstatten.

Frau Anna Brändli, 40 Jahre alt, eine gesund aussehende Bäuerin mittlerer Grösse, soll schon von Jugend auf oft an Kopfschmerz gelitten haben, der keine Stelle besonders bevorzugte und im Laufe des letzten Jahres eher an Intensität und Häufigkeit abnahm.

Sechs Wochen nach dem letzten Wochenbette, das vor einem Jahre stattfand, bemerkte sie ein allmähliges Herab-

Monatsbl. f. Augenhdlke. 1869. 13

Johann Friedrich Horner: Ueber eine Form von Ptosis. Klin. Monatsbl. Augenheilkd., 7:193–198, 1869. (Courtesy of the Library of the College of Physicians of Philadelphia)

nerves in animals, and by Claude Bernard in 1858, but Horner's name has become a part of the syndrome of miosis, narrowing of the palpebral fissure, and retraction of the globe. Klumpke, working in Vulpian's laboratory, showed in 1885 that these signs were the result of section of the lower roots (eighth cervical and first dorsal nerves), but that section of the sixth and seventh cervical nerves did not produce the lesion. She localized it to the communicating rami of the first dorsal.

Horner had been a pupil of Albrecht von Graefe and practiced in Zurich. He was instrumental in enforcing a law for the prevention of ophthalmia neonatorum, which was passed by the authorities in Switzerland in 1865.

After Amici developed the achromatic lens for the microscope in 1818, and much later, after the Abbe condenser was invented in 1886, there was a great interest in microscopy. Improved staining techniques were

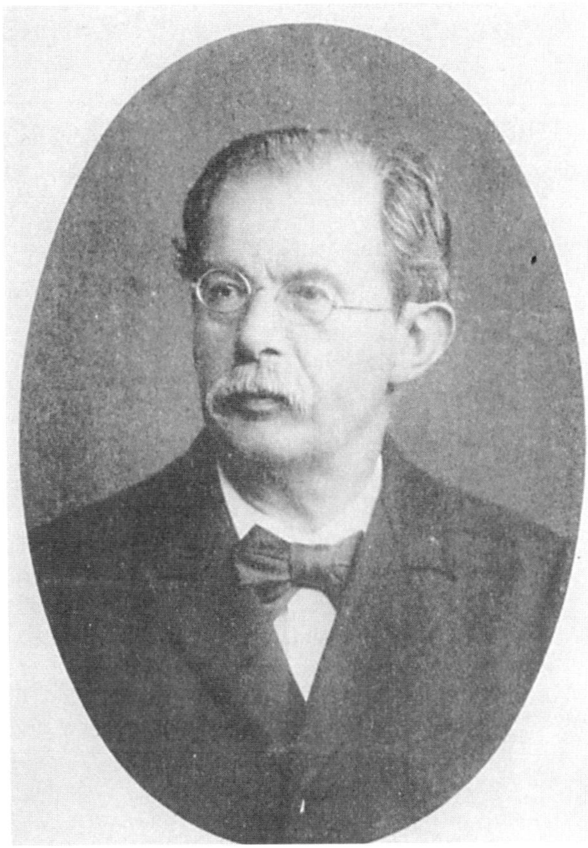

Friedrich Daniel von Recklinghausen. (From Beilage Munch. Med. Wochenschr., *50*[2]:147, 1903. Courtesy of the Library of the New York Academy of Medicine)

developed, and some men became interested in the field of physicochemical changes. These were men who were already well grounded in embryology and anatomy and who were now ready to study the pathological processes. Virchow, of course, was one of the pioneers, and it was one of his students whose name was given to a disease occasionally seen manifested in the upper extremity.

Friedrich Daniel von Recklinghausen (1833–1910) described the multiple fibromas along peripheral nerves, often associated with nevi, in 1882. But early in his career, while working in Virchow's laboratory, he made an important contribution to the study of lymphatics, a work that resulted from the development of a staining technique using silver salts.

Recklinghausen was born in Westphalia and studied at Bonn and Würzburg before taking his degree at Berlin, where, as Volkmann had

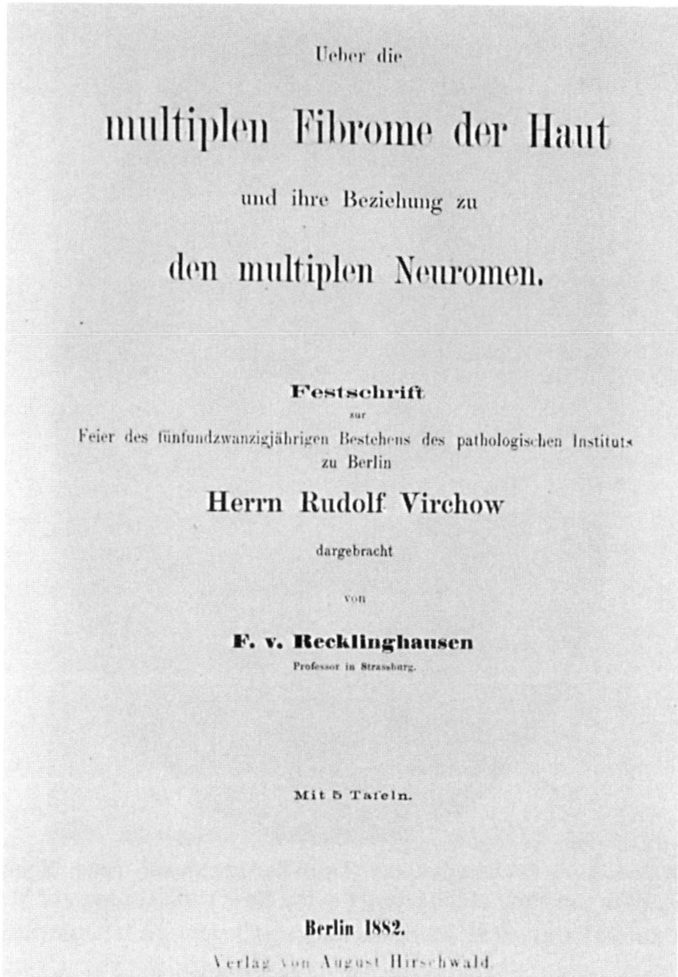

Ueber die

multiplen Fibrome der Haut

und ihre Beziehung zu

den multiplen Neuromen.

Festschrift

zur

Feier des fünfundzwanzigjährigen Bestehens des pathologischen Instituts
zu Berlin

Herrn Rudolf Virchow

dargebracht

von

F. v. Recklinghausen

Professor in Strassburg.

Mit 5 Tafeln.

Berlin 1882.

Verlag von August Hirschwald.

Friedrich Daniel von Recklinghausen: Ueber die multiplen Fibrome der Haut und ihre Beziehung zu den multiplen Neuromen. Berlin, August Hirschwald, 1882. (Courtesy of the Library of the College of Physicians of Philadelphia)

done a few years earlier, he defended his thesis in Latin. After several years as Virchow's assistant, he went directly to the professorship of pathological anatomy at Königsberg and then Würzburg.

When, in 1872, at the end of the Franco-Prussian War, Strassburg became a part of Germany, its university was completely reorganized. Recklinghausen was chosen to reestablish a faculty of medicine. This he did, and the school became an outstanding teaching center. Later, he also

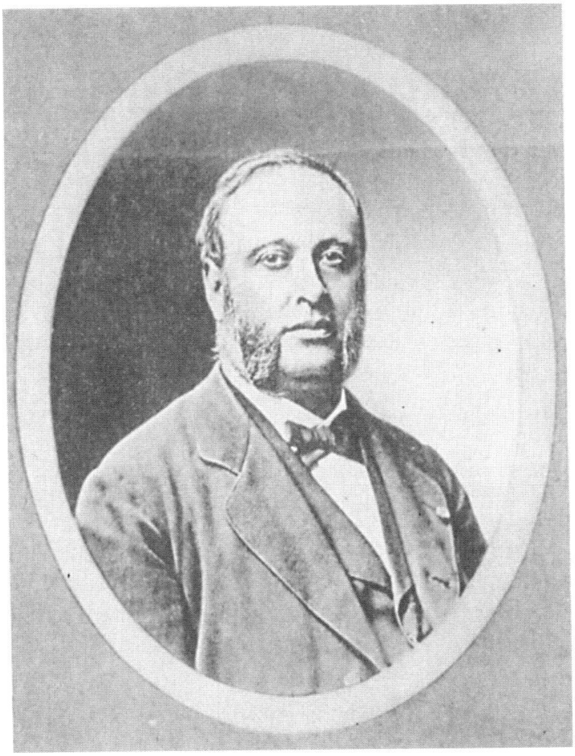

Maurice Raynaud. (Courtesy of the Library of the New York Academy of Medicine)

took on the duties of university rector. He chose to remain in Strassburg when he was offered the chair and Cohnheim's laboratory at Leipzig.

He made many original studies, and with Naunyn he founded the *Archiv für Experimental Pathologie and Pharmakologie*. He gave the name of hemochromatosis to the disease first described by Trousseau, described osteitis fibrosa cystica with associated parathyroid tumor, and published the classic on neurofibromatosis.

Recklinghausen was one of the leaders in demonstrative pathology, but was not particularly interested in the experimental phase nor in the new bacteriological work being started. He was interested in many other things, publishing articles on microphotography; lesions of the retina; spina bifida; myomas of the uterus as a source of bleeding; and many reports of observations at the cellular level, such as the response of leukocytes in the inflammatory process, phagocytosis, and embolic phenomena.

He was a good lecturer, using clear demonstrations, and was a demanding teacher, emphasizing detailed observations and logical conclusions. His influence as a teacher spread widely through Europe.

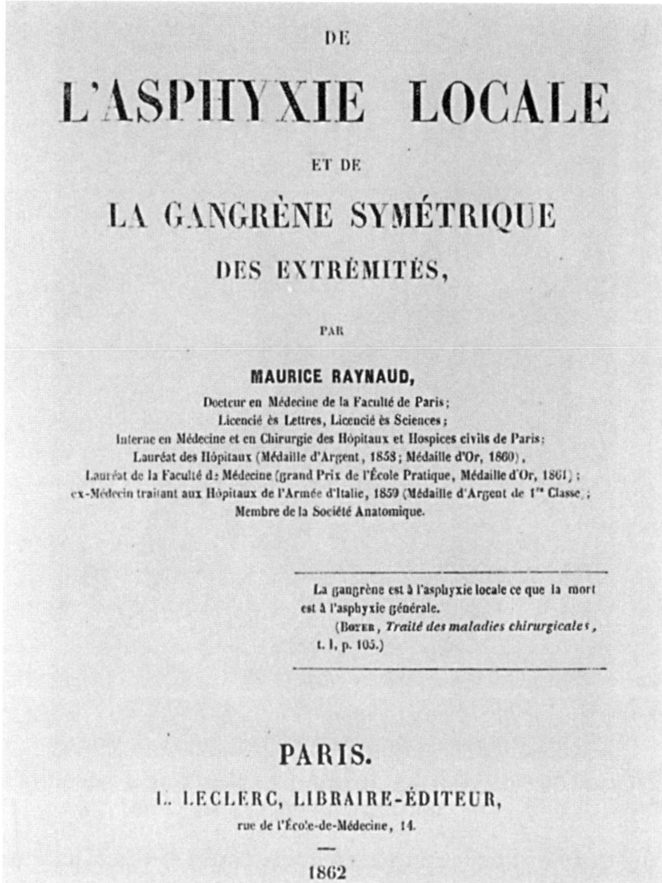

DE

L'ASPHYXIE LOCALE

ET DE

LA GANGRÈNE SYMÉTRIQUE

DES EXTRÉMITÉS,

PAR

MAURICE RAYNAUD,

Docteur en Médecine de la Faculté de Paris;
Licencié ès Lettres, Licencié ès Sciences;
Interne en Médecine et en Chirurgie des Hôpitaux et Hospices civils de Paris;
Lauréat des Hôpitaux (Médaille d'Argent, 1858; Médaille d'Or, 1860),
Lauréat de la Faculté de Médecine (grand Prix de l'École Pratique, Médaille d'Or, 1861);
ex-Médecin traitant aux Hôpitaux de l'Armée d'Italie, 1859 (Médaille d'Argent de 1re Classe);
Membre de la Société Anatomique.

La gangrène est à l'asphyxie locale ce que la mort est à l'asphyxie générale.
(BOYER, *Traité des maladies chirurgicales*, t. I, p. 105.)

PARIS.

L. LECLERC, LIBRAIRE-ÉDITEUR,
rue de l'École-de-Médecine, 14.

1862

Maurice Raynaud: De l'Asphyxie Locale et de la Gangrène Symétrique des Extrémités. Paris, L. Leclerc, 1862. (Courtesy of the Library of the College of Physicians of Philadelphia)

At the same time in France, born a year later, **Maurice Raynaud** (1834–1881), in his inaugural thesis, described a new syndrome. Dupuytren had been called a "meteor" in science by Balzac, and young Raynaud, in a short life, was another, flashing through the skies. His first contribution in 1863 was a major one, and the description he gave of the first twenty-five patients is a classic in medical writing. Later, he included more patients and reported it again in 1874. Both papers were published in English by the Sydenham Society.

In his studies he noted the lack of signs of major arterial disease and postulated as a cause a reflex mechanism at the arteriolar level. A postmortem study of the limb of one of the patients showed, by injection, a normal arterial pattern. One case report is a classic description of scleroderma.

Raynaud graduated from the University of Paris, where his father was a professor. He trained in Paris hospitals and qualified in medicine in 1862. Although he never received a senior academic post, either in medicine or in medical history, which may have been his real desire, he was made an officer of the Legion of Honor and a member of the Academy of Medicine. He died at the age of 47 of a heart attack.

Raynaud's interest in medical history centered on the seventeenth century, the time of Molière; his thesis for a degree in letters, published the same year as his medical one, was on the physicians of that early period. Molière, in *The Imaginary Invalid,* had satirized the medical profession.

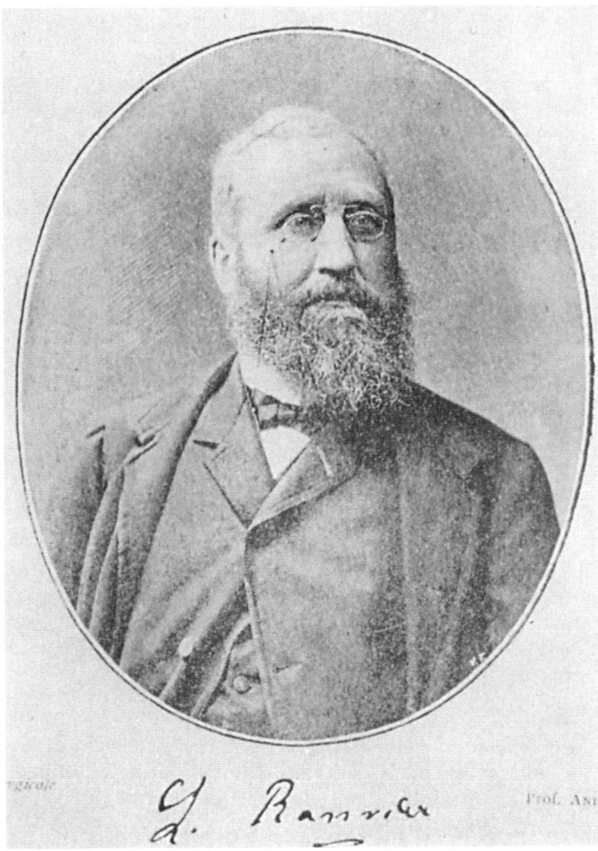

Louis Antoine Ranvier. (From Ferrannini [ed.]: Eleventh congrée internationale de medecin, Rome. Numero souvenir. Les grande medécines contemporains. Ital. Med.-Chir. [Naples], *1*, 1893–1894. Courtesy of the Library of the New York Academy of Medicine)

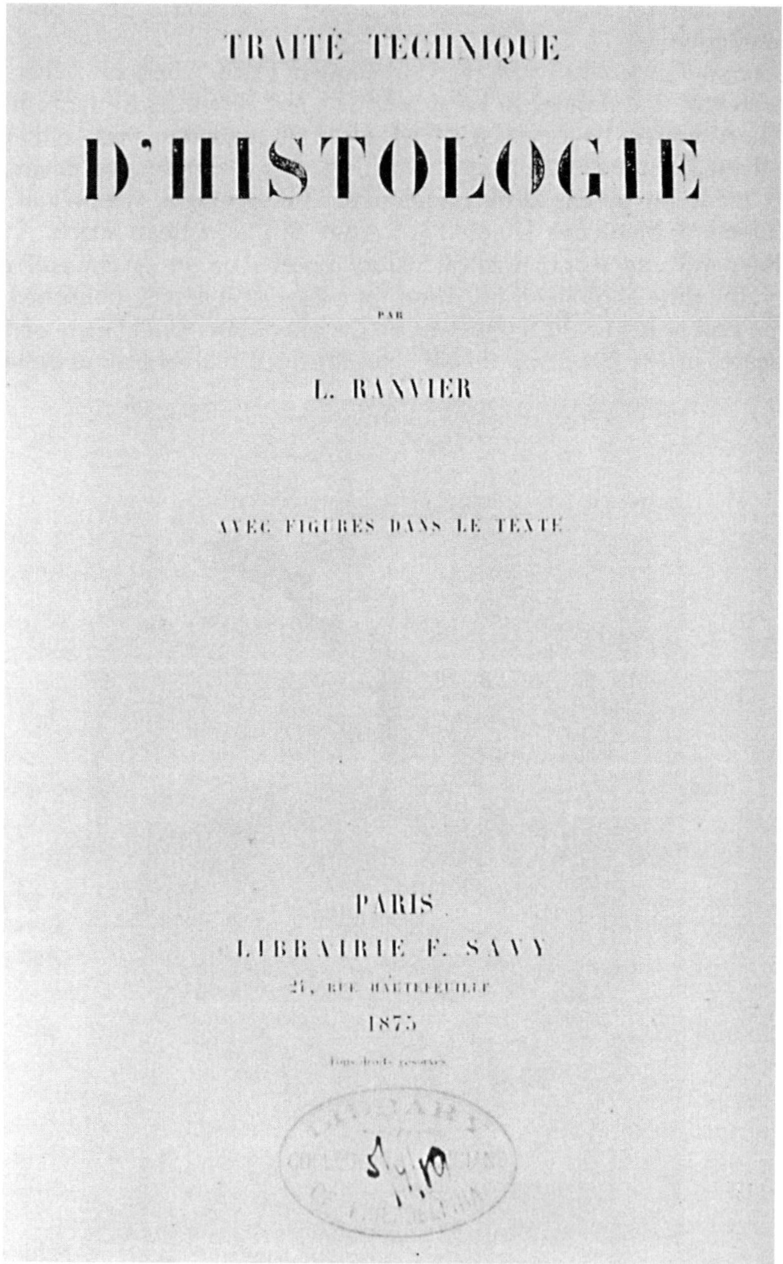

TRAITÉ TECHNIQUE

D'HISTOLOGIE

PAR

L. RANVIER

AVEC FIGURES DANS LE TEXTE

PARIS

LIBRAIRIE F. SAVY

24, RUE HAUTEFEUILLE

1875

Tous droits réservés

Louis Antoine Ranvier: Traité Technique d'Histologie. Paris, Librairie F. Savy, 1875. (Courtesy of the Library of the College of Physicians of Philadelphia)

One of the characters in the play was said to represent Dr. Guy Patin, the then dean of the faculty of medicine. The popularity of the play and the criticisms of the profession that followed were said to have been responsible for many improvements in medical training during subsequent years. Molière (1622–1673) died during a performance of the play. In 1973, on the tricentennial of Molière's death, the medical students of Paris put on a modern version; this time, instead of attacking blood letting, enemas, and purges, they focused attention on unnecessary transplantations and the uncontrolled use of antibiotics.

Just as Recklinghausen in Germany was developing pathology as a field of special interest, the study of microscopic anatomy was developing in France. **Louis Antoine Ranvier** (1835–1922) is recalled as being the describer of the node of Ranvier, which marks the division between one Schwann cell and another; but he made many other studies on nerves, as

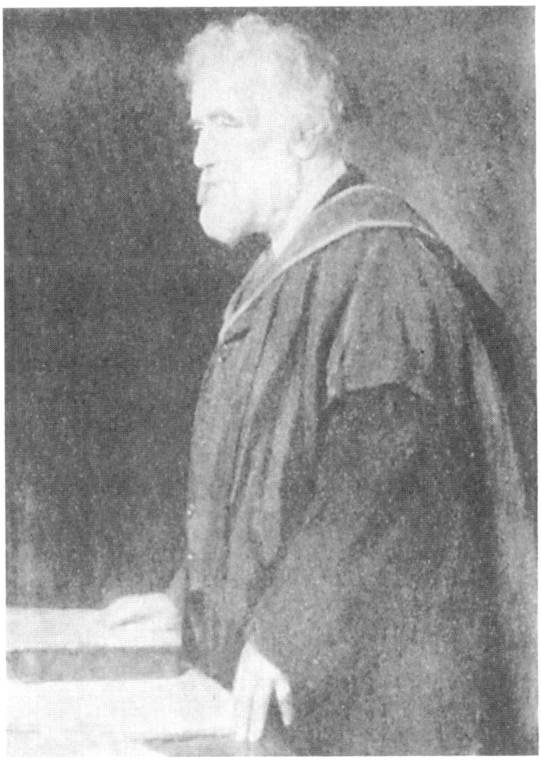

John Cleland. (From Comrie: History of Scottish Medicine. vol. 2. London, Bailliere, Tindall, and Cox, 1932. Courtesy of the Library of the New York Academy of Medicine)

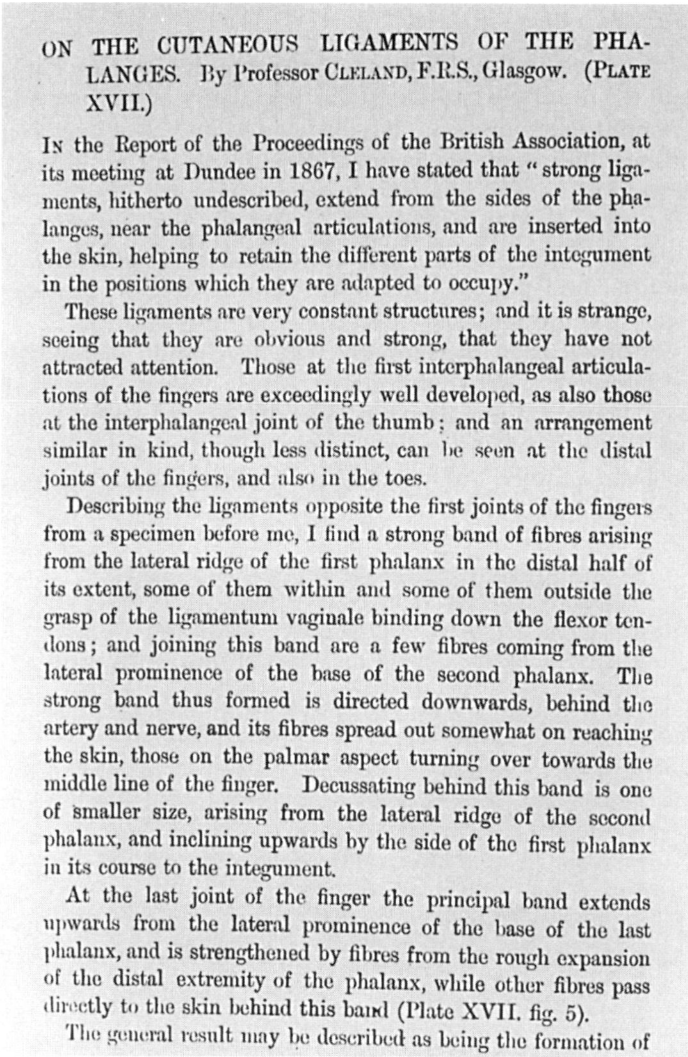

ON THE CUTANEOUS LIGAMENTS OF THE PHALANGES. By Professor CLELAND, F.R.S., Glasgow. (PLATE XVII.)

IN the Report of the Proceedings of the British Association, at its meeting at Dundee in 1867, I have stated that "strong ligaments, hitherto undescribed, extend from the sides of the phalanges, near the phalangeal articulations, and are inserted into the skin, helping to retain the different parts of the integument in the positions which they are adapted to occupy."

These ligaments are very constant structures; and it is strange, seeing that they are obvious and strong, that they have not attracted attention. Those at the first interphalangeal articulations of the fingers are exceedingly well developed, as also those at the interphalangeal joint of the thumb; and an arrangement similar in kind, though less distinct, can be seen at the distal joints of the fingers, and also in the toes.

Describing the ligaments opposite the first joints of the fingers from a specimen before me, I find a strong band of fibres arising from the lateral ridge of the first phalanx in the distal half of its extent, some of them within and some of them outside the grasp of the ligamentum vaginale binding down the flexor tendons; and joining this band are a few fibres coming from the lateral prominence of the base of the second phalanx. The strong band thus formed is directed downwards, behind the artery and nerve, and its fibres spread out somewhat on reaching the skin, those on the palmar aspect turning over towards the middle line of the finger. Decussating behind this band is one of smaller size, arising from the lateral ridge of the second phalanx, and inclining upwards by the side of the first phalanx in its course to the integument.

At the last joint of the finger the principal band extends upwards from the lateral prominence of the base of the last phalanx, and is strengthened by fibres from the rough expansion of the distal extremity of the phalanx, while other fibres pass directly to the skin behind this band (Plate XVII. fig. 5).

The general result may be described as being the formation of

John Cleland: On the cutaneous ligaments of the phalanges. J. Anat. Physiol., *12*:526–527, 1878. (Courtesy of the Library of the New York Academy of Medicine)

well as on the muscular and osseous sytems. His work on the technique of histology is a classic.

Ranvier was born in Lyon in 1835, and he went to school and was graduated in Paris. Here he started a private laboratory with a colleague, Cornil, to teach histology to medical students. This drew the attention of Claude Bernard, and in 1867 Ranvier headed the first laboratory of histology at the Collège de France, becoming a professor 5 years later. He described himself as being an experimental histologist.

One of his student recalled that he created in them a profound respect, a "shade of a bit" of fear, and infinite admiration. His work culminated in the splendid *Traité technique d'histologie*, a classic in its time.

In a memoir, Nageotte wrote of how Ranvier retired to an estate in the country, where he "lived with the honors and titles he had accepted but never sought." He gave to science his youth and maturity, but reserved his old age for the earth that he had never ceased to love. When he died at the age of 87, he left a part of his estate to the town of Thélys, near Roanne, for the building of a sanatarium for tuberculosis.

In the British Isles there were two men in this era whose names are familiar to us in our field of surgery.

John Cleland (1835–1925) described the cutaneous ligaments of the finger, first in 1867, but in a more complete form in 1877, in which appeared the drawing by the author, so often repeated in others' works. This description should be read by anyone interested in surgery of the hand—it is brief and clear—and should be followed by the study of the modern monograph of Lee Milford.

Cleland was a most interesting man, and we use his name with fond remembrances of a remarkable individual. He was born in Perth, Scotland, the only child of a physician who died of typhoid fever and who left his widow with a young son. Moving to Edinburgh for his education, Cleland completed his course through medical school there. But he was only 20, and since no one was allowed to graduate until reaching the age of 21, he spent a year of study in France and Germany. Goodsir had stimulated his interest in anatomy, and on his tour he must have made contact with those men whose work was in both anatomy and surgery (often the two chairs were combined). These would have included Thiersch at Erlangen, Esmarch at Kiel, and Denonvilliers at Paris. Returning to Edinburgh, Cleland spent several years as assistant in anatomy and senior demonstrator. Then he accepted the chair of anatomy and physiology at Queen's College in Galway. Here he was active in teaching but also in performing surgery at the hospital. He wrote many articles and was editor of the seventh edition of *Quain's Anatomy*.

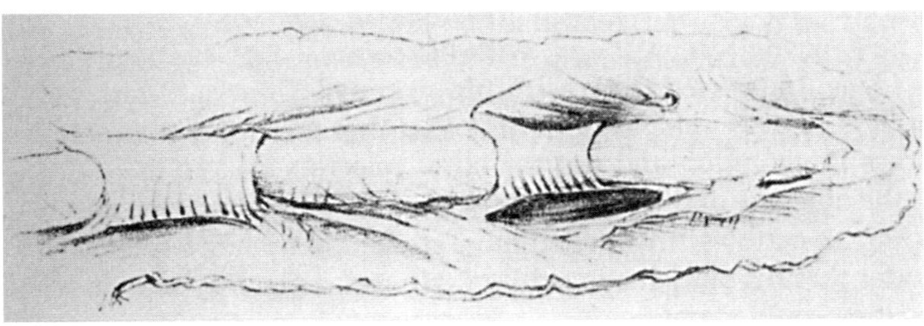

John Cleland: On the cutaneous ligaments of the phalanges. J. Anat. Physiol., *12*:526–527, 1878. (Courtesy of the Library of the New York Academy of Medicine)

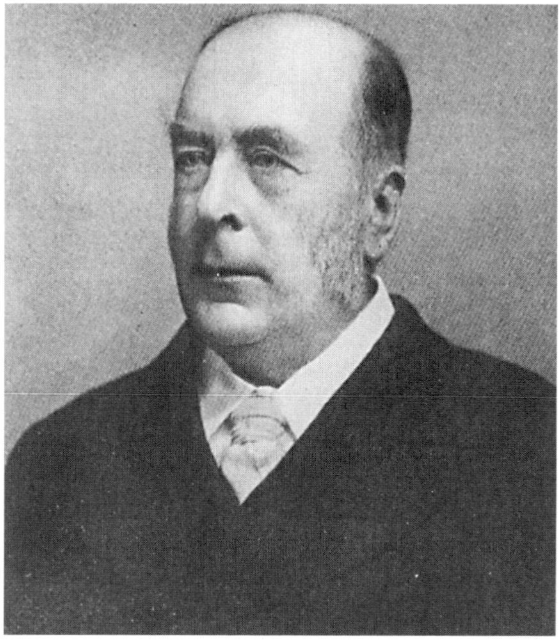

Edward Halloran Bennett. (From McNealy, R. W., and Lichtenstein, M. E.: Bennett's fracture and other fractures of the first metacarpal. Surg. Gynecol. Obstet., 56:197–201, 1933. Reproduced by permission of Surgery, Gynecology & Obstetrics. Courtesy of the Library of the College of Physicians of Philadelphia)

In 1877 he returned to Scotland, and in Glasgow he held the chair of anatomy. For more than 30 years he was the leading anatomist in Scotland. He created a marvelous collection of anatomical specimens and saw them installed in a special museum. His students described him as having a virile personality, with a massive head, a big-framed body, and a short-fused temper, which was immediately followed by deep contrition. When he laughed, there was a period of shortness of breath.

As a teacher, he was liked by his students. He was full of spirit, and his humor was boisterous. During a lecture he might seize upon some small point and take off on a lengthy discourse far removed from the subject. But he kept their interest and, with his command of language and positive ideas, impressed them with his sincerity. Darwin's work bothered him, and he was outspoken in his belief that there was a "determinate" process in evolution and not the blind selection that so many believed was the outcome of the Darwinian theory. A keen observer, a stimulating teacher, an earthy scholar; what more could one wish in a teacher? It is no wonder that his students loved him. He was a giant upon whose shoulders they could stand.

He was an artist of above-average ability, and he could write poetry: "Eternal Truth; clear browed like morn arises, throw back the clouds of error rolling in, and deign to guide an earnest wanderer."

Fractures of the Metacarpal Bones.—Dr. E. H. Bennett exhibited a series of united fractures of the metacarpal bones, with the object of determining the character and site of the most frequent fracture of these bones. He said: Every systematic treatise on surgery and the special treatises on fractures all contain some account of these injuries, but in few are any exact details to be found. The author of the "First Lines," S. Cooper, asserts that "the carpal and metacarpal bones can be broken only by great direct violence, as by gunshot wounds, the action of machinery on the parts, or the passage of the wheel of a heavy carriage over them." Beyond these compound fractures of the bones of the hand he recognises none. Sir A. Cooper mentions, apart from the compound injuries indicated in the passage I have quoted from the "First Lines," the occurrence of fracture of the distal extremity of the metacarpal, "which is called the head," as a simple injury. Boyer, taking a wider view, discusses the question of the relative frequency of simple fractures of the metacarpals in the individual bones, and assigns the premier position to the fifth metacarpal, while he states that, arguing *à priori*, we should expect to find the first most commonly broken, only for its free movement. To correct this uncertainty we find Malgaigne first giving statistical information, which proves the first bone to be equal in its liability to simple fracture to all the others taken together. His numbers are, however, too small for any final conclusion.

The following passage by Mr. Hulke exposes the facts most clearly:—

"The statements that have hitherto been made as to the comparative liability of the different bones of the series to fracture are very unsatis-

Edward Halloran Bennett: Fractures of the metacarpal bones. Dublin J. Med. Sci., *73*:72–75, 1882. (Courtesy of the Library of the College of Physicians of Philadelphia)

He retired in 1908, with many honors. He died some years later, leaving one son. An anonymous obituary notice in the *Glasgow Medical Journal* closes with these words: "He was a man; take him for all in all; we shall not look upon his like again."

Our other man of this time is **Edward Halloran Bennett** (1837–1907), Irish born and educated, first an anatomist and then a surgeon. Quiet and dignified, he was a trained observer. He collected specimens of fractures and is remembered for his description of the intra-articular fracture of the base of the first metacarpal bone.

In 1882 he reported five specimens of healed fractures of the base of the first metacarpal, pointing out that the major fragment, the shaft, was the one that was displaced. He remarked on how much disability this produced, even when cared for promptly. He later added other examples of the same lesion.

Bennett was born in Cork and was graduated from Trinity College in Dublin in 1859. Appointed demonstrator in anatomy, he succeeded Barton as head of the department 5 years later. He was a strong personality, blunt and outspoken in criticism, but always fair and not unkind. Apparently of a retiring nature, he loved teaching and was a great favorite of the students. McNealy described him as being "dignified without pedantry, and cultured without arrogance." His work on fractures, all done

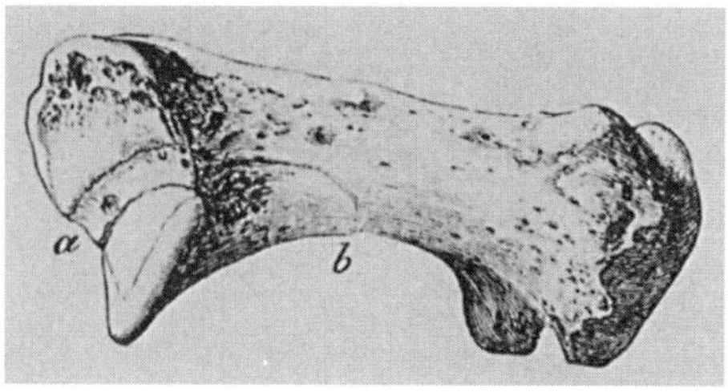

The characteristic site of the intra-articular fracture, the major portion of the metacarpal being displaced dorsally. Edward Halloran Bennett: Fractures of the metacarpal bones. Dublin J. Med. Sci., 73:72–75, 1882. (Courtesy of the Library of the College of Physicians of Philadelphia)

before Röntgen's discovery of the x-ray, represents the best clinical observation and perseverance in follow-up, which characterized so many of the giants of those times.

The importance that Bennett gave to this "simple" fracture, as he called it, has been well proven. Today we know that only a most accurate reduction and fixation, with anatomical restoration of the joint surface, will result in healing with minimum disability.

When Duchenne, in 1855, shortly after Faraday's discovery, reported the findings of the use of electricity in the treatment of paralytic disorders, there was a 15-year-old boy in the Black Forest of Germany, the son of a woodsman, who was to become one of the world's leading neurologists. At 17, he would enter the University of Heidelberg and would make it world famous.

Wilhelm Heinrich Erb (1840–1921) is remembered for his description, in 1873, of the upper brachial palsy, in which he pointed out that Duchenne had noted it in the newborn; thus the two names are usually associated in defining this lesion of the fifth and sixth cervical roots. Erb's report of four cases included one of a traumatic neuritis following the carrying of a heavy load on the head, a second subsequent to a fall on the shoulder, another of unknown cause, and the fourth from pressure of a metastatic carcinoma in the supraclavicular glands. The constant finding of paralysis limited to the deltoid, biceps, brachialis and brachioradial muscles led him to localize the lesion in the upper two roots, as distinguished from lesions in the more distal parts of the plexus, lesions which were better known at that time. In the cases of birth palsy, he pointed out the diagnostic value of the palsy of the infraspinatus in localizing the lesion.

During Erb's time, clinical neurology was developing in other countries. Charcot, Marie, and Vulpian in Paris, and Little and Gowers in England all contributed to the study of diseases of the nervous system;

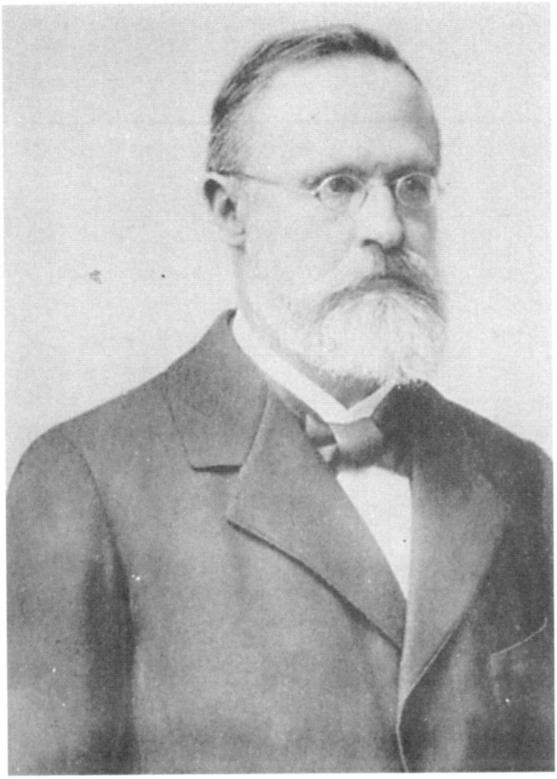

Wilhelm Heinrich Erb. (Courtesy of the Library of the New York Academy of Medicine)

but Erb, with Teutonic thoroughness, established the present form of the neurological examination. He was an investigator, but above all a teacher, imbuing in his students, by example, the need for thoroughly detailed examinations and recording of the findings.

Erb started in internal medicine, taking his degree at Munich. At Heidelberg he fell under the influence of Friedreich (ataxia) and was to be converted to neurology. Erb had 273 publications, two thirds of which dealt with neurology. He is responsible for pointing out the use of pupillary and patellar reflexes in diagnosis. The term *tendon reflex* was coined by him. Erb's contributions were important in introducing neurology into the medical curriculum and making it an acceptable specialty.

He was convinced that tabes dorsalis resulted from syphilis long before Schaudinn discovered the spirochete, or Wassermann the test. Following Duchenne, Erb became extremely interested in electricity as a diagnostic and therapeutic measure. Erb's point and Erb's phenomenon come from

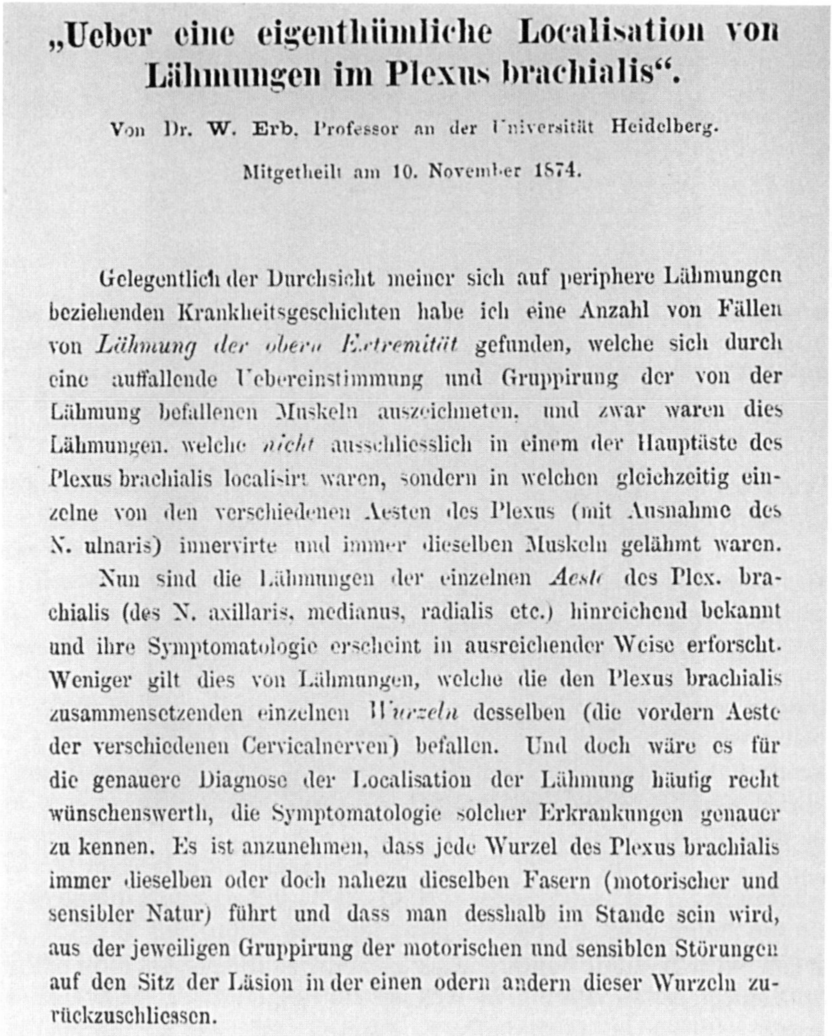

„Ueber eine eigenthümliche Localisation von Lähmungen im Plexus brachialis".

Von Dr. W. Erb, Professor an der Universität Heidelberg.

Mitgetheilt am 10. November 1874.

Gelegentlich der Durchsicht meiner sich auf periphere Lähmungen beziehenden Krankheitsgeschichten habe ich eine Anzahl von Fällen von *Lähmung der obern Extremität* gefunden, welche sich durch eine auffallende Uebereinstimmung und Gruppirung der von der Lähmung befallenen Muskeln auszeichneten, und zwar waren dies Lähmungen, welche *nicht* ausschliesslich in einem der Hauptäste des Plexus brachialis localisirt waren, sondern in welchen gleichzeitig einzelne von den verschiedenen Aesten des Plexus (mit Ausnahme des N. ulnaris) innervirte und immer dieselben Muskeln gelähmt waren.

Nun sind die Lähmungen der einzelnen *Aeste* des Plex. brachialis (des N. axillaris, medianus, radialis etc.) hinreichend bekannt und ihre Symptomatologie erscheint in ausreichender Weise erforscht. Weniger gilt dies von Lähmungen, welche die den Plexus brachialis zusammensetzenden einzelnen *Wurzeln* desselben (die vordern Aeste der verschiedenen Cervicalnerven) befallen. Und doch wäre es für die genauere Diagnose der Localisation der Lähmung häufig recht wünschenswerth, die Symptomatologie solcher Erkrankungen genauer zu kennen. Es ist anzunehmen, dass jede Wurzel des Plexus brachialis immer dieselben oder doch nahezu dieselben Fasern (motorischer und sensibler Natur) führt und dass man desshalb im Stande sein wird, aus der jeweiligen Gruppirung der motorischen und sensiblen Störungen auf den Sitz der Läsion in der einen odern andern dieser Wurzeln zurückzuschliessen.

Wilhelm Heinrich Erb: Ueber eine eigenthümliche Localisation von Lähmungen im Plexus brachialis. Verh. Naturhist. Med. Vereins Heidelberg, *1*:130–139, 1874–1877. (Courtesy of the Library of the New York Academy of Medicine)

this interest, and he described the reaction of degeneration. He failed to demonstrate any value of electricity in the treatment of mental disease, with the methods then available.

He was a hard taskmaster, but expected no more from others than he would do himself. Respected, rather than loved, by his students, he had a quick temper and a vocabulary that was quite foreign to the academic circle of his day. He was the traditional professor—proud, austere, and brusque, with an air of detachment about him. Immaculately dressed and full-bearded, and with narrow metal-rimmed glasses, he was feared by all except his patients. All of his biographers remarked on the solicitous care he gave everyone, from the peasant on the ward to the grand duke in his private practice. To them he was known as *der Grosse Zauberer,* a great charmer.

He succeeded Friedreich at Heidelberg and retired in 1907, after 27 years as the dean of German neurologists. On his seventieth birthday, the city of Heidelberg erected a statue of him near the hospital and named a street after him.

For many years he suffered from attacks of tachycardia and arrhythmia and had some gall stones removed surgically. His last years were full of sorrow. He had four sons; one, a physician, and another died in adult life, and a third son was killed on the western front in World War I. He was grief-stricken at seeing his fatherland destroyed by war. Weakened by an intestinal infection, he was attending a concert, listening to Beethoven's *Eroica,* his favorite symphony, when he collapsed, fell into a coma, and died. He was a giant of the nineteenth century.

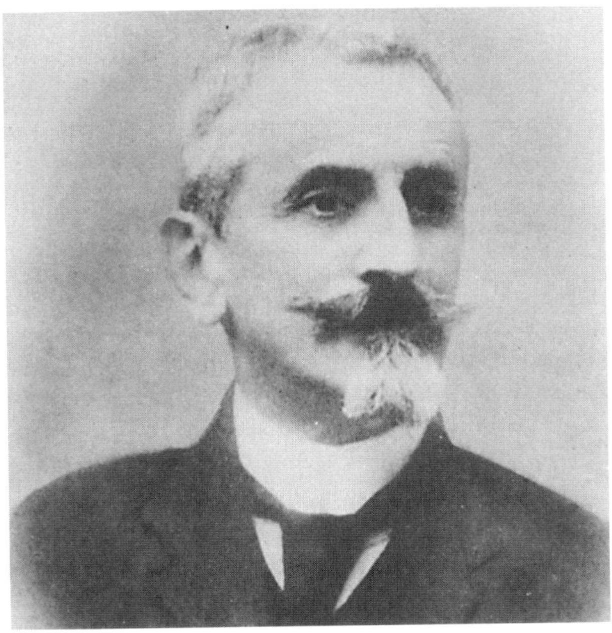

Corrado Parona, who, with his brother Ernesto, found hookworm ova in feces. See text for a discussion of their brother Francesco. (From Riv. Parassitol., *12,* 1951. Courtesy of the Library of the New York Academy of Medicine)

408

operare sollecitamente ed a distanza anche maggiore di quanto suole farsi ordinariamente. In quanto ad operare sollecitamente non è sempre in nostro potere; o perchè i malati ripugnano a farsi mozzare la lingua, e temporeggiano; o perchè il morbo viene e cresce insidioso e senza gravi minaccie in principio, d'onde lusinghe e speranze; e molto spesso perchè cadono nelle mani di chi non seppe a tempo apprezzare la gravezza del morbo. Da altra parte la osservazione ha anche dimostrato, che il cancro della lingua recidiva più frequentemente e più sollecitamente che quello, a cose pari, di altri organi. Dunque in queste amputazioni dovrassi essere ancora più larghi, più generosi: onde la rarità anche maggiore dei casi, nei quali sarà permesso di farne la remozione attraverso la sola apertura orale.

Dell' oncotomia negli ascessi profondi diffusi dell'avambraccio; *Nota del dott.* FRANCESCO PARONA.

L'argomento, sul quale intendo parlare, non lo reputo immeritevole che venga preso in considerazione dai pratici, avvegnacchè esso si raggira intorno ad una malattia altrettanto frequente, quanto difficile a curarsi. Io accenno agli ascessi profondi dell'avambraccio, la cura dei quali preoccupò le menti di insigni chirurghi, la cui valentia fu spesso inefficace ad impedire infausti risultamenti.

Le difficoltà che si incontrano nella cura di tale malattia sono attestate dal Chassaignac, dal Nelaton, dal Gosselin e da altri, e recentemente il Doibeau, nel pregevole suo lavoro sulla patogenia e cura dei flemmoni profondi dell' avambraccio, ebbe esplicitamente a dichiarare: *che tali flemmasie sono sempre gravi, difficili a curarsi e troppo sovente cagione di morte all'ammalato.*

Senza escludere affatto l'influenza, che lo stato generale dell'ammalato può avere sull'andamento ed esito della malattia, io penso che, per molta parte almeno, vi concorrano le condizioni anatomiche della regione ammalata, nonchè il modo col quale gli ascessi profondi dell'avambraccio vengono localmente trattati.

Infatti nella regione anteriore inferiore dell' avambraccio le raccolte di pus, che vi si formano profondamente, non sono, mas-

Francesco Parona: Dell'oncotomia negli ascessi profondi diffusi dell'avambraccio. Ann. Univers. Med. Chir. (Milan), *237*:408–414, 1876. (Courtesy of the National Library of Medicine, Bethesda, Maryland)

An Italian orthopaedist described the space between the pronator quadratus and the digital flexors in 1876, and noted the location of the incisions for drainage of pus from this antebrachial space. **Francesco Parona** (1842–1908) was born in Lodi of an old family that was well known in the Pavia region. He was the second of seven boys; one became a lawyer, one a businessman, one a professor of geology, and four became doctors of medicine. Ernesto and Corrado made names for themselves in the finding of hookworm ova in the feces. Francesco, after graduating at Pavia in 1865, worked with Bottini, who was an early

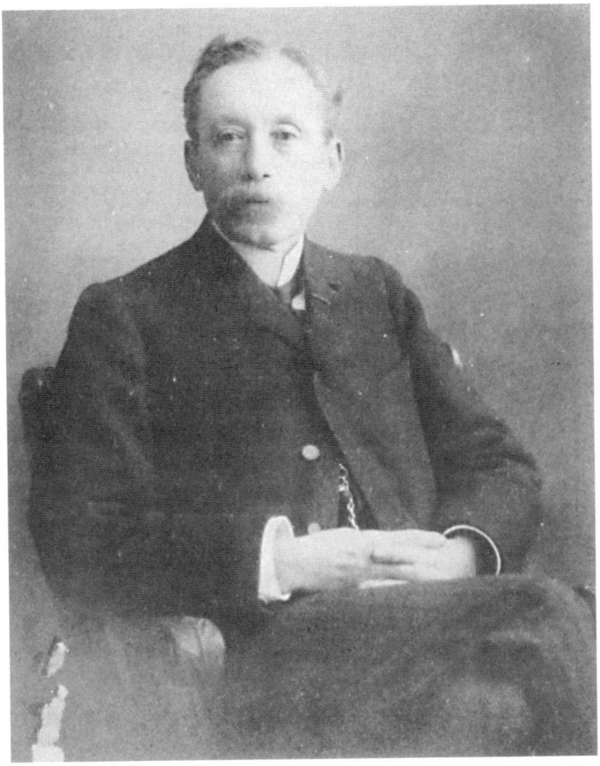

Jacques Louis Reverdin. (Courtesy of the Library of the New York Academy of Medicine)

advocate of Lister's phenol spray, at Hospital Novara. Francesco succeeded Bottini in 1871 as director of the surgical service.

The name of **Jacques Louis Reverdin** (1842–1929) is not used much today, though his report of the epidermal skin graft has been noted (see Wolfe). He was a Swiss who studied in Paris and whose inaugural thesis was on internal urethrotomy, perhaps influenced by his teacher, Guyon. He practiced in Genf, was surgeon to the local hospital, and was then professor of pathology and surgical medicine from 1876. His paper on epidermal grafts was published in 1872, but as was noted before, the graft included a part of the corium as well and today would be called a thin split-graft. He was better known for his reports on surgery of the thyroid gland, published in 1883.

Switzerland at this time was the center of thyroid study. Emil T. Kocher (1841–1917) only a year older, had been professor at Berne since 1872, and in 1878 did his pioneer operation, thyroidectomy. His assistant was Fritz de Quervain, whom we will meet later, with his description of

— 493 —

Greffe épidermique — M. REVERDIN lit un travail renvoyé à une commission composée de MM. Guyon, Chassaignac, Després.

COMMUNICATIONS

Lithotritie périnéale. — M. DOLBEAU. Messieurs, au mois de janvier 1863, j'ai pratiqué, pour la première fois, à Paris, une opération à laquelle j'ai cru devoir donner le nom de lithotriti[illegible]

[illegible] Mon [illegible] guéri très [illegible]

[illegible] la première fois qu'on [illegible] du crâne sur une certaine étendue. La guérison est restée complète.

M. GUYON fait un rapport verbal sur le travail suivant de M. Reverdin.

Greffe épidermique. — Expérience faite dans le service de M. le docteur Guyon, à l'hôpital Necker. — Messieurs, la communication que j'ai l'honneur de faire à la Société de chirurgie a trait à une question de pathologie bien vulgaire, en appa-

— 512 —

rence bien connue, mais qui présente cependant encore quelques points obscurs et intéressants à élucider. Je veux parler de la cicatrisation des plaies par seconde intention.

Tous les chirurgiens savent que si, dans la très-grande majorité des cas, les plaies arrivées à la période de granulation se cicatrisent par leurs bords, dans quelques cas exceptionnels on voit des îlots d'épiderme se former à la surface d'une plaie, plus ou moins loin de ces bords; que la formation de ces îlots centraux a sur la longueur de la cicatrisation une influence remarquable et bien connue; ils l'abrégent considérablement.

Ce fait constaté et admis, reste l'interprétation; et là-dessus on n'est pas d'accord : les uns, et Biltroth est très-affirmatif sur ce point, croient que toujours alors une mince couche, si mince fût-elle, de la couche profonde de l'épiderme, du réseau de Malpighi, est restée en place quelque part; ils se basent sur ce fait que c'est surtout dans des cas de brûlures qu'on observe la formation des îlots centraux.

D'autres pathologistes ne regardent point ces conditions comme indispensables.

J'ai eu précisément, il y a quelque temps, l'occasion d'observer un fait de cette nature; il s'agissait d'un ouvrier mécanicien qui avait eu le pouce droit broyé; il en résulta la nécessité de retrancher tout ce pouce jusqu'à l'articulation métacarpo-phalangienne; quand la cicatrisation eut commencé, nous vîmes se former au centre de cette plaie plusieurs îlots épidermiques qui hâtèrent singulièrement le travail de réparation.

Quelque temps après, ayant à observer une plaie étendue dont la cicatrisation était fort lente, me souvenant du malade dont je viens de parler, l'idée me vint de tenter l'expérience qui fait le sujet de cette communication.

Le malade sur lequel elle a été pratiquée est un homme de 35 ans, qui, le 16 octobre dernier, en tombant d'une échelle, essaya de se retenir avec le coude gauche fléchi à une barre de fer; la peau fut coupée au niveau du pli du coude, décollée dans toute son épaisseur jusqu'au milieu de l'avant-bras, et forma ainsi un grand lambeau qui ne tarda pas à se mortifier dans son entier. La surface mise à nu était formée par le tissu cellulaire sous-cutané, et à la partie externe du membre par l'aponévrose, éraillée par places. Cette plaie se mit bientôt à bourgeonner, mais ce n'est que le 14 novembre qu'on commença à distinguer sur ses bords un petit liséré épidermique. Les jours suivants le liséré s'étendit lentement.

Jacques Louis Reverdin: Greffe épidermique. Bull. Soc. (Imperial) Chir. Paris, *10*(2):493, 511, 512, 1869. (Courtesy of the National Library of Medicine, Bethesda, Maryland)

stenosing tenosynovitis of the radial styloid. It was Kocher who found that removal of the thyroid gland resulted in myxedema and whose studies led to a better understanding of the role of the ductless glands. Kocher received the Nobel Prize in 1909.

The influence of a man can spread widely through his students, and there are many examples, such as Langenbeck, who trained Billroth, Esmarch, and Trendelenburg. Another was Johannes Müller, from whose laboratories came the studies of Schwann. Among many others, W. J. Little went there to study for his medical degree. Paget, in London, used techniques of anatomical study that had been worked out in Müller's department. One of Müller's students with Schwann was Henle, who went on to become professor at Göttingen, where he attracted students interested in microscopic anatomy. One of these is our source for the next eponym.

Friedrich Sigmund Merkel (1845–1919) described the Merkel disc, that particular type of nerve ending in the skin. He was born in Nürnberg, the

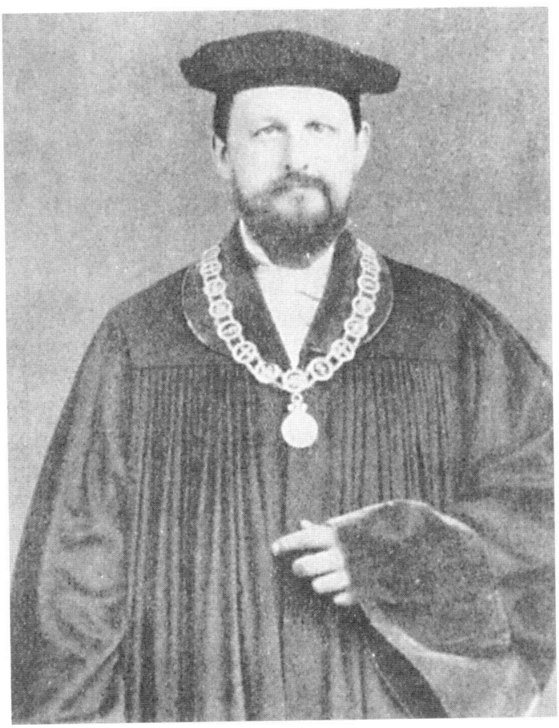

Friedrich Sigmund Merkel. (From Schumacher, G. H., and Heinzgünther, W.: Anatomia Rostochiensis. Berlin, Akademie Verlag, 1970. Courtesy of the Library of the New York Academy of Medicine)

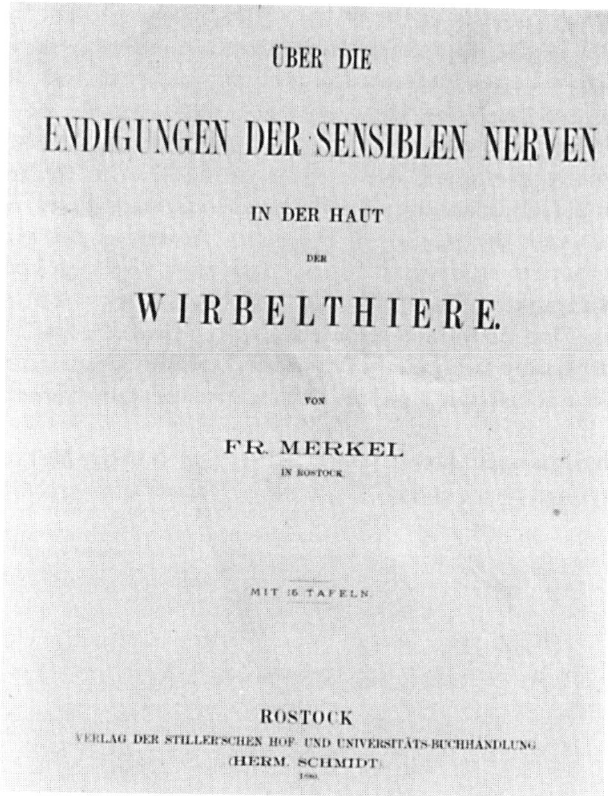
ÜBER DIE

ENDIGUNGEN DER SENSIBLEN NERVEN

IN DER HAUT

DER

WIRBELTHIERE.

VON

FR. MERKEL

IN ROSTOCK

MIT 15 TAFELN.

ROSTOCK

VERLAG DER STILLER'SCHEN HOF- UND UNIVERSITÄTS-BUCHHANDLUNG

(HERM. SCHMIDT)

Friedrich Sigmund Merkel: Über die Endigungen der Sensiblen Nerven in der Haut der Wirbelthiere. Rostock, Verlag der Stiller'schen Hof- und Universitäts-Buchhandlung, 1880. (Courtesy of the National Library of Medicine, Bethesda, Maryland)

son of a pharmacist, and, as so many students at that time, went from school to school, depending on which professor was most popular at the time. He started at Erlangen, but, developing an interest in microscopic anatomy, went to Göttingen to work under Henle. While carrying on his regular medical studies, he worked in the laboratory and published a series of observations. After graduating from Erlangen, his original school, he returned to be prosector to Henle. Apparently, he became not only a good investigator but also married Henle's daughter, Anna. When he was invited to both Basel and Rostock, he chose the latter and remained there for 11 years. When Henle died, Merkel returned to Göttingen and, as professor, remained until his death from a stroke in 1919.

Merkel's first work was on the anatomy of the eye, including studies of the retina and of the muscles of the iris. The work in which he described the sensible nerve endings was published in 1880, while he was at Rostock. He introduced many new techniques in microscopic anatomy, especially the use of xylol. Other studies were done in macroscopic anatomy and included a handbook of topographic anatomy. He did some anatomical studies from the artist's point of view and wrote a biography of Henle.

He was a good lecturer, documenting his demonstrations with practical applications of the anatomy for the surgeon and physician. He was respected by the students far more than were Erb or Meissner, for he was not the austere chief or the difficult personality. He was heartbroken by the war; two sons, one an officer and the other a talented artist, were both killed in action. He believed that life consisted of constant indefatigable work and should come to an end with a slow, easy death; this, he believed, rather than war, was the plan of all creation.

Merkel's name is well remembered for his work in anatomy (the improvements in technique), and although his eponym remains with this simple nerve ending, we can say that he has a rightful place among the giants of medicine.

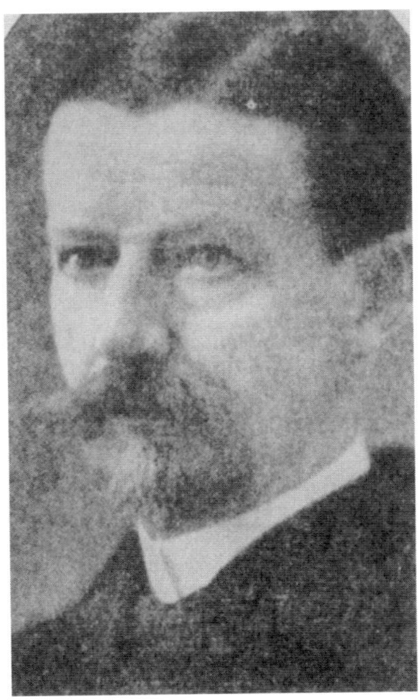

Otto Wilhelm Madelung. (From the doctor's page. J. Organotherapy, *18*[5]:269, 1934. Courtesy of the Library of the New York Academy of Medicine)

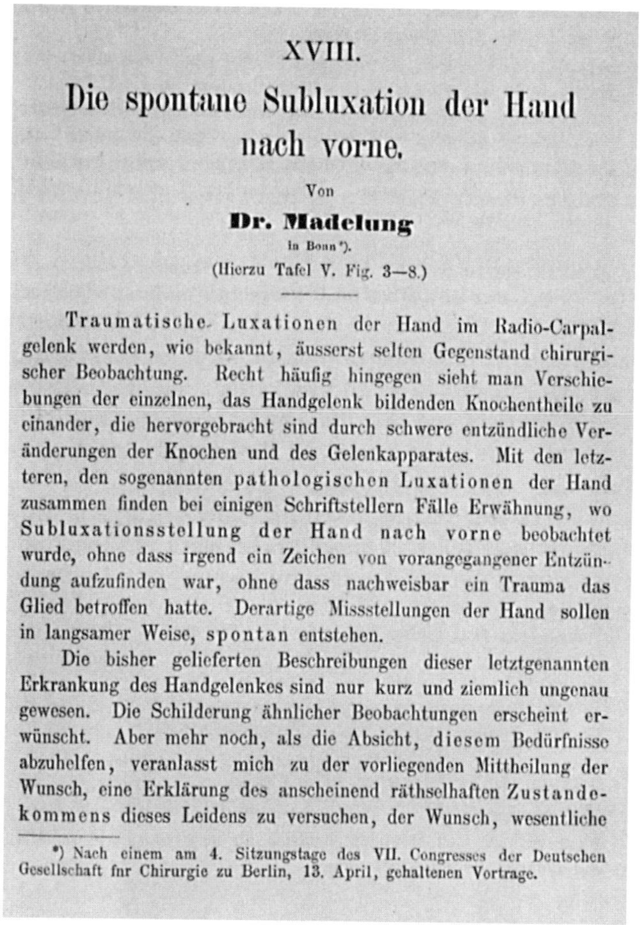

XVIII.

Die spontane Subluxation der Hand nach vorne.

Von

Dr. Madelung

in Bonn*).

(Hierzu Tafel V. Fig. 3—8.)

Traumatische Luxationen der Hand im Radio-Carpalgelenk werden, wie bekannt, äusserst selten Gegenstand chirurgischer Beobachtung. Recht häufig hingegen sieht man Verschiebungen der einzelnen, das Handgelenk bildenden Knochentheile zu einander, die hervorgebracht sind durch schwere entzündliche Veränderungen der Knochen und des Gelenkapparates. Mit den letzteren, den sogenannten pathologischen Luxationen der Hand zusammen finden bei einigen Schriftstellern Fälle Erwähnung, wo Subluxationsstellung der Hand nach vorne beobachtet wurde, ohne dass irgend ein Zeichen von vorangegangener Entzündung aufzufinden war, ohne dass nachweisbar ein Trauma das Glied betroffen hatte. Derartige Missstellungen der Hand sollen in langsamer Weise, spontan entstehen.

Die bisher gelieferten Beschreibungen dieser letztgenannten Erkrankung des Handgelenkes sind nur kurz und ziemlich ungenau gewesen. Die Schilderung ähnlicher Beobachtungen erscheint erwünscht. Aber mehr noch, als die Absicht, diesem Bedürfnisse abzuhelfen, veranlasst mich zu der vorliegenden Mittheilung der Wunsch, eine Erklärung des anscheinend räthselhaften Zustandekommens dieses Leidens zu versuchen, der Wunsch, wesentliche

*) Nach einem am 4. Sitzungstage des VII. Congresses der Deutschen Gesellschaft für Chirurgie zu Berlin, 13. April, gehaltenen Vortrage.

Otto Wilhelm Madelung: Die spontane Subluxation der Hand nach vorne. Langenbecks Arch. Klin. Chir., 23:395–412, 1879. (Courtesy of the Library of the College of Physicians of Philadelphia)

When, after the Franco-Prussian War, Strassburg was returned to German control, the faculty of the school was reconstituted under the leadership of Recklinghausen, who made it a center for teaching and research. He drew his faculty from many places and in 1894, he asked **Otto Wilhelm Madelung** (1846–1926) to become the professor of surgery. In 1878 Madelung had described a deformity of the wrist occurring in young women, probably due to a defect in the development of the distal radial epiphysis. This report, without x-ray, was done while he was an assistant in Bonn, and his description is clear and unmistakable in defining a particular lesion, so that we recognize Madelung's deformity as a specific entity. It was not this relatively minor contribution that resulted in the invitation to Strassburg, but his work in general surgery. His major work was in abdominal surgery, intestinal suture, and the advocacy of early laparotomy in trauma. He covered all the fields of surgery, writing on surgery of the thyroid, rhinoplasty, varicose veins, colostomy, and echinococcus disease. He described a posterior approach to the shoulder joint and an easy method of suturing tendons (1882), and he wrote on the etiology and treatment of Dupuytren's contracture (1875) as well as on Sayre's method of treating vertebral disease (1879). In 1874 he visited England and the United States.

Madelung, the son of a merchant, was born in Gotha and studied in Bonn, Berlin, and Tübingen. After his army service and his travel, he spent most of the time in Bonn, succeeding his professor there; but in 1881 he went to Rostock, where Merkel was head of anatomy.

It was only in 1894 that he went to Strassburg and stayed there until the end of World War I, when the town again was reverted to the French and all the faculty was relieved. Fritz Lange, later to be in Munich, was one of his assistants. Madelung retired to Göttingen, where he died of a stroke 2 months after his eightieth birthday. Georg Perthes wrote Madelung's obituary, closing with these words, "All in all, a man to whom German surgery can point with pride."

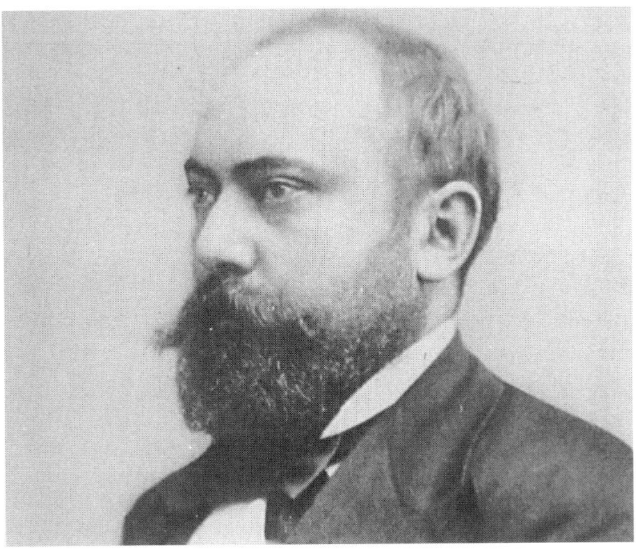

Carl Nicoladoni. (From Nicoladoni, C.: Anatomie und Mechanismus der Skoliose. Berlin, Urban & Schwarzenberg, 1909. Courtesy of the Library of the New York Academy of Medicine)

XXVIII.

Daumenplastik und organischer Ersatz der Fingerspitze (Anticheiroplastik und Daktyloplastik).

Von

Professor Dr. C. Nicoladoni

in Graz (Oestreich).

(Mit 6 Figuren.)

Der Gedanke, den in seinen Phalangen verloren gegangenen Daumen als lebendiges und bewegliches Glied wiederzuersetzen, eröffnet ein fruchtbares Feld einer neuartigen Plastik, wie ein von mir in dieser Absicht, mit, wenn auch nur theilsweisem Erfolge, operirter Fall zeigt.

Ich habe in einer früheren Publication: Wiener med. Klinik, 1897, darauf hingewiesen, dass es gelingt, einen Daumen, der die Haut des ganzen Thenars und der beiden Phalangen durch Abschälung verloren hat, so mit Brusthaut nach Handschuhart zu bedecken, dass das sonst verloren gewesene Glied gebrauchsfähig und beweglich erhalten werden kann.

Ich habe ferner gezeigt, dass auf einen Stumpf, welcher den Metacarpus I und einen Theil der I. Phalanx enthält, ein häutiger Daumen aus der Brust, nach Art eines Handschuhdaumenstückes überpflanzt werden kann, wenn nur am Thenar ein hinreichendgrosses Stück desselben Wurzel gefasst hat.

Durch Einpflanzung eines entsprechend langen und dicken Tibiastückes in den neugebildeten häutigen Daumen sollte letzterer steif und widerstandsfähig genug gemacht werden, um als neu geschaffenes Glied zum Fassen und Festhalten verwendet werden zu können.

Carl Nicoladoni: Daumenplastik und organischer Ersatz der Fingerspitze (Anticheiroplastik und Daktyloplastik). Arch. Klin. Chir., *61*:606–614, 1900. (Courtesy of the Library of the College of Physicians of Philadelphia)

Carl Nicoladoni (1847–1902) has nothing named after him, but he was one of the pioneers in surgery of the hand and deserves mention for his work on tendon transfers and tendon sutures and for the pollicization of a toe. He lived only 55 years and spent all of his life in Austria, but he made many contributions. He was born in Vienna, completing his education there in 1871. He became an assistant to Dumreicher at Innsbruck and succeeded him in the professorship 10 years later. He was the first to operate on an esophageal diverticulum and was the first to describe torsion of the spermatic cord. He wrote papers on nerve endings in the joint capsules and on intestinal resections in strangulated hernia. He did a fundamental study of torsion of the spine in scoliosis. He suggested the operation of gastroenterostomy. In 1895, he went to Graz as a professor. He died there in 1902.

Otto Sprengel (1852–1915), in 1891, described the deformity that we call by his name. This uncommon lesion results from a failure of the scapulae to descend from their original high position in embryonic life.

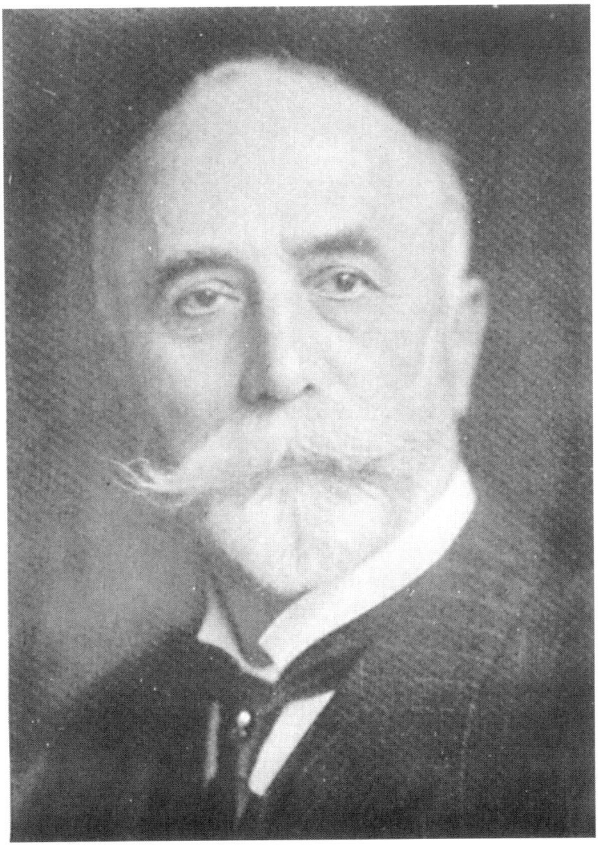

Otto Sprengel. (From Deutsche Gesellschaft für Chirurgie. Zentralbl. Chir., 1926. Courtesy of the Library of the New York Academy of Medicine)

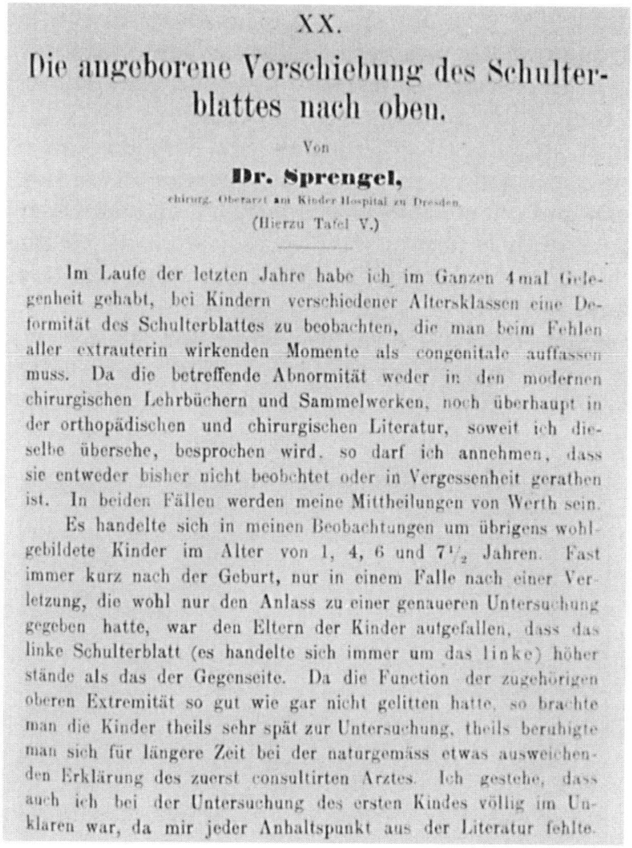

XX.

Die angeborene Verschiebung des Schulterblattes nach oben.

Von

Dr. Sprengel,

chirurg. Oberarzt am Kinder-Hospital zu Dresden.

(Hierzu Tafel V.)

Im Laufe der letzten Jahre habe ich im Ganzen 4 mal Gelegenheit gehabt, bei Kindern verschiedener Altersklassen eine Deformität des Schulterblattes zu beobachten, die man beim Fehlen aller extrauterin wirkenden Momente als congenitale auffassen muss. Da die betreffende Abnormität weder in den modernen chirurgischen Lehrbüchern und Sammelwerken, noch überhaupt in der orthopädischen und chirurgischen Literatur, soweit ich dieselbe übersehe, besprochen wird, so darf ich annehmen, dass sie entweder bisher nicht beobachtet oder in Vergessenheit gerathen ist. In beiden Fällen werden meine Mittheilungen von Werth sein.

Es handelte sich in meinen Beobachtungen um übrigens wohlgebildete Kinder im Alter von 1, 4, 6 und $7^1/_2$ Jahren. Fast immer kurz nach der Geburt, nur in einem Falle nach einer Verletzung, die wohl nur den Anlass zu einer genaueren Untersuchung gegeben hatte, war den Eltern der Kinder aufgefallen, dass das linke Schulterblatt (es handelte sich immer um das linke) höher stände als das der Gegenseite. Da die Function der zugehörigen oberen Extremität so gut wie gar nicht gelitten hatte, so brachte man die Kinder theils sehr spät zur Untersuchung, theils beruhigte man sich für längere Zeit bei der naturgemäss etwas ausweichenden Erklärung des zuerst consultirten Arztes. Ich gestehe, dass auch ich bei der Untersuchung des ersten Kindes völlig im Unklaren war, da mir jeder Anhaltspunkt aus der Literatur fehlte.

Otto Sprengel: Die angeborene Verschiebung des Schulterblattes nach oben. Arch. Klin. Chir., *42*:545, 1891. (Courtesy of the Library of the College of Physicians of Philadelphia)

Again we have an example of an eponym resulting from a contribution that was minor, when compared with the major field of interest of the author. Sprengel was a general surgeon, and though he also wrote on traumatic coxa vara, he spent some years in Dresden at the Children's Hospital, where he described the shoulder lesion (others think Eulenburg did it first in 1863).

Sprengel was born in Mecklenburg province and is said to have carried his native accent all his life. He was an assistant to Volkmann at Halle, before going to Dresden. Here a family tragedy occurred; his wife and only child died of some infectious disease. He went to Braunschweig and became an exponent of early surgery for appendicitis and advocated an

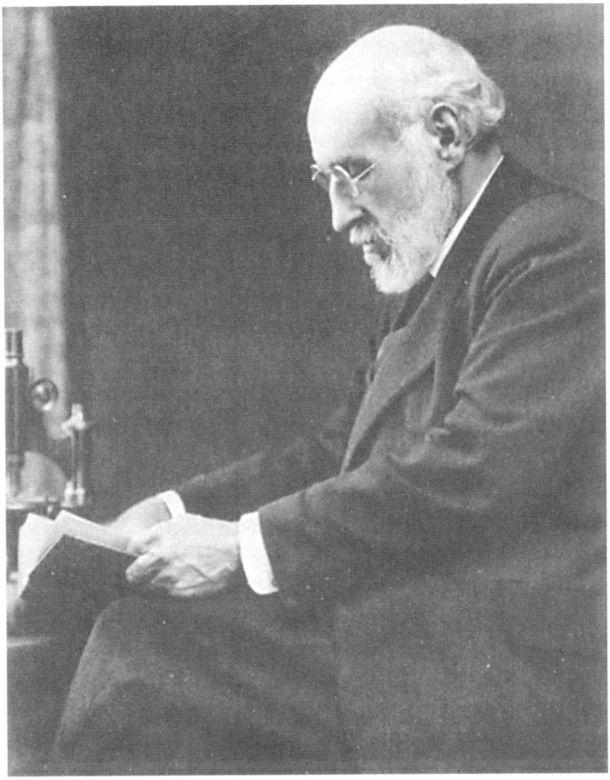

Santiago Ramón y Cajal. (From Ramón y Cajal, S.: Degeneration & Regeneration of the Nervous System. [vol. 1] Translated and edited by Raoul M. May. London, Oxford University Press, 1928. Courtesy of the Library of the New York Academy of Medicine)

oblique incision, rather than one in the midline, because he thought that it produced less of a scar.

He was a prominent member of the German Surgical Society and was to be its president in 1915. In his work as a surgeon, however, he developed an infection from some contamination during an operation on a wounded soldier. Although there is no record of what part this involved, several months of suffering followed, and he died in January, 1915.

It hardly seems possible that in 1873, in the latter half of the nineteenth century, a man could graduate as a doctor, spend a year in the army service in Cuba, where malaria and dysentery were epidemic, and yet never see a microscope. Yet that is what happened to a young Spanish doctor, **Santiago Ramón y Cajal** (1852–1934), who later would share with

Golgi the Nobel Prize for his detailed studies of the nerve cell and would become one of the world's most renowned neurohistologists.

Spain had long passed its golden age, when its king had been emperor of the Holy Roman Empire. It had squandered its riches from the New World, the Hapsburg line had degenerated, and Napoleon had come and gone. Spain had settled back behind the Pyrenees, a mental as well as a physical barrier, and scientific study was a rarity. Müller's laboratory in Berlin was already famous, Schleiden and Schwann had proposed the cell theory in 1838, Pacini in Italy had described the corpuscle in 1835, and in 1850 Waller in England had published the results of his experiments on the frog's tongue. Yet this 23-year-old Aragonese physician, the son of a professor of anatomy at Zaragoza, coming to Madrid for his doctoral examination, had never even seen, much less used, the instrument that was to make him famous. We have nothing in our field of surgery of the hand which specifically relates to Ramón y Cajal; yet he was a giant, and we owe him much for his work, his writings, and his examples.

Santiago's father, Justo Ramón y Cassasus, was a "surgeon of the second class" in a remote mountain village, but was so determined to become a fully accredited physician that he finally got his diploma from the University of Zaragoza. A most unusual man, he insisted that Santiago would become a physician. But Santiago's sole interest seemed to be in drawing. Even this talent was decried by local critics, and, being labeled a poor student, he was apprenticed first to a barber and then to a shoemaker. Still, only drawing and sketching appealed to him, and the father undertook to educate the boy, teaching him to read and write and giving him an understanding of mathematics, French, and geography. Father and son now started a study of the human skeleton (using bones from a nearby cemetery), and Santiago's drawing ability led to such a high quality in the sketches that later, when he qualified at Zaragoza, a serious consideration was given to the publication of these as an anatomic atlas.

Ramón y Cajal's university days were not marked by any brilliant records in academics, but he did become the champion "strong man" in the gymnasium. This came about when he discovered that another student had stronger arms and wrists as a result of regular exercises. Not to be outdone, Ramón y Cajal started a planned program of exercises for 2 hours daily, eventually succeeding in outperforming his rival. Much later, in his writings, he was to remark on this and noted that too much physical effort lessened the powers of thought, as he had found it to be in his own case, and noted the general lack of intense thought among the more athletic types. (How many All-Americans in sports have made their mark in science?)

After graduation, his army service in Cuba was done, and he returned in poor health. After suffering a severe pulmonary hemorrhage, he spent a year in the mountains, during which he furthered his interest in photography. He developed a faster gelatin plate by a process that some think might have made him a fortune, if properly exploited.

When he went to Madrid for his examination and saw a microscope for the first time, he could not resist the challenge. He purchased one with a maximum magnification of 180 power, for the equivalent of $140.00, to be paid in four installments. Along with a microtome, also purchased, and a book of instructions, he returned to Zaragoza as director of the anatomical laboratory.

His papers on general histological sujects were well received in local circles. Offered the chair of anatomy at Valencia, he accepted, but found himself involved in a cholera epidemic, and his work was focused on bacteriology. The people of Valencia were so appreciative of his work that he was made a gift of the best Zeiss microscope available. Soon he was offered the post in Barcelona, and here he came into contact with a psychiatrist, Dr. Luis Simarro, at the university who introduced him to Golgi's work on a staining method for nerve tissues. Ramón y Cajal improved the staining methods and published his reports, first in Spanish, then in other European journals.

Traditionally, Spanish workers in the sciences did not publish their works outside their own country, and other Europeans treated their work lightly. Ramón y Cajal's break with the tradition was criticized, but when an opportunity came to demonstrate his findings before the German Society of Anatomists, he made a great impression on the listeners, and Kölliker, then dean of German histology, put the seal of approval on his work.

The story of his experience with chess, while he was in Barcelona, illustrates the type of man he was. It seems that his interest in the game became almost an addiction. He would play four matches simultaneously, extending over 2 or 3 days. Finally realizing that too much time and effort was being expended, he took 1 week off from all work, defeated every one of his strongest opponents, and then quit the game completely for 25 years.

Finally he was offered the professorship in Madrid, and here he attracted pupils from all over the world.* His fame spread throughout the world. He was given the Moscow Prize in Paris in 1920 and the Helmholtz Medal of Prussia, and he received honorary degrees from Cambridge and Oxford. He was a house guest of Sherrington, and he and his wife visited the United States in 1892 for a series of lectures at Clark

*Wilder Penfield wrote a moving tribute to Ramón y Cajal in the Archives of Neurology and Psychiatry, *16*:213–220, 1926, describing his first visit to Ramón y Cajal.

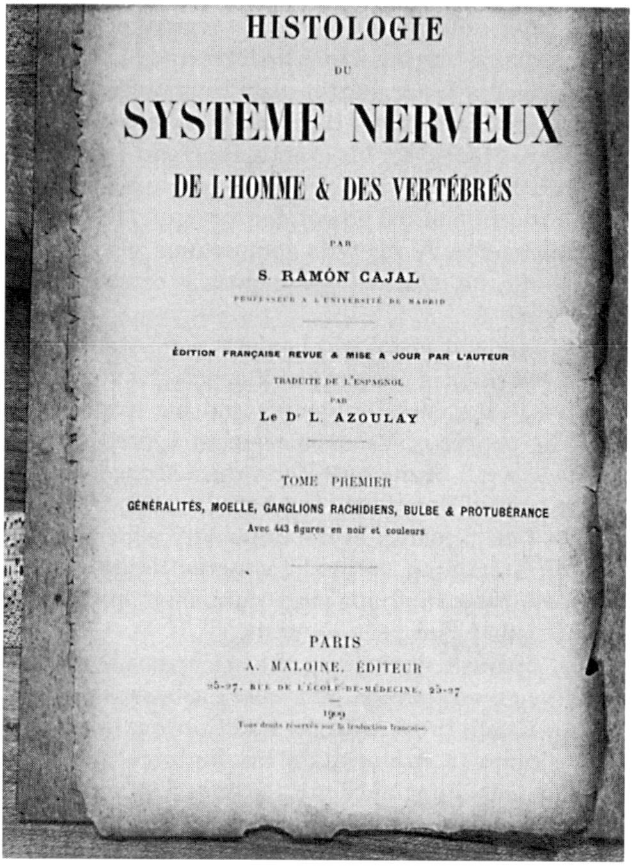

HISTOLOGIE

DU

SYSTÈME NERVEUX

DE L'HOMME & DES VERTÉBRÉS

PAR

S. RAMÓN CAJAL

PROFESSEUR A L'UNIVERSITÉ DE MADRID

ÉDITION FRANÇAISE REVUE & MISE A JOUR PAR L'AUTEUR

TRADUITE DE L'ESPAGNOL

PAR

Le Dr L. AZOULAY

TOME PREMIER

GÉNÉRALITÉS, MOELLE, GANGLIONS RACHIDIENS, BULBE & PROTUBÉRANCE

Avec 443 figures en noir et couleurs

PARIS

A. MALOINE, ÉDITEUR

25-27, RUE DE L'ÉCOLE-DE-MÉDECINE, 25-27

1909

Tous droits réservés pour la traduction française.

Santiago Ramón y Cajal: Histologie du Système Nerveux de l'Homme & des Vertébrés. Paris, A. Maloine, 1909. (Courtesy of the Library of the New York Academy of Medicine)

University in Worcester, Massachusetts. He shared the Nobel Prize with Golgi in 1906.

His investigations continued and included studies of the neuroglia as well as the neurofibrils. His manual of pathological anatomy went through seven editions, the last in 1922.

He fell in love with Madrid, taking long walks in the countryside and using his camera to photograph the surrounding scenes, which were so different from those of the mountain village of his youth. He strove to improve the scientific life of Spain, writing a classic monograph on the rules and precepts that should apply to scientific investigation and reports. He declined the post of minister of public instruction.

He was a philosopher as well as a scientist, writing essays as well as a lighter work titled *Charlas de Café* (*charlas* means light talk, chatterings, or even gossip), in which he recorded the anecdotes and aphorisms of his day as they were discussed among his friends. These discussions are a part of what is called the *tertulia*, a meeting of a group of men that is usually held in the late afternoon over a cup of coffee at a local cafe, where the discussion focuses on topics of the day or any subject that one wishes. Ramón y Cajal called these periods his "diastoles"—periods of relaxation from the strenuous "systoles" of work.

A few of his sayings are illustrative of his philosophical bent. "Grey matter abounds in countries with grey skies." "The saddest thing about old age is that its future is behind it." "We disdain and hate from lack of self comprehension and we understand in proportion as we study ourselves."

Ramón y Cajal's work continued up to the last year of his life, including 295 publications (most with his own illustrations), an autobiography, and more than twenty other books. He died at 82, one of the giants of medicine. Although we have no disease, sign, or procedure by his name in our field of surgery, there is hardly a city in Spain without an *Avenida* (avenue) de Ramón y Cajal, the scientific genius of new Spain.

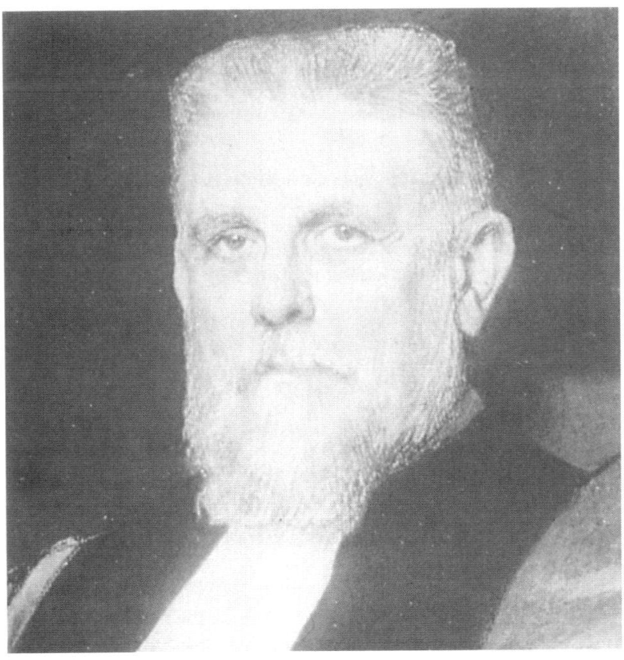

Pierre Marie. (Courtesy of the Library of the New York Academy of Medicine)

trou de la méninge, nettement arrondi, à l'emporte-pièce, avait le caractère des orifices méningés congénitaux que l'on a parfois signalés.

Il y avait donc chez cet homme, sur un petit espace, toute une série, peut-on dire, de déhiscences congénitales : déhiscence de la paroi postéro-supérieure du sinus sphénoïdal, déhiscence de la lame quadrilatère, déhiscence de la méninge elle-même (1). Sans doute existait-il aussi un certain degré d'inflammation, mais cette inflammation avait pu être tardive, modérée, et ainsi s'expliquait peut-être pour une bonne part l'intégrité relative de la glande pituitaire elle-même.

Quoi qu'il en soit, des faits de ce genre nous paraissaient mériter d'être signalés par le fait qu'ils révèlent un mode d'infection possible, et peut-être pas très rare, de la glande pituitaire, à savoir la voie des sinus sphénoïdaux.

VI. Atrophie isolée de l'éminence thénar d'origine névritique. Rôle du ligament annulaire antérieur du carpe dans la pathogénie de la lésion, par MM. PIERRE MARIE et FOIX.

L'atrophie isolée non progressive des petits muscles de la main est un syndrome relativement fréquent, car depuis le mémoire que nous avons publié sur ce sujet dans la *Nouvelle Iconographie de la Salpêtrière* (2), mémoire qui comportait dix observations personnelles, nous en avons observé encore une dizaine de cas.

Ce syndrome peut relever de causes multiples, névrite radiculaire ou non radiculaire, et ces petits foyers limités à la corne antérieure, que nous avons qualifiés de foyers de *téphromalacie antérieure*.

Dans ce dernier cas, il s'agit presque toujours de sujets syphilitiques.

Cliniquement, l'on peut distinguer trois types de ces atrophies isolées non progressives : un type thénarien pur, un type hypothénarien plus ou moins pur, un type thénaro-hypothénarien diffus, le plus fréquent.

Nous n'avons pas eu l'occasion d'observer d'atrophie pure hypothénarienne, mais simplement des cas à prédominance hypothénarienne. Par contre, il est assez fréquent d'observer des cas d'atrophie thénarienne pure, et dans ces cas l'on voit ordinairement (dans tous les cas par nous observés) que l'atrophie respecte le muscle adducteur du pouce, frappant ainsi *exclusivement le territoire du médian*.

Nous ne croyons pas que ce soit là une raison suffisante pour admettre comme démontrée *l'origine névritique de la lésion*, car nous avons constaté la même intégrité de l'adducteur dans un cas de poliomyélite antérieure aiguë. C'est là cependant un argument considérable en faveur de l'origine périphérique, et il s'agissait d'une lésion du nerf médian dans le cas, avec autopsie, dont nous allons donner ici le résumé.

Il devient alors malaisé de comprendre pourquoi, dans ces cas, l'atrophie musculaire frappe exclusivement les muscles thénariens, respectant les muscles innervés par le médian dans le reste du membre supérieur.

La disposition de la lésion dans notre cas permet d'en apporter une explica-

(1) Fait à remarquer, le canal cranio-pharyngien, qui constitue une déhiscence beaucoup plus commune, faisait ici absolument défaut ; sa situation aurait pourtant été exactement entre les déhiscences de la paroi antérieure et à la paroi postérieure de la selle turcique.

(2) PIERRE MARIE et FOIX, Atrophie isolée non progressive des petits muscles de la main. *Nouvelle Iconographie de la Salpêtrière*, septembre et novembre 1912, n°s 5 et 6.

Pierre Marie: Atrophie isolée de l'eminence thénar d'origine névritique. Rôle du ligament annulaire antérieur du carpe dans la pathogénie de la lésion. Rev. Neurol. (Paris), 26:647–649, 1913. (Courtesy of the Library of the College of Physicians of Philadelphia)

The clinical differentiation of various neurological diseases has almost been a prerogative of French neurology. Charcot, of course, was the leader, and his favorite pupil was **Pierre Marie** (1853–1940), who succeeded him as dean of the neurologists. In 1913, Marie and Charles Foix, his agrégé and lecturer, described the findings at an autopsy of bilateral thenar atrophy due to compression of the median nerves in the carpal tunnels. Paget had reported a case, in 1853, of compression of the nerve by callus of a fracture of the distal radius. This lesion described by Marie and Foix was not treated surgically until 1941 by Woltman, and Seddon reported two cases in 1945. Today this lesion is common, and the operation is done frequently. One should read the work of George Phalen for an extensive review of the symptoms and treatment.*

Marie, of course is remembered for many things, such as Charcot-Marie-Tooth disease (Howard Henry Tooth [1856–1925] also described it independently the same year in England). Marie also is remembered for the Marie-Strümpell ankylosing spondylitis, the first description of acromegaly, hypertrophic pulmonary osteoarthropathy, and cleidocranial dysostosis, and for calling attention to the tremor of Basedow's disease. Marie was a shrewd clinician and diagnostician, not much interested in experimental neurology, as were Vulpian and Déjèrine, his contemporaries in Paris.

Marie was born in Paris of a wealthy family and first studied law. After changing to medicine, he became an intern, and in 1878 he came under the influence of Charcot. He was made chief of the clinic and the laboratory for Charcot and progressed to professor agrégé. His lectures became very popular. His apparently authoritarian manner was accentuated by a square-cut beard and hair style. Percival Bailey, who went to Paris as a student in 1921, described Marie as being dignified and courteous to all, including the patients. He had a great facility in stirring up controversy and argument and in getting people to debate their ideas vigorously. At one time he was professor of pathological anatomy, but only clinical work interested him. He was so sensitive to formalin that a fixed specimen of brain tissue could only be viewed through a window.

He retired in 1925 to an estate on the south coast of France, but his last years were tragic. First his wife died, then his daughter died of appendicitis, and finally his only son, studying botulism at the Pasteur Institute, contracted the disease and died.

The study of diseases of the nervous system was not confined to France. Erb in Germany had systematized the examination and recording of findings and had described many syndromes. A young English physi-

*Phalen, G. S.: The carpal tunnel syndrome. Clinical evaluation of 598 hands. Clin. Orthop., *83*:29–40, 1972.

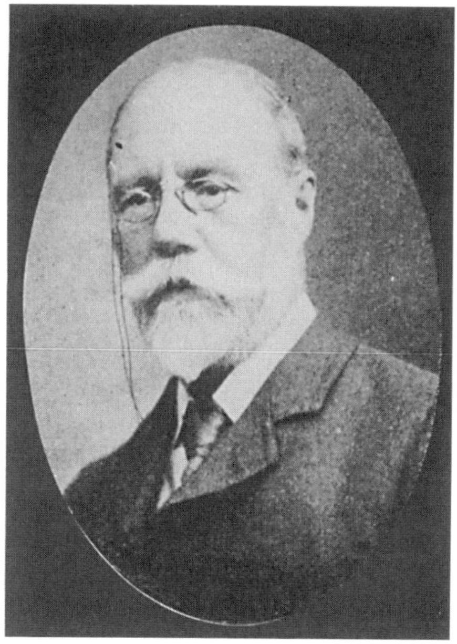

Charles Edward Beevor. (From Foreign guests. JAMA, *50*:1795, 1908. Copyright 1908, American Medical Association. Courtesy of the Library of the New York Academy of Medicine)

cian, after his travels to Leipzig, Berlin, and Paris, returned to make some major contributions to the anatomy of the brain, especially the localization of function and the intricate blood supply of the cerebrum. But this man, **Charles Edward Beevor** (1854–1908), is of interest to us for a maneuver called Beevor's sign. He described how, in a clawhand from intrinsic paralysis, the long finger extensor muscles can extend the interphalangeal joints when hyperextension of the metacarpophalangeal joints is prevented. Simple pressure on the dorsum of the proximal phalanx demonstrates this and proves that the long extensors are capable of full finger extension, providing that the metacarpophalangeal joints are not allowed to hyperextend. We also know that if the long extensors are paralyzed, as in a radial palsy, the intrinsic muscles can extend the interphalangeal joints, although their action is more efficient when the metacarpophalangeal joints are extended.

The function of the intrinsic muscles has been studied for many years, and much acrimonious debate has gone on concerning one or another's theories or concepts. Paraphrasing Steindler, there is no place in medicine for personal attacks or chauvinistic attitudes. The discussion of a problem is not an adversary contest, and decisions should be based on

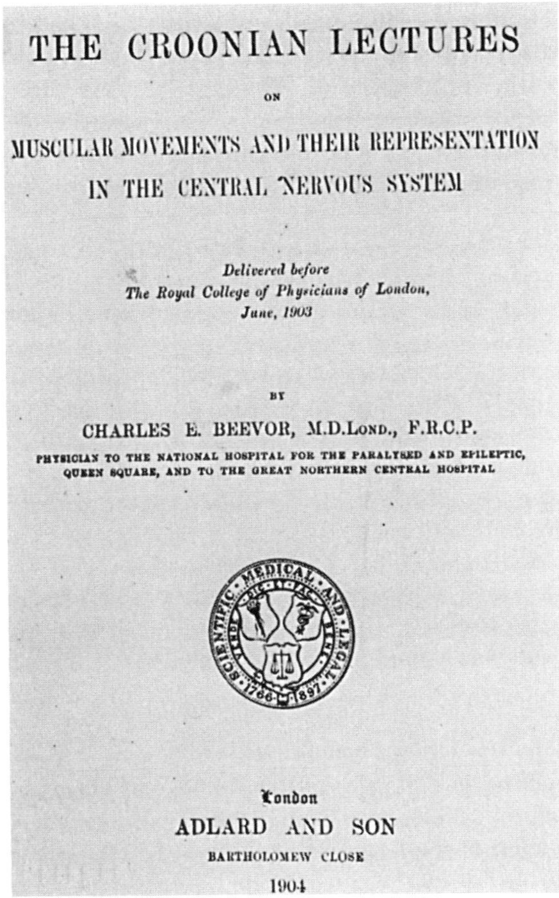

THE CROONIAN LECTURES

ON

MUSCULAR MOVEMENTS AND THEIR REPRESENTATION IN THE CENTRAL NERVOUS SYSTEM

Delivered before
The Royal College of Physicians of London,
June, 1903

BY

CHARLES E. BEEVOR, M.D.Lond., F.R.C.P.

PHYSICIAN TO THE NATIONAL HOSPITAL FOR THE PARALYSED AND EPILEPTIC, QUEEN SQUARE, AND TO THE GREAT NORTHERN CENTRAL HOSPITAL

London
ADLARD AND SON
BARTHOLOMEW CLOSE
1904

Charles Edward Beevor: Muscular Movements and Their Representation in the Central Nervous System (The Croonian Lectures, 1903). London, Adlard and Son, 1904. (Courtesy of the Library of the Los Angeles County Medical Association)

conclusions that are developed from a study of the facts and in accordance with logical principles. Too many reports today read more like those of propagandists than of scientists.

Beevor was a careful observer, and his work with Horsley on localization of function in the brain led him to agree with Hughlings Jackson that the brain knows nothing of muscles, only movements.

Beevor was born in London in 1854, the oldest son of Charles Beevor, a surgeon. He was graduated from University College in London and took his Bachelor of Medicine degree in 1878, his Doctor of Medicine degree in 1881, and his membership in the Royal College of Physicians in 1882. He spent several months traveling, first to Vienna, where he was apparently interested in diseases of the throat and the eye. Soon he was in Leipzig and worked with Cohnheim and Weigert, studying the technique of microscopy and the staining of sections. Erb was there, as a professor, and must have influenced Beevor, because he continued in his neurological studies in Berlin, and then in Paris with Charcot, Marie, and Déjèrine.

Returning to England, he was appointed to the National Hospital for the Paralysed and Epileptic, where he remained all his life. Here Horsley was one of his clinical clerks, and later the two joined efforts in a 4-year study on the representation of movement in the cortex, work which was later described in the Croonian Lecture of 1903. Another study involved the arterial supply of the brain, in which simultaneous injection of the five main arteries with different-colored gelatin solutions displayed the variations as well as the overlapping of the blood supply to important areas, thus disproving the then-held theory that the arrangement of the blood supply had a functional significance. Beevor's study was the first to describe the blood supply to all parts of the brain.

Beevor was a careful worker, cautious in his conclusions and precise in recording his observations. He was apparently held in high esteem by his colleagues and was valued for his clinical work as well as his scientific endeavors. His lectures and writing provided evidence of marked literary ability.

He lectured in the United States in 1908, to the American Medical Association meeting in Chicago, to the American Neurological Society, and in Philadelphia, New York, and Boston. He was president of the neurological section of the Royal Society of Medicine, when, on the day following the award dinner of the Society, he died unexpectedly of coronary occlusion.

When Madame Klumpke described her studies and experimental work on the form of paralysis due to lesions of the lower part of the brachial plexus, she began the report with a review of the previous works of Erb and Duchenne and referred to a contemporary study, a thesis published from the same department and service of Professor Vulpian.

Thus we meet **Henri François Secrétan** (1856–1916), whose name we now apply to a peculiar form of swelling on the dorsum of the hand. In his thesis of 1885, he had verified the studies of Erb and Duchenne and reported instances of paralysis from various causes, including a cervical spine abscess.

Henri Secrétan was the son of a philosopher, Charles, and was born in Switzerland in 1856. He first took up the study of law, but changed to medicine, going from Genf to Pisa, and finally to Paris, where he graduated and took his hospital training. Although his later work did not

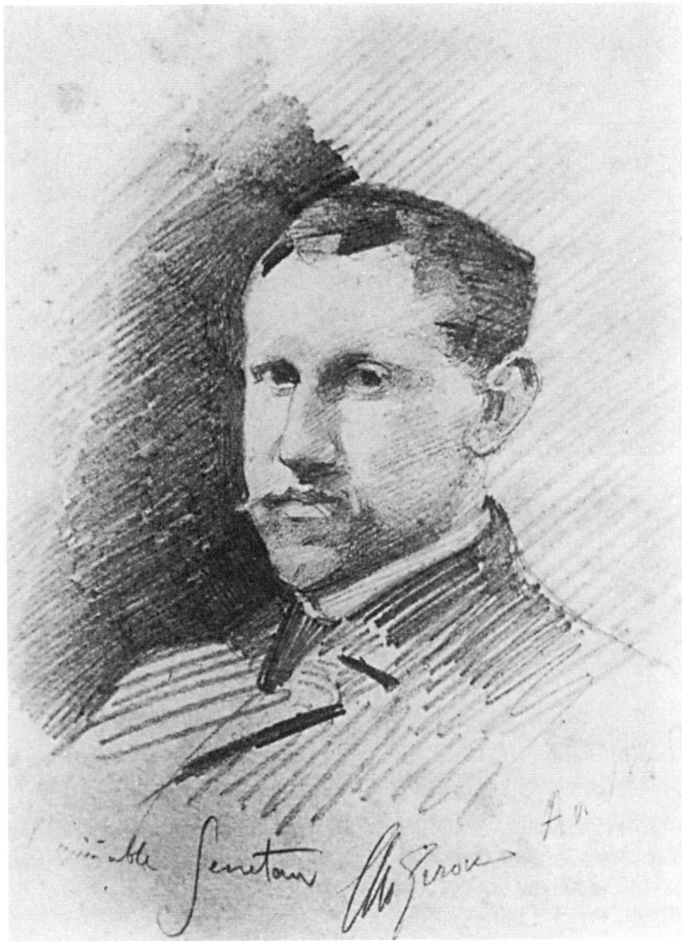

Henri François Secrétan. (Courtesy of the Bibliothèque Cantonale et Universitaire, Lausanne, Switzerland)

deal with neurology, the training he received in Paris in careful observation and logical thinking must have helped in his later work in the field of insurance against work accidents, which was his special interest. Vulpian's laboratory was one of the great research centers, and Déjèrine, Klumpke, Foix, Nageotte, Tinel, Barré, and later Spiller are listed among the students of that school.

Secrétan returned to Switzerland in 1885 and practiced in Lausanne as a specialist in insurance and accident work. He was the editor of the journal *Revue Suisse des Accidents du Travail.* He died in 1916.

Œdème dur et hyperplasie traumatique du métacarpe dorsal.

Par le Dr Henri SECRÉTAN.

Dans une note précédente[1], nous avons proposé d'isoler sous le nom d'*atrophie traumatique* une conséquence éloignée de la contusion en masse d'un doigt, nous nous proposons maintenant de donner une description spéciale d'une forme de la contusion du métacarpe dorsal dont les signes pathognomoniques sont les suivants : Œdème dur du dos du métacarpe, gêne de la flexion des doigts, durée de la lésion qui peut persister plusieurs semaines et souvent plusieurs mois.

Cette lésion me paraît mériter une place à part dans le groupe des contusions. Elle n'est pas exceptionnelle, puisque j'en ai noté onze cas récents, mais elle n'est pas assez connue et expose à de graves fautes dans le pronostic et dans le traitement des contusions de la main.

Je vais donner tout d'abord l'observation de deux cas récents dont je suis actuellement la marche.

OBS. I. — T., âgé de 35 ans, manœuvre à la canalisation de Chailly, travaillait à la pelle dans un fossé étroit sous les yeux de son contremaitre qui l'excitait à hâter sa besogne.

En ramenant vivement sa pelle à lui, après avoir lancé la terre sur le bord du fossé, sa main gauche qui tenait le bout du manche a heurté violemment la paroi opposée de la tranchée, qui contenait de grosses racines saillantes. L'accident date du 21 mai, à six heures du soir. Il désirait continuer son travail d'autant plus que, sa main ne présentant pas traces

[1] Voir le numéro du 20 juin.

Henri François Secrétan: Oedème dur et hyperplasie traumatique du métacarpe dorsal. Rev. Med. Suisse Romande, *21*:409–416, 1901. (Courtesy of the Library of the College of Physicians of Philadelphia)

In his work appearing in 1901, he reported nine cases of what he called hard edema and traumatic hyperplasia of the dorsum of the metacarpus. The important observation he made was that this process was caused by a single violent contusion, resulting in an exudate that infiltrated the soft tissues and the extensor tendons. He noted that there were no bony lesions or hematomas and that flexion of the fingers was impaired, but the thumb was not involved. The process disappeared slowly, requiring 3 or 4 months. In one case, a partial excision of the mass resulted in persistent ulceration and induration for more than 6 months. His description of the mass in the usual case was quite graphic, noting that the feeling imparted to the examining finger is similar to that of a tightly packed pillowcase. One of the cases involved the dorsum of the foot.

In England during this latter part of the nineteenth century there was a

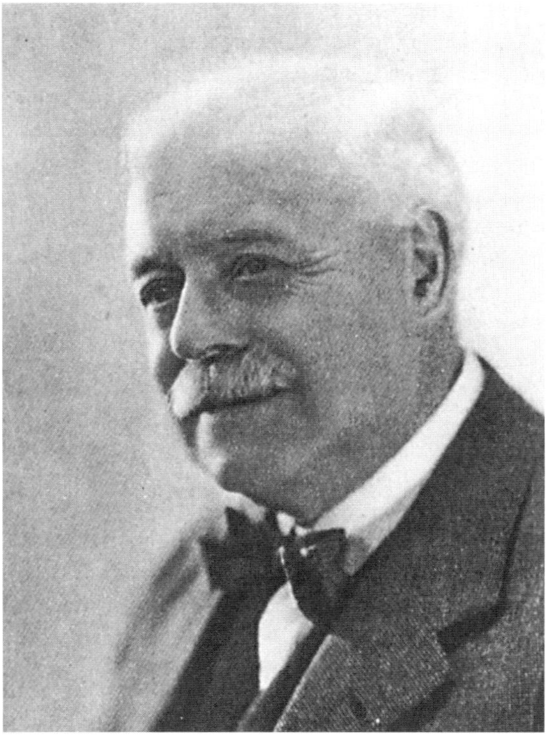

Sir Robert Jones. (From Cave, E. F.: Sir Robert Jones lecture. Twins [extra] ordinary: the knee and the elbow. Bull. Hosp. Joint Dis., *26*:127–140, 1965. Courtesy of the Library of the College of Physicians of Philadelphia)

man who contributed so much to reconstructive surgery and to that of the upper extremity and whose personality was so outstanding that Leo Mayer said he was one of the two "great" men he had ever known.

Sir Robert Jones (1858–1933) is responsible for orthopaedic surgery as a specialty, but to those of us in surgery of the upper extremity, his work on tendon transfers is reason enough to consider him one of the giants. He had the ability to organize his thoughts and experiences, and in 1921 he gave us the four basic rules of tendon transfer: (1) the joints must be as mobile as possible; (2) the muscle and tendon must have sufficient strength to carry out the action; (3) the muscle and tendon must traverse a straight course from origin to insertion, not obliquely or around an angle; and (4) the transplant must be attached under slight tension. These were fundamental rules, and although—as with all rules—these are exceptions, these are the bases of all the work done on tendon transfers.

Jones's operation is the transfer of pronator teres to radial wrist exten-

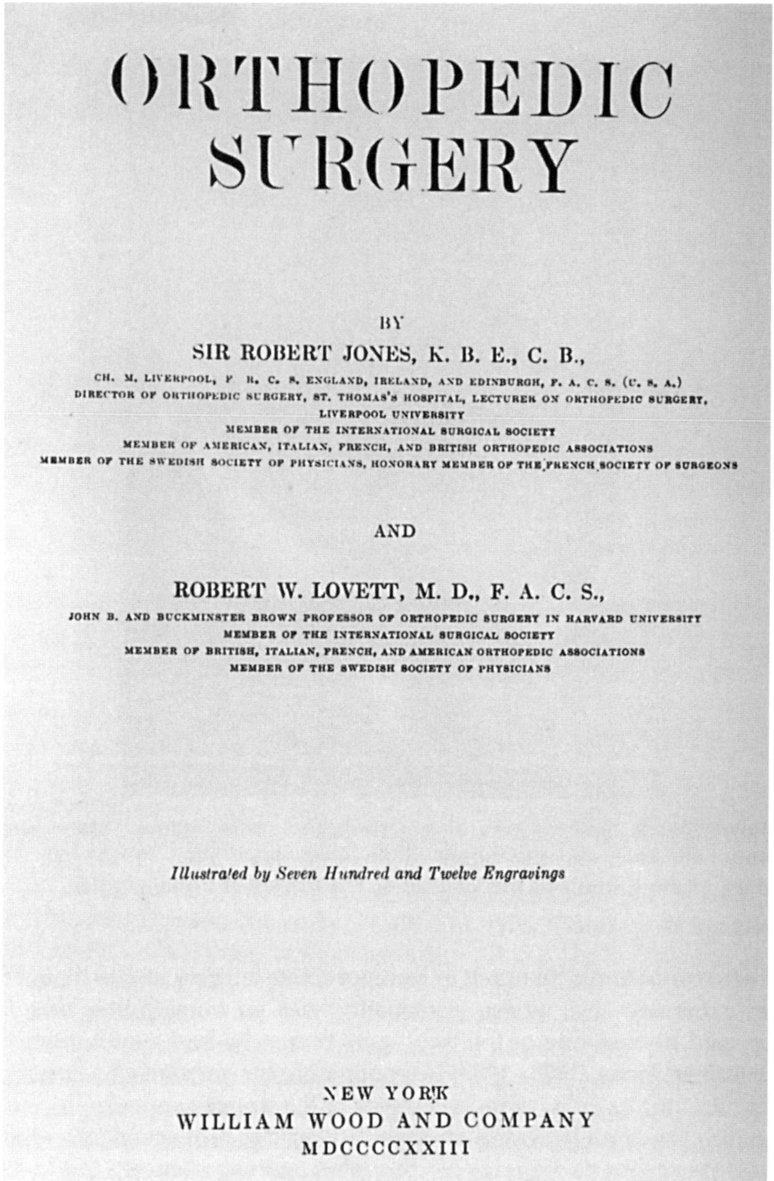

ORTHOPEDIC
SURGERY

BY

SIR ROBERT JONES, K. B. E., C. B.,

CH. M. LIVERPOOL, F. R. C. S. ENGLAND, IRELAND, AND EDINBURGH, F. A. C. S. (U. S. A.)
DIRECTOR OF ORTHOPEDIC SURGERY, ST. THOMAS'S HOSPITAL, LECTURER ON ORTHOPEDIC SURGERY,
LIVERPOOL UNIVERSITY
MEMBER OF THE INTERNATIONAL SURGICAL SOCIETY
MEMBER OF AMERICAN, ITALIAN, FRENCH, AND BRITISH ORTHOPEDIC ASSOCIATIONS
MEMBER OF THE SWEDISH SOCIETY OF PHYSICIANS, HONORARY MEMBER OF THE FRENCH SOCIETY OF SURGEONS

AND

ROBERT W. LOVETT, M. D., F. A. C. S.,

JOHN B. AND BUCKMINSTER BROWN PROFESSOR OF ORTHOPEDIC SURGERY IN HARVARD UNIVERSITY
MEMBER OF THE INTERNATIONAL SURGICAL SOCIETY
MEMBER OF BRITISH, ITALIAN, FRENCH, AND AMERICAN ORTHOPEDIC ASSOCIATIONS
MEMBER OF THE SWEDISH SOCIETY OF PHYSICIANS

Illustrated by Seven Hundred and Twelve Engravings

NEW YORK
WILLIAM WOOD AND COMPANY
MDCCCCXXIII

Sir Robert Jones, and Robert W. Lovett: Orthopedic Surgery. New York, William Wood and Company, 1923. (Courtesy of the Library of the Los Angeles County Medical Association)

sors in the treatment of radial palsy. Before this, the wrist extensors had either been tenodesed or were simply shortened, or even disregarded entirely while attention was paid to the digital extension. This operation, by providing wrist extension independent of the digital action, was a most important advance in the treatment of radial palsy. Many years later, Zachary showed the importance of retaining one of the wrist flexors to provide the necessary control of the wrist.

Our present views on tendon transfers are the result of the work of many men. A basic study was done by Mayer and Bielsalski in Berlin, just prior to World War I. The names of Georg Perthes, Fritz Lange, Vulpius, and Nicoladoni all appear in the history of this important phase of hand surgery. Steindler, with his encyclopedic knowledge of the German literature, added to the study of the principles involved, and Bunnell applied them to the upper extremity. In developing the operation for opposition and using the pulley principle, Bunnell showed an exception to the third rule of Jones, demonstrating a way to alter the direction of pull of a tendon by an anatomic means.

Robert Jones was first a general surgeon, having been apprenticed at age 16 to his uncle, Hugh Owen Thomas, in Liverpool. Jones went to medical school in Edinburgh and practiced with his uncle until the latter's death in 1891. By 1905 Jones had restricted his practice to orthopaedics and, with Agnes Hunt, set up the center at Oswestry. His reputation spread through his writings, but also through visitors, mainly from abroad. The Mayo brothers, Lovett from Boston, and many others made the grand tour of British surgery—to Jones in Liverpool, Moynihan in Leeds, and Stiles in Edinburgh, all renowned teachers and surgeons.

An original thinker, an unusually adept surgeon, and a remarkable personality, Jones attracted people from all over; however, his real value was not recognized by his own confreres until after he was a member of French, Swedish, German, Italian, and American orthopaedic societies.

World War I provided him with an opportunity to show his great organizational ability and his ways of getting people to work together. He was responsible for a plan of treatment beginning with first aid at the front to care in specialized centers. Starting with a unit at Shepherds Bush, which was staffed by an enthusiastic group, among which were many Americans, the system grew until, at the end of the war 30,000 beds were under his administration as head of the orthopaedic department of the war office.

After the war he helped to form the British Orthopaedic Association and a national plan for the detection and treatment of cripples. He died in early 1933 of a heart attack while visiting his son-in-law, Frederick Watson, a well-known author.

Jones was a great surgeon, innovative and original. He published many papers, but it was his ability to organize and express his ideas and thoughts into principles, along with a personality that made it a pleasure for others to work with him toward his ideals, that sets him apart. He

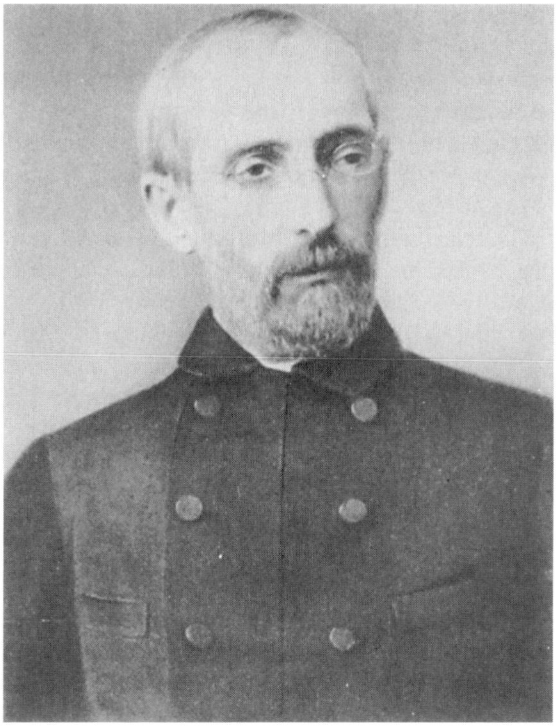

Hugh Owen Thomas. (From Koch, S. L., and Mason, M. L.: Purposeful splinting following injuries of the hand. Surg. Gynecol. Obstet., *68*:1–16, 1939. Reproduced by permission of Surgery, Gynecology & Obstetrics. Courtesy of the Library of the New York Academy of Medicine)

recognized the importance of segregating cases of similar type to provide the most expert care. Gillies did this for maxillofacial injuries, and Bunnell did it for hand cases during World War II. Again, talent and opportunity combined to make a man famous and commanding of our respect and admiration.

Hugh Owen Thomas (1834–1891) was the uncle of Robert Jones. Thomas, of course, is one of the legendary figures in orthopaedics. He was a graduate of a medical school, but his father was a "bone-setter," the seventh in line in the family. Thomas had studied in Edinburgh, London, and Paris and was practicing at 11 Nelson Street, a place that became a shrine of orthopaedic surgery. He was an advocate of uninterrupted rest, and he made his own splints; the Thomas splint became well known by its use in World War I. Thomas also used passive hyperemia to stimulate healing, calling it, "damming," and introduced it in 1873, long before Bier, whose name has become attached to it.

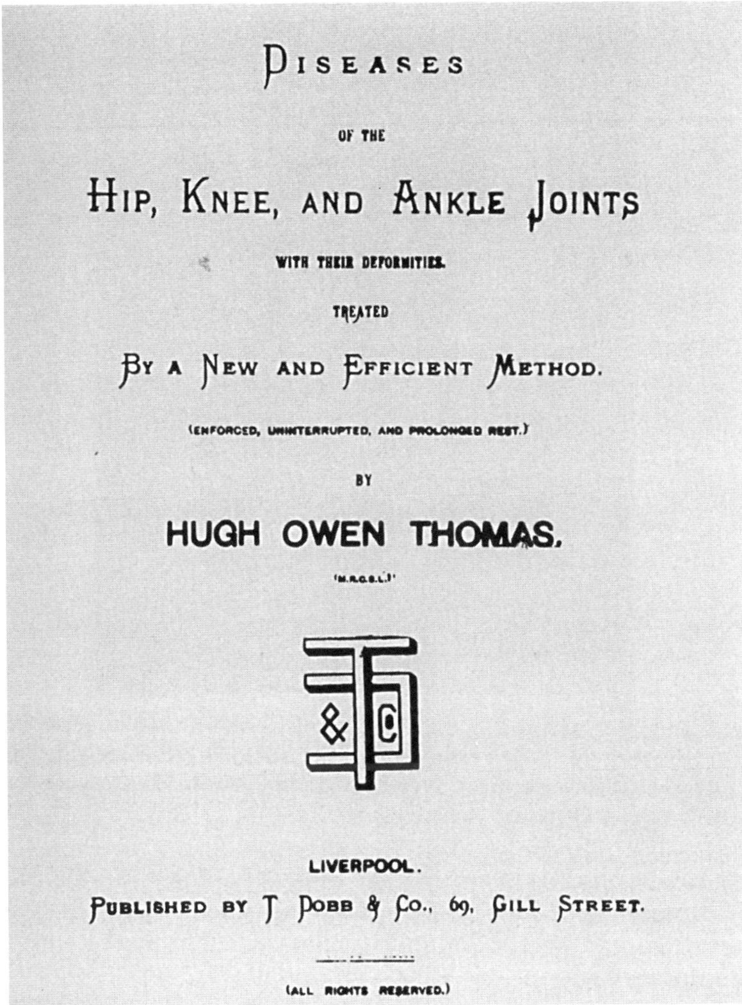

DISEASES

OF THE

HIP, KNEE, AND ANKLE JOINTS

WITH THEIR DEFORMITIES.

TREATED

BY A NEW AND EFFICIENT METHOD.

(ENFORCED, UNINTERRUPTED, AND PROLONGED REST.)

BY

HUGH OWEN THOMAS.

(M.R.C.S.L.)

LIVERPOOL.

PUBLISHED BY T. DOBB & CO., 69, GILL STREET.

(ALL RIGHTS RESERVED.)

Hugh Owen Thomas: Diseases of the Hip, Knee, and Ankle Joints. ed. 2. Liverpool, T. Dobb & Co., 1876. (Courtesy of the Library of the New York Academy of Medicine)

One woman's name appears in the list of eponyms relating to the upper extremity. **Augusta Klumpke** (1859–1927) described the type of brachial palsy resulting from damage to the lower roots of the plexus in 1885, while still an extern at the hospital in Paris. It was a decade after Duchenne and Erb had identified the upper plexus lesion from damage to the fifth and sixth roots, which is now known by their names. Her

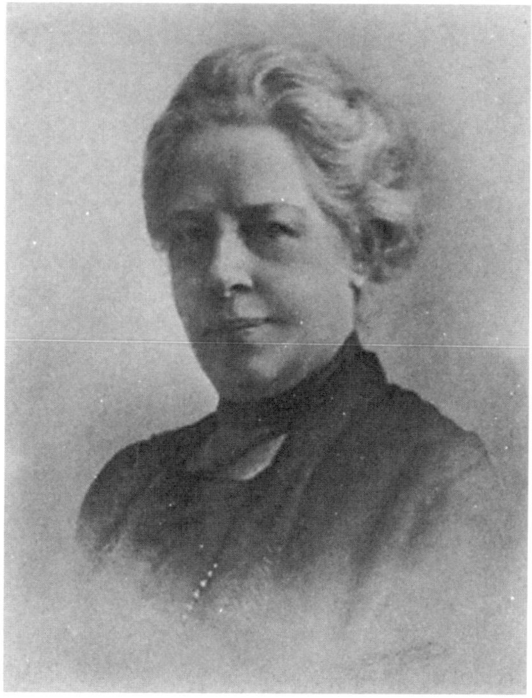

Augusta Klumpke. (From Éloge de Madame Dejerine-Klumpke. Discours Prononcé a la Séance du 1er Décembre 1927 de la Société de Neurologie de Paris par le Professeur Gustave Roussy, Président de la Société. Courtesy of Mme. le Docteur Y. Sorrel-Dejerine, Paris, France)

descriptions were complete, and she carefully pointed out the different types of paralyses and the oculopupillary signs that occur with the lesion of the lower roots. This oculopupillary sign was confirmed by experimental studies on dogs.

She was born in San Francisco, and at the age of 11, the family moved to Lausanne, Switzerland, to provide a better education for the four girls. One of her sisters became an accomplished musician, another an artist, and a third a doctor of science. In 1877 the girls went to Paris, and Augusta tried to enroll as a medical student, against the objections of the faculty, particularly the head of neurology, Vulpian. She persisted, won admission, and became the first woman extern, then intern, in the hospital—surprisingly on Vulpian's service, where she did her important work. She was only 26 and an extern when she wrote the paper on brachial palsy. The paper was fully documented and carefully acknowledged the works of Duchenne, Erb, Hutchison, Landouzy, and Déjèrine, the latter to become her husband in 1888. One of her references was to a

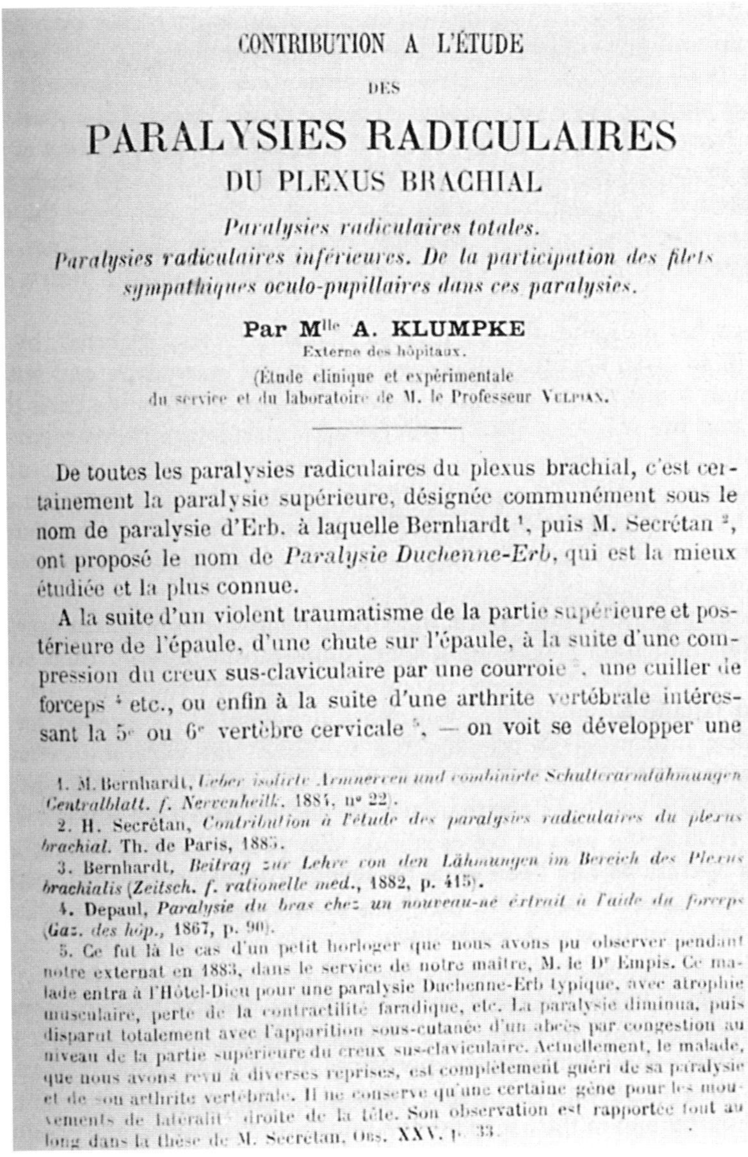

CONTRIBUTION A L'ÉTUDE

DES

PARALYSIES RADICULAIRES

DU PLEXUS BRACHIAL

Paralysies radiculaires totales.
Paralysies radiculaires inférieures. De la participation des filets sympathiques oculo-pupillaires dans ces paralysies.

Par Mlle A. KLUMPKE
Externe des hôpitaux.
(Étude clinique et expérimentale du service et du laboratoire de M. le Professeur VULPIAN.

De toutes les paralysies radiculaires du plexus brachial, c'est certainement la paralysie supérieure, désignée communément sous le nom de paralysie d'Erb. à laquelle Bernhardt [1], puis M. Secrétan [2], ont proposé le nom de *Paralysie Duchenne-Erb*, qui est la mieux étudiée et la plus connue.

A la suite d'un violent traumatisme de la partie supérieure et postérieure de l'épaule, d'une chute sur l'épaule, à la suite d'une compression du creux sus-claviculaire par une courroie [3], une cuiller de forceps [4] etc., ou enfin à la suite d'une arthrite vertébrale intéressant la 5e ou 6e vertèbre cervicale [5], — on voit se développer une

1. M. Bernhardt, *Ueber isolirte Armnerven und combinirte Schulterarmlähmungen* (*Centralblatt. f. Nervenheilk.* 1884, n° 22).
2. H. Secrétan, *Contribution à l'étude des paralysies radiculaires du plexus brachial.* Th. de Paris, 1885.
3. Bernhardt, *Beitrag zur Lehre von den Lähmungen im Bereich des Plexus brachialis* (*Zeitsch. f. rationelle med.*, 1882, p. 415).
4. Depaul, *Paralysie du bras chez un nouveau-né extrait à l'aide du forceps* (*Gaz. des hôp.*, 1867, p. 90).
5. Ce fut là le cas d'un petit horloger que nous avons pu observer pendant notre externat en 1883, dans le service de notre maître, M. le Dr Empis. Ce malade entra à l'Hôtel-Dieu pour une paralysie Duchenne-Erb typique, avec atrophie musculaire, perte de la contractilité faradique, etc. La paralysie diminua, puis disparut totalement avec l'apparition sous-cutanée d'un abcès par congestion au niveau de la partie supérieure du creux sus-claviculaire. Actuellement, le malade, que nous avons revu à diverses reprises, est complètement guéri de sa paralysie et de son arthrite vertébrale. Il ne conserve qu'une certaine gêne pour les mouvements de latéralité droite de la tête. Son observation est rapportée tout au long dans la thèse de M. Secrétan, Obs. XXV, p. 33.

Augusta Klumpke: Contribution a l'étude des paralysies radiculaires du plexus brachial. Rev. Médecine, 5:591–616, 1885. (Courtesy of the Library of the New York Academy of Medicine)

thesis on radicular paralysis, done in 1885 by Henri Secrétan, who had been a student in Vulpian's laboratory and had trained in experimental neurology.

Madame Déjèrine-Klumpke became a leading figure in her own right, but combining her talents with those of the brilliant Joseph Jules Déjèrine (1849–1917) gave rise to a series of important works, especially the pioneer study of the localization of function in the brain. Their *Anatomy of the Nervous System* (1894), based on a study of serial sections of the whole brain, organized the study of brain anatomy; it was a study that was needed, to straighten out the chaos that had resulted from the discoveries of the neuron theory and the works of Ramon y Cajal, Golgi, and His. The Déjèrines' students included Foix, Spiller, Nageotte, Barré, and Tinel.

When her husband died in 1917—exhausted, it was reported, by his work in an army hospital—she continued in her researches, and with a daughter, Madame Sorrel-Déjèrine, also a former intern of the Paris hospitals and the wife of a doctor, she set up a foundation in his memory, consisting of a laboratory, museum, and library for neurological study.

Madame Déjèrine-Klumpke was a remarkable woman, respected and loved by her colleagues and students. Her funeral was held in the American Church in Paris, and she was buried in Père Lachaise cemetery with her husband.

Chance plays a part in having something named after one in surgery. If it is the right time and there is some opportunity present, then some minor contribution becomes important. Such was the case with **Sir Harold Jalland Stiles** (1863–1946), who, in our field, is recalled for an operation involving the transfer of a sublimis tendon to the extensor apparatus, to overcome the claw deformity. The operation he did was not a good one; it was not done many times, and no follow-up reports were given. In fact, the idea of the operation was proposed long before, and similar operations had been done by several German surgeons, notably Lexer. In Stiles's report, the incisions shown are atrocious, violating every principle in which we believe. Yet his name is usually coupled with that of Bunnell to indicate a method of correcting the claw deformity. Stiles's work appeared in a book co-authored with Forrester-Brown, *Treatment of Injuries of the Peripheral Spinal Nerves,* a work that was a direct result of their war experiences. It was well received because at that time there was an intense interest in the surgical treatment of nerve injuries and in the use of tendon transfers to overcome the paralytic states.

It is unfortunate that this is so, for this contribution is minor compared with two of his major achievements. He was one of the pioneers in transplantation of the ureters and was personally responsible for introducing steam sterilization and aseptic surgery into Edinburgh, the home of Listerism.

Stiles was born in Lincolnshire, England, where his father and grandfather were both general practioners. At the age of 15, he started as an

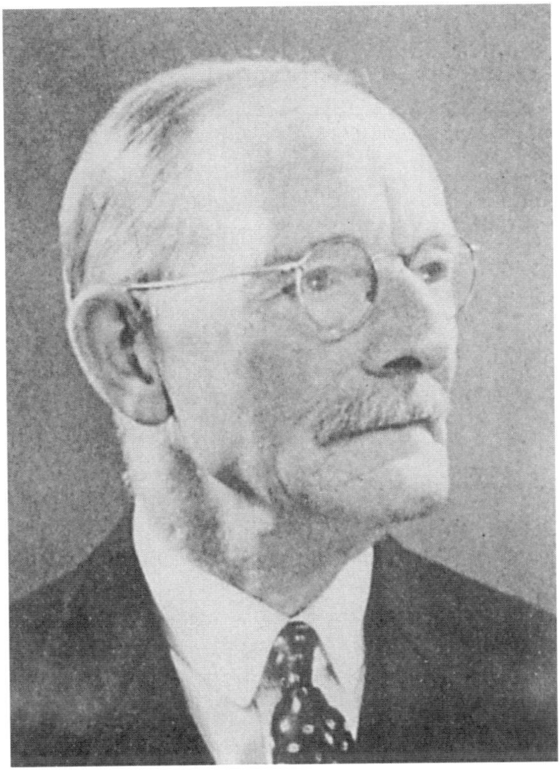

Sir Harold Jalland Stiles. (From Edinburgh J. Med., 53, 1946. Courtesy of the Library of the New York Academy of Medicine)

apprentice with his father and quickly showed an intense interest in anatomy. His father sent him to Edinburgh to medical school because of the reputations of Syme and Lister. He graduated at the age of 18 with first-class honors and a scholarship and worked at the Royal Infirmary under Stewart and Chiene. Not wishing to return to general practice, he became a junior assistant in surgery, a demonstrator in anatomy, and a tutor to students.

Stiles set up a laboratory for bacteriology and surgical pathology in the surgical department, one of the first. Even though it had been 35 years since Waller's work and 20 years after Koch, the use of the microscope was new to surgeons. Stiles improved the fixation method for tissues, using a paraffin embedding method known to the embryologists. He made some notable studies on carcinoma of the breast, enough to gain him the Walker Prize of the Royal College of Surgeons in 1895.

At this time, Kocher was the prominent surgeon in Berne, and Stiles

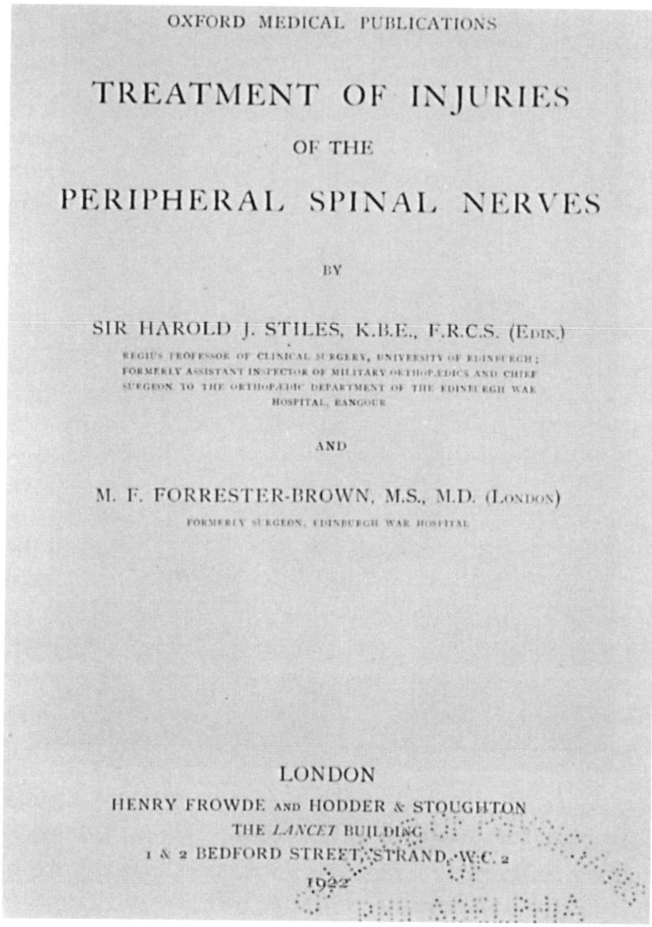

OXFORD MEDICAL PUBLICATIONS

TREATMENT OF INJURIES

OF THE

PERIPHERAL SPINAL NERVES

BY

SIR HAROLD J. STILES, K.B.E., F.R.C.S. (EDIN.)

REGIUS PROFESSOR OF CLINICAL SURGERY, UNIVERSITY OF EDINBURGH;
FORMERLY ASSISTANT INSPECTOR OF MILITARY ORTHOPÆDICS AND CHIEF
SURGEON TO THE ORTHOPÆDIC DEPARTMENT OF THE EDINBURGH WAR
HOSPITAL, BANGOUR

AND

M. F. FORRESTER-BROWN, M.S., M.D. (LONDON)

FORMERLY SURGEON, EDINBURGH WAR HOSPITAL

LONDON

HENRY FROWDE AND HODDER & STOUGHTON

THE *LANCET* BUILDING

1 & 2 BEDFORD STREET, STRAND, W.C. 2

1922

Sir Harold Jalland Stiles, and M. F. Forrester-Brown: Treatment of Injuries of the Peripheral Spinal Nerves. London, Henry Frowde and Hodder & Stoughton, 1922. Courtesy of the Library of the College of Physicians of Philadelphia)

spent 6 months there, where he translated Kocher's *Textbook of Operative Surgery* into English. Here Stiles saw aseptic treatment being carried out; later he was instrumental in introducing it into Edinburgh.

After being appointed to the Children's Hospital, Stiles did his work on ureteral transplants, and he was able also to have a service for surgery of adults in another hospital. He firmly believed that bovine tuberculosis was a cause of disease in children, thus opposing Koch's view that this was a disease restricted to animals.

166 SURGERY OF THE PERIPHERAL NERVES

ligament, so that this may need to be partly divided in order to expose them satisfactorily.

The skin is now undermined on the radial border of the forearm between the two wounds in order to allow the extensors to reach the flexor aspect ; care must be taken that there is no kinking of the tendons and that the radial vessels are not injured. The transplant is finished on the lines described above under 'General principles'. It is simplest to suture the dorsal wound before fixing the tendons. If this is done, the surgeon's gloves and forceps must be well rinsed, or changed in order not to carry organisms from the skin in among the tendons.

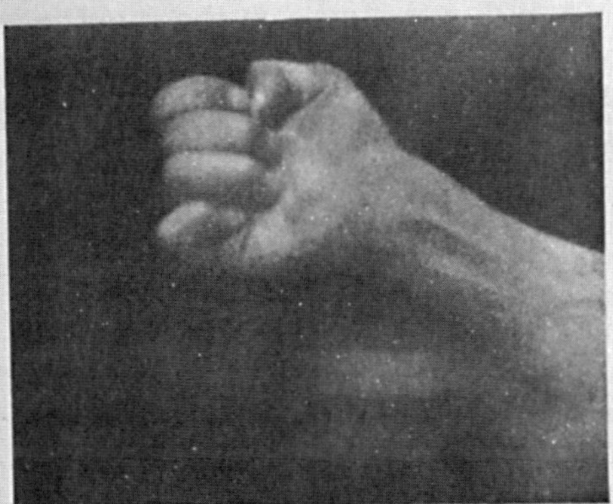

FIG. 53.—Flattening of the hand when all the thenar muscles are paralysed.

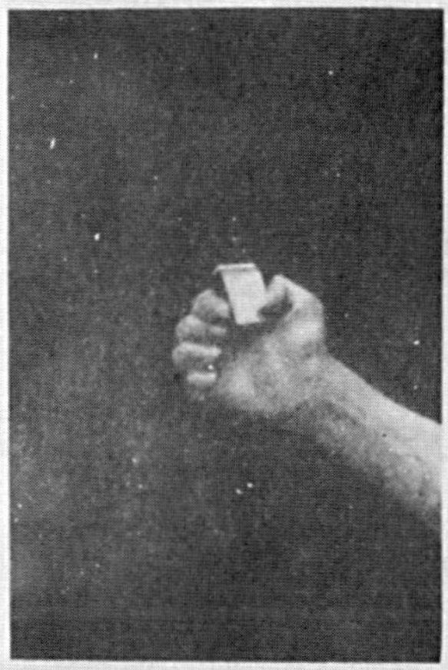

FIG. 54.—Loss of the pincer action of the thumb ; grip by long flexor only, aided by long extensor, which together give a pseudo-adduction.

(3) Transplantation to Compensate for Loss of the Intrinsic muscles of the Hand.

No satisfactory transplant appears to have been devised to replace the intrinsic thumb muscles, whose loss makes that digit almost useless, as it falls back into line with the other digits and is unable to be opposed to them for picking up objects. Fortunately this function can be largely restored by the operation of arthrodesis of the first carpo-metacarpal joint, as devised by Major Baldwin, U.S.A., who pointed out that the functioning position of the thumb for almost all purposes is one in which the first and second metacarpals meet at an angle of 60° ; so that if the joint is fixed at this angle, the loss of the muscles which normally bring

Sir Harold Jalland Stiles, and M. F. Forrester-Brown: Treatment of Injuries of the Peripheral Spinal Nerves. p. 166. London, Henry Frowde and Hodder & Stoughton, 1922. Courtesy of the Library of the College of Physicians of Philadelphia)

Soon after 1905, he visited the Mayo Clinic and thus began a warm friendship with Dr. William Mayo. Many surgeons who came to the British Isles often spent some time with Robert Jones in Liverpool, Stiles in Edinburgh, and Berkeley Moynihan in Leeds. At the meeting of the American Surgical Association in Denver in 1911, Stiles's paper was on his method of ureteral transplantation.

He was a good conversationalist and companion, always active and seemingly always with a full head of steam. His surgery was anatomic. He said he had never touched a knife in his first 10 years of practice, except in the dissecting room. Applied anatomy in the operating room might be a simple way of describing his surgery.

During the First World War he was a consultant, wrote the monograph referred to above, and was knighted for his work. He became regius professor in 1919, but resigned in 1925 and moved to the country. He lived for another 21 years, having taken up geology first and then, when declining strength prevented the necessary field trips, the study of botany. He was 83 when he died.

THE LATE NINETEENTH CENTURY

Visible deformities in the newborn have usually been reported in some term that is descriptive of the lesion, such as clubfoot, clubhand, and harelip, often in a Greek or Latin form. Syndactylism, brachyphalangia, and similar diagnoses are simply descriptive terms of the condition present, made to sound more scientific by the use of a "classical" language. Some observers, however, have noted certain patterns or associations of these lesions, and thus a syndrome. Often these will then become known by the name of the describer.

Eugène Apert (1868–1940) was the first to describe a combination of face and hand deformity, an acrocephalosyndactyly. The first patient with this combination was seen in 1896, but the report was not published until 1906.

Apert was one of France's best-known pediatricians and, after interning in the Paris hospitals, had written his thesis on the purpuric diseases. He soon showed interest in the pediatric diseases, especially in the congenital problems, such as chondroplasias and glandular disturbances. One of his reports described seventeen cases of hirsutism, adiposity, and genital dysplasia, and an autopsy of one showed a tumor of the adrenal cortex. He was one of the organizers of the Eugenic Society and wrote extensively on hereditary disease. He died suddenly at age 72, apparently without any prior signs of illness.

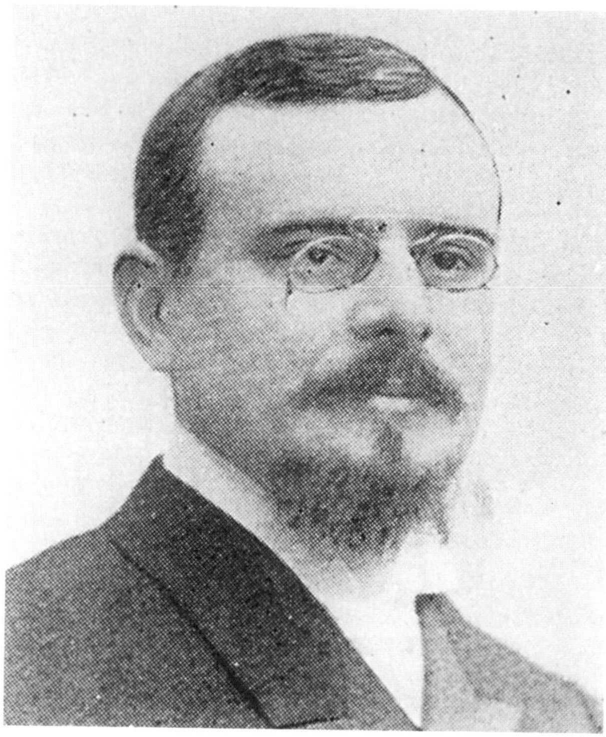

Eugène Apert. (From Gedda, L.: Studio dei Gemelli. Rome, Edizioni Orizzonte Medico, 1951. Courtesy, Library of the College of Physicians of Philadelphia)

Little was done in the way of treatment of this congenital deformity (Apert's syndrome) until reconstructive surgery was developed. A recent review by Flatt, Hoover, and Weiss* best defines the aim of treatment and some of the procedures that can be carried out.

Stenosing tenosynovitis of the sheath of the extensor pollicis brevis and abductor pollicis longus at the radial styloid occurs frequently, is usually diagnosed early, and responds well to proper treatment. It fell to **Fritz de Quervain** (1868–1940) to describe this entity, treat it successfully by surgery, and report a 1-year follow-up of the first case. This was done in 1895, just after he had started practice in surgery in a Swiss watchmak-

*Flatt, A. E., Hoover, G. H., and Weiss, M. S.: The hand and Apert's syndrome. J. Bone Joint Surg., *52A*:878–895, July, 1970.

Il s'agit ici d'une démence secondaire surajoutée à une aphasie primitive dont M. le Dr Lenoir a pu faire l'examen durant plusieurs mois, examen dont il a bien voulu nous communiquer le sommaire établi par M. P. Camus, son interne :

« Aphasie complexe sensorielle et motrice avec légère hémiparésie « droite, troubles visuels secondaires (hémianopsie gauche bilatérale « homonyme). »

Le malade, agraphique et aphasique complet à l'entrée à l'asile, était en outre agnosique (ex : il prenait son urinoir pour son carafon et cherchait à boire à même).

Décédé quatre mois après l'entrée par suite d'ictus final, il présenta à l'autopsie des foyers multiples de la région frontale mais avec prédominance marquée dans la région de Broca.

Concomitance des lésions de la zone de Wernicke, avec extension maximum dans la région pariétale postéro-inférieure, ainsi que des lésions capsulaires gauches d'apparence plus récente et moins ocreuse (cause probable de l'ictus terminal). L'hémisphère droit présente un foyer lacunaire du bras postérieur de la capsule interne (volume d'un pois) et un ramollissement en bloc de tout le pôle occipital inférieur en dessous de la scissure calcarine.

De l'acrocéphalosyndactylie,

par M. E. Apert.

Je propose le nom d'*acrocéphalosyndactylie* pour désigner un type tératologique compatible avec l'existence et bien caractérisé par la coexistence des deux particularités suivantes : 1° *Crâne tout en hauteur, aplati en arrière et parfois aussi sur les côtés, saillant au contraire d'une façon exagérée à la région frontale supérieure* ; 2° *Syndactylie des quatre extrémités.* Dans les neuf cas de ce type tératologique complexe, que j'ai pu recueillir, les déformations de la tête et des extrémités sont de même sens et presque identiques. Il n'y a que des différences d'intensité.

J'ai observé un cas de cette curieuse malformation en 1896, à l'hôpital des Enfants-Malades, quand j'étais l'interne de M. Grancher, chez une petite fille de quinze mois hospitalisée salle Husson. Je n'ai plus eu depuis personnellement occasion d'en revoir d'autres, mais j'ai rencontré dans différentes publications des descriptions détaillées de malformations si identiques à celles de cet enfant qu'on pourrait croire qu'il s'agit des mêmes sujets, n'étaient les différences d'âge, de sexe et de lieu. Ces observations sont celles de Troquart, *Mémoires et Bulletins de la Société de chirurgie de Bordeaux*, 1886, p. 69 ; de Béno, *la Syndactylie*

Eugène Apert: De l'acrocéphalosyndactylie. Bull. Soc. Med. Hop. Paris, 23:1310–1330, 1906. (Courtesy of The Francis A. Countway Library of Medicine, Boston, Massachusetts)

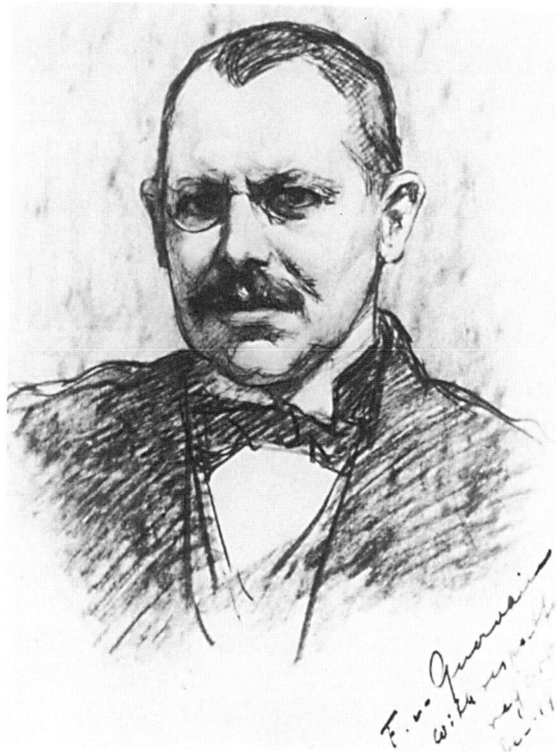

Fritz de Quervain. (Courtesy of the Library of the College of Physicians of Philadelphia)

ing center. His name is fixed to the syndrome, and seldom is other than his name listed in diagnostic files, so specific is its use.

De Quervain was born in Sion, Switzerland, of a family that had been in Switzerland for 200 years. His father was a Protestant pastor. De Quervain was fluent in German and French and is said to have been an excellent lecturer, with clear, elegant, and precise diction. He was graduated at Berne, where Kocher and Langhans were professors. One of his projects was with Kocher on the problem of endemic goiter. He practiced surgery for several years, and then he returned to Kocher's service, where he collaborated with Kocher on the *Encyclopedia of Surgery*. In 1907 his textbook *Surgical Diagnosis* came out. It went through nine German editions and was translated into many languages. He lived in Basel from 1910 to 1918, but returned to succeed Kocher as professor at Berne.

De Quervain's interest in goiter never lessened. He founded a Swiss

Ueber eine Form von chronischer Tendovaginitis.

Von Dr. **F. de Quervain** in La Chaux-de-Fonds.

Wenn auch die chronischen Sehnenscheidenentzündungen mit Recht immer mehr als tuberculös aufgefasst werden, so gibt es doch Formen, welche weder den klinischen Erscheinungen noch dem anatomischen Befunde nach der Tuberculose zugezählt werden dürfen. Als solche werden angeführt: die Tendovaginitis chronica sicca (als Analogon der Arthritis sicca), die Tendosynovitis prolifera urica, die seröse nicht tuberculöse Tendosynovitis. Ausser der letztern, gewiss oft doch der Tuberculose verdächtigen Form hat die nicht tuberculöse chronische Tendovaginitis wohl nur selten zu chirurgischen Eingriffen Veranlassung gegeben und wird daher in den meisten Lehr- und Handbüchern der Chirurgie nur kurz oder gar nicht erwähnt. Es mag desshalb gerechtfertigt sein, einige Fälle mitzutheilen, welche, obwohl noch am ehesten der Tendosynovitis sicca zugehörend, sich doch von dem für dieselbe[1]) entworfenen Bilde erheblich entfernen, und bei denen sich die chirurgische Behandlung als sehr zweckmässig erwiesen hat.

Der klinischen Besprechung dieser Form von Tendovaginitis seien die Krankengeschichten in Kürze vorausgeschickt:

1) Den ersten Fall hatte ich Gelegenheit, als I. Assistent der chirurgischen Klinik in Bern zu beobachten und zu operiren. Herr Prof. *Kocher* hat mir dessen Verwerthung gütigst gestattet.

Frau L., 55 Jahre alt, die sich neben der Besorgung ihrer Haushaltung mit Holzauflesen beschäftigte, bemerkte im October 1893, dass die Bewegungen des rechten Daumens allmählig schmerzhaft wurden. Der Schmerz localisirte sich hauptsächlich auf das distale Radiusende und strahlte von da auf den Vorderarm aus. Er wurde zeitweise so heftig, dass Patientin keine Greifbewegungen ausführen konnte. In ihrer Arbeit wurde sie dadurch erheblich gestört. Von Schwellung, Hautröthung, Crepitation bemerkte

[1]) *Nicaise*, Gaz. méd. 1872, p. 98.

Fritz de Quervain: Ueber eine Form von chronischer Tendovaginitis. Korrespondenz Blatt Schweiz. Aertze, 25:389–394, 1895. (Courtesy of the Library of the College of Physicians of Philadelphia)

goiter commission and was instrumental in introducing iodized salt into Switzerland. He was a general surgeon and was careful and exacting like Kocher, insisting on complete case reports and follow-up studies.

Harvey Williams Cushing (1869–1939) was not only one of the pioneers in brain surgery but was also an accomplished writer and scientific investigator. He was a master technician and developed many of the operative approaches in brain surgery as well as techniques to improve his surgical results. In one of his papers, a report of a minor technical change, he described the use of a pneumatic tourniquet to prevent bleeding from a scalp incision. What is of interest to hand surgeons is that incidentally he mentioned that the pneumatic cuff (from the blood pressure apparatus) had been used for operations on the upper extremity that were done under cocaine anesthesia. This was probably the first report of the use of a tourniquet with pneumatic pressure of measurable degree. But of greater interest was his description of the use of a large tire pump to inflate the cuff quickly before the veins became distended, and although he apparently did not use it, he suggested connecting the cuff to a central pressure supply.

Some form of tourniquet must have been used in prehistoric times. Subsequently, various forms of compression of the vessels were de-

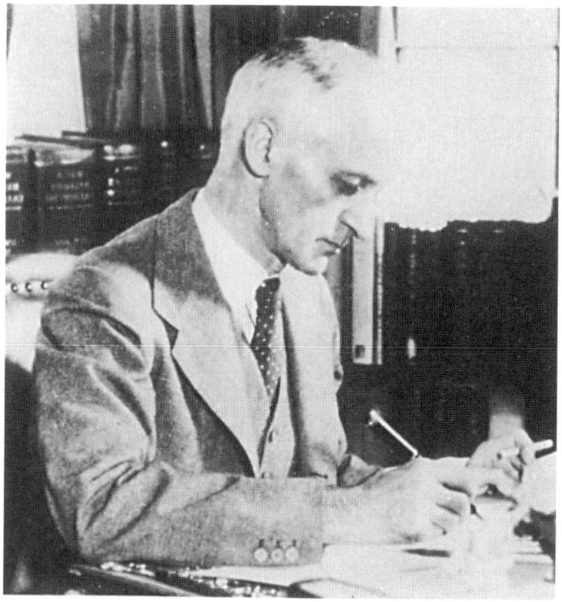

Harvey Cushing. (Courtesy of the Library of the New York Academy of Medicine)

veloped, such as the screw tourniquet, and then the Esmarch tourniquet, which persisted to the twentieth century. Pneumatic tourniquets had been tried by Perthes, but Cushing's use of the inflatable cuff, a part of the apparatus for measuring blood pressure, was a real advance, and our modern operative tourniquet is but an extension of his idea.

Cushing was born in 1869 in Cleveland, Ohio, of a family of physicians. This area of Ohio was known as the Western Reserve of New England and had been settled by families from that area of the original colonies. Cushing went to Yale and then to Harvard Medical School, graduating in 1895. Interning at the Massachusetts General Hospital, he illustrated his case histories with sketches of patients and recorded blood pressure during anesthesia. Cushing had gone to Europe and returned with the new Riva-Rocci sphygmomanometer.

Cushing was at Johns Hopkins Hospital for 4 years, under the famous William S. Halsted, who used cocaine as an anesthetic so much that he became addicted. Here Cushing became interested in neurosurgery. He then went to Berne with Kocher, where he did an experimental study of the relationship of blood pressure and intracranial pressure. He spent a short time with Sir Charles Scott Sherrington, England's great physiologist, and then he returned to Johns Hopkins to develop neurological surgery. One of the reasons for using the pneumatic tourniquet was to control the bleeding from the craniotomy wounds, which

THE MEDICAL NEWS.

A WEEKLY JOURNAL OF MEDICAL SCIENCE.

VOL. 84. NEW YORK, SATURDAY, MARCH 26, 1904. NO. 13.

ORIGINAL ARTICLES.

PNEUMATIC TOURNIQUETS: WITH ESPECIAL REFERENCE TO THEIR USE IN CRANIOTOMIES.

BY HARVEY CUSHING, M.D.,

OF BALTIMORE;

ASSOCIATE PROFESSOR OF SURGERY, THE JOHNS HOPKINS UNIVERSITY.

SURGEONS and neurologists alike are familiar with the postoperative palsies of the extremities consequent upon the too energetic and prolonged application of an elastic tourniquet. Out of a considerable number of pressure paralyses, which have come under the writer's observation during the past two years, eight of them have thus originated. The greater number of these were of the brachial type, the tourniquet having been employed to render bloodless the field at the elbow usually for resections of the joint. A thin, flabby arm, especially in these cases of joint disease and in spite of all precautions, lends itself readily to such an injury as the poorly protected nerves are easily compressed against the hard shaft of the humerus. The skilful application of the old type of rubber tourniquet, varying it for the individual so that it exerts a compression just sufficient to shut off the arterial supply and yet not enough to harm the nerve trunks, is an art rarely acquired even by an adept hospital orderly, who may have had years of experience.

There remain other objections to its employment. One of these concerns the technic of the operation. The tourniquet usually occupies a position on the borderline of the aseptic field, and when once applied must remain so until the completion of the operation. If once relaxed, and in certain procedures, in amputations or plastic operations on aneurismal sacs for example this may be necessary in order to see whether there is a continuance of any arterial bleeding, it is most difficult to readjust the tourniquet again, should this be desirable, without dislocating all of the clean surroundings, towels, etc., at the wound. A still further drawback from an elastic band, when tightly applied, is the ensuing vasomotor palsy, evidenced by the flushing of the extremity peripheral to the site of application. In a major amputation this produces the "wet stump" oftentimes so annoying to an operator inasmuch as it necessitates drainage which otherwise might have been avoided.

Pain is another objection. In many operative procedures on the extremities, preferably carried out under local anesthesia, the temporary cessation of the local circulation is of great assistance. Patients, however, can endure the discomfort of an elastic tourniquet for a very brief period. It is furthermore a common surgical practice, and one, I think, of questionable merit, to apply an elastic ligature, when necessary to control hemorrhage, in cases of traumatic lacerations of the extremities and to wait until the "shock" from the original traumatism wears away. Such a practice, from afferent impulses of pain due to the tourniquet alone, may add not a little to the already existing vascular depression.

Thus the possibility of paralysis, the difficulties of observing the best technic during the application, removal and especially of reapplication, and the pain when no general anesthetic is administered are all familiar drawbacks to the common form of elastic tourniquet. I think they may be avoided in large measure by the use of tourniquets of another sort.

The suggestion of an inflatable tourniquet doubtless originated in the use of the distensible armlet of the Riva-Rocci blood-pressure apparatus. On one or two occasions I had utilized the apparatus itself as a means of shutting off the circulation during cocaine operations on the hand, by holding the pressure slightly above that of the registered systolic arterial pressure. Objections are self-evident. Although the pressure of the armlet is relatively painless, its slow distention by shutting off the veins before the arteries, causes such an engorgement as to render a clean dissection most difficult. Consequently a similar armlet, though broader, of less distensible rubber and of such quality that it would stand boiling, was constructed, and by connecting it with a bicycle pump of sufficient size one or two quick strokes of the piston sufficed to fill it. Such an arrangement I have made use of many times for cocaine operations on the extremities with the greatest satisfaction. The tourniquet may be adjusted but not blown up until the moment of beginning the operation, and by palpating a peripheral artery one can tell easily when a sufficient degree of inflation has been reached.* When operating on minor cases without an assistant I have used a small bicycle foot-pump, the tourniquet either being adjusted well above the operative field before "cleaning up" or, having been boiled, placed around the member within the aseptic field just before operating. In similar fashion a larger and stronger form of cylinder than those which I have had constructed would answer for use on a muscular thigh or leg.

There is a further and a therapeutic use to which this form of peripheral construction could well be put though I have had little personal experience with this particular variety of tourni-

* It would be a refinement, of course, to insert a manometer in the course of the tube connecting tourniquet and pump, and, after measuring the tension necessary to obliterate the systolic pressure, to carry the pressure in the tourniquet slightly above this point. In a large operating room this could be conveniently and accurately done by having a tank of compressed air by which the tension could be instantly carried to the required number of millimeters of mercury.

Harvey Cushing: Pneumatic tourniquets: with especial reference to their use in craniotomies. Med. News, *84*:577–580, 1904. (Courtesy of the Library of the New York Academy of Medicine)

was always a problem. Cushing used anything for hemostasis; he was instrumental in developing the Bovie electrocoagulation unit and pioneered the use of suction. Horsley had devised bone wax, and Cushing, being a follower of the black silk school of Halsted, pulled the suture through a bit of wax to make it glide more easily through the tough scalp. He removed his first brain tumor in 1902 and reached the 2,000th in 1931, choosing for the latter operation a patient with a pituitary adenoma, the problem of his early research and the basis for one of his most carefully written monographs. It was in 1912 that he reported fifty cases of pituitary adenoma.

In 1912 the new Peter Bent Brigham Hospital in Boston was built, near the Harvard Medical School and Children's Hospital. Cushing became the first surgeon-in-chief, with Henry Christian in medicine, S. Burt Wolbach in pathology, and Merrill Sosman in radiology. The "Brigham" became the mecca for all those interested in neurosurgery. Cushing's students included many who would become leaders in their own areas. Percival Bailey, Norman Dott, Eric Oldberg, Gilbert Horrax, Carl Rand, and many others were among his students.

Cushing was an advocate of better postgraduate education and the residency system, with proper grounding in surgery and the laboratory. He was not tall, but was "wiry," brisk, and well organized. During his most active surgical period, he wrote the biography of Sir William Osler, for which he received the Pulitzer Prize. Although there was no doubt about who was "chief," Cushing was not the *geheimrat*. He had a remarkable sense of humor and was considerate of his patients. His hobby was medical history, and his library became famous. After receiving a particulary high fee for the removal of some intracranial tumor, he would purchase some rare volume, thus, as he said, "consecrating" the sum received. After retirement from Harvard, he returned to Yale and left to its library his collection of historical volumes of inestimable value. His unfinished study of Vesalius was completed by the distinguished physiologist, John Fulton, who also wrote a biography of Cushing.

Cushing had one son, who died while attending Yale, and two daughters, the eldest of whom resembled her father in many ways. She married James Roosevelt, whose father became President of the United States in 1933.

Cushing was a great practical joker. I recall a meeting at which he introduced a visiting doctor from some unheard-of European university. The professor proceeded to give a lecture, in the most garbled English, illustrated with a film demonstrating the technique of esophagoscopy, which terminated in a big ovation when the surgeon extracted a long chain of sausages from what appeared to be a patient. When the last scene faded out and the lights came on, there was no sign of the visitor, and no discussion followed. Richard Meagher, then one of the residents in surgery, had played the part of the visitor and, properly attired in a cutaway coat and an artificial beard, to go with his natural mustache, had convinced most of us, up to the last scene, that it was real.

Cushing had a keen eye and missed little that was going on in the hospital. On one occasion I found a note in my mailbox from the "chief" saying that he had seen an article of mine about Thomas Dover (of Dover's powder) and Robinson Crusoe in the *New England Journal of Medicine*. The note called attention to a current exhibit of Daniel Defoe's work in the Boston Public Library.

Cushing had a distinguished record in the First World War, and he kept copious notes of the many and varied wounds of the brain and of the techniques developed for treating them. His results in the treatment of brain tumors may never be surpassed. He was a master surgeon.

The discovery of the x-ray in 1895 opened up a whole new field of investigation. It made possible the early diagnosis of many lesions of the skeleton, heretofore described clinically and verified only by autopsy.

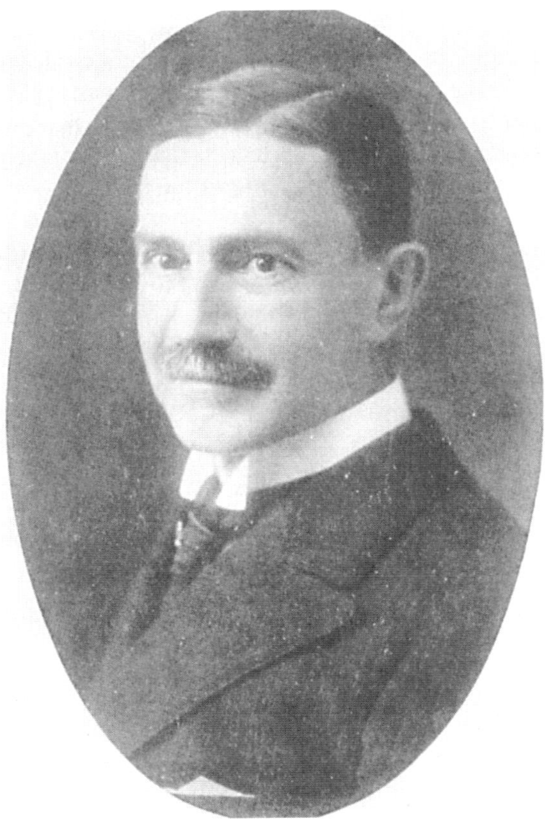

Georg Clemens Perthes. (From Beilage Munch. Med. Wochenschr. 74[1]:384, 1927. Courtesy of the Library of the New York Academy of Medicine)

Georg Clemens Perthes's (1869–1927) name is attached to the juvenile coxitis and is usually combined with those of Legg and Calvé. In the field of surgery of the upper extremity, we use his name for a method of tendon transfer for radial palsy, a method that was very commonly used for many years, but that is now superseded by more detailed techniques. But Perthes did much more. He was a surgeon with interests in many fields, including the use of the newly discovered radiation.

Perthes was born in Mörs in the Rhineland. His father was a teacher in the local secondary schools, and when his mother died, presumably of tuberculosis, his father went to Davos in Switzerland and started a school for children with lung disease. Georg grew up there until his father was called to Bonn. His father died, leaving Georg in the care of a maiden aunt, Agnes Perthes. It was through her grandfather, a dealer in books in Hamburg, that he met Trendelenburg, who would influence him to study medicine. Perthes later became Trendelenburg's assistant, following him from Bonn to Leipzig in 1895. He went to several medical schools (in Freiburg, Berlin, and Bonn), which was a common practice. From 1900 to 1901 he was in China as a surgeon with a German army unit, where he did a radiological study of the bound feet of the Chinese women.

When Trendelenburg went to Leipzig to replace Thiersch, he encouraged his young assistant, Perthes, to attend the congresses and enter into the discussions. One of Perthes's confreres described the contrast between the professor, who had an open, happy disposition, and the serious mien of Perthes; yet there was a warm understanding and respect between them. Perthes was said to have been Trendelenburg's favorite student and was deeply appreciated by Trendelenburg.

In his early work, Perthes developed a suction-catheter drainage method for empyema, and he also used it to drain abscesses of soft tissues. This tubing was also filled with air, to be used as a pneumatic cuff, which he said he used for operations done on the arm or leg under conduction anesthesia. Thus, perhaps Perthes should get the credit for the pneumatic tourniquet, although Cushing showed how the pressure could be controlled and maintained at the desired level.

Early in his career, Perthes had recognized the effect of the roentgen ray on epithelial cell growth and its destructive effect on warts, skin cancer, and metastatic cancer of the breast. He experimented with the effect of the rays on cells of plants and the chromatin of the nucleus. He used x-ray as a treatment after operation for mammary carcinoma. He was one of the pioneers of x-ray therapy.

He was also interested in problems involving the bones and joints, as was his teacher, Trendelenburg. While in Leipzig, Perthes described the osteochondritis now known by his name, developed a procedure for treatment of habitual dislocation of the shoulder, and performed os-

Über plastischen Daumenersatz insbesondere bei Verlust des ganzen Daumenstrahles.

Von

Prof. **Perthes**-Tübingen.

Mit 18 Abbildungen im Text.

(Eingegangen am 20. Januar 1921.)

Literatur.

1. v. Arlt, Wien. klin. Wochenschr. 1917. 15. — 2. Burkard, Otto, Münch. med. Wochenschr. 1916. 1407. — 3. v. Eiselsberg, Verhandl. d. Deutsch. Ges. f. Chir. 29. Kongr. Teil II. 1900. 493. — 4. Hohmann, Zeitschr. f. orthop. Chir. **37**. 414. — 5. Hörhammer, Münch. med. Wochenschr. 1915. 1681. — 6. Derselbe, Münch. med. Wochenschr. 1917. 1115. — 7. Hueck, Deutsche Zeitschr. f. Chir. **153**. 321. — 8. Klapp, Deutsche Zeitschr. f. Chir. **118**. 479. — 9. Klemm, Arch. f. klin. Chir. **96**. 181. — 10. Kraft, Wien. klin. Wochenschrift 1906. 1443. — 11. Krause, Fedor, Berl. klin. Wochenschr. 1906. 1527. — 12. Lauenstein, Deutsche med. Wochenschr. 1888. 612. — 13. Luksch, Verhandl. d. Deutsch. Ges. f. Chir. 1903. Teil I. 221. — 14. Derselbe, Wien. klin. Wochenschr. 1903. 916. — 15. Derselbe, Münch. med. Wochenschr. 1916. 881. — 16. Machol, Bruns Beitr. z. klin. Chir. **114**. 180. — 17. Manasse, Deutsch. med. Wochenschr. 1920. 352. — 18. Meyer, Herm., Bruns Beitr. z. klin. Chir. **119**. 386. — 19. Müller, Walther, Bruns Beitr. z. klin. Chir. **120**. 599. — 20. Mühsam, Berl. klin. Wochenschr. 1918. 1045. — 21. Muskat, Arch. f. Orthop. u. Unfallchir. **16**. 255. — 22. Neuhäuser, Berl. klin. Wochenschr. 1916. 1287. — 23. Nicoladoni, Wien. klin. Wochenschr. 1897. 663. — 24. Derselbe, Arch. f. klin. Chir. **61**. 606. — 25. Derselbe, Arch. f. klin. Chir. **69**. 695. — 26. Noeßke, Münch. med. Wochenschrift. 1909. 1403. — 27. Derselbe, Münch. med. Wochenschr. 1915. 1085. — 28. Payr, vgl. Hörhammer. 1917. — 29. Quetsch, Berl. klin. Wochenschr. 1918. Nr. 33. — 30. Ritter, Berl. klin. Wochenschr. 1918. Nr. 44. — 31. Rietz, Referat a. d. schwed. Zentralbl. f. Chir. 1918. 536. — 32. Schepelmann, Zeitschr. f. orthop. Chir. **34**. 174. — 33. Derselbe, Ebenda. **35**. — 34. Derselbe, Ebenda. **39**. 181. — 35. Schmidt, Walther, Deutsch. Zeitschr. f. Chir. **145**. 420. — 36. Spitzy, Wien. klin. Wochenschr. 1917. 1502. Münch. med. Wochenschr. 1917. 1622. — 37. Derselbe, Verhandl. d. Deutsch. orth. Ges. 14. Kongr. Wien. 1918. Zeitschr. f. orth. Chir. **38**. 134. — 38. Wierzejewsky, Münch. med. Wochenschrift. 1919. 19.

Trotzdem der Krieg den Chirurgen vielfachen Anlaß gegeben hat, sich mit dem plastischen Ersatz des verloren gegangenen Daumens zu befassen, ist die Frage, welche Methode im allgemeinen die besten Aussichten bietet, keineswegs geklärt. Vor allem sind die Erfahrungen über Daumenplastik bei gleichzeitigem Verlust von Daumen und Daumenmetakarpus noch spärlich. Gerade diese letzteren Fälle stellen aber Anforderungen ganz besonderer Art. Das sind die Gründe, welche die Wiedergabe unserer Erfahrungen an 6 in den Jahren

Archiv für orthopädische und Unfall-Chirurgie. Bd. XIX. 14

Georg Clemens Perthes: Über plastischen Daumenersatz insbesondere bei Verlust des ganzen Daumenstrahles. Arch. Orthop. Unfall-Chir., *19*:198–214, 1921, J. F. Bergmann Verlag, Munich. (Courtesy of the Library of the College of Physicians of Philadelphia)

teotomies for clubfeet, knock-knees, and bowlegs. For loss of a thumb, he created a deep cleft between the first and second metacarpals to restore grasp.

He was very active in World War I and, after service at the front, was stationed in a hospital that had many cases of severe peripheral nerve disease. In a handbook on war surgery, he wrote a section on the indications for nerve surgery, including the techniques and the functional recovery seen after suture. He also wrote a monograph on injuries of the jaw.

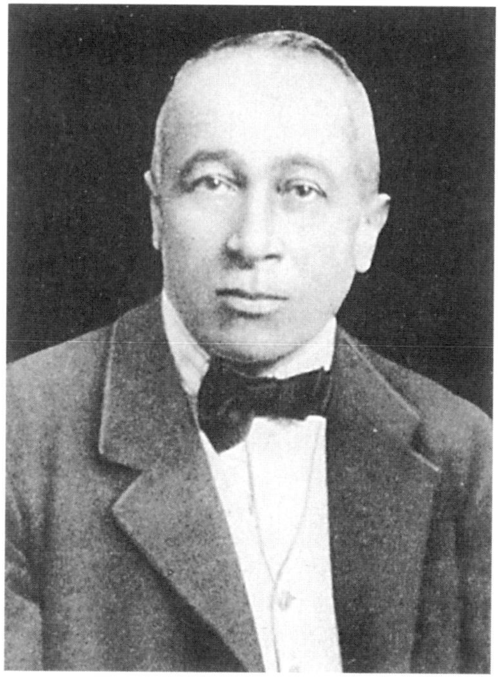

Robert Kienböck. (From Korad Weiss: In memoriam, Robert Kienböck. Radiol. Austriaca, *8*[2]:109, 1955. Courtesy of the Library of the New York Academy of Medicine)

He later returned to Bonn as a professor. While on a holiday during Christmas in Arosa, Switzerland, he died suddenly of a stroke.

Perthes was described as being "solid and absolutely reliable," outspoken in discussion, but deeply respected. Perthes contributed much to surgery, and we honor him by using his name for a disease process and for an operative procedure; however, would he not remind us that it was on Trendelenburg's shoulders that he stood to see that much ahead?

About the same time, **Robert Kienböck** (1871–1953) would use the newly discovered x-rays to establish diagnostic and therapeutic radiology as a special field of study. His paper on lunate malacia, from which we derive the eponym Kienböck's disease, was written in 1910. Here also, the disease process is so characteristic in appearance and the etiology so obscure that describing the condition simply as a disease by this man's name will mean that it is universally understood.

Kienböck, the son of an attorney, was born in Vienna and completed all his education there. He then spent a year in Paris and London. Back in Vienna as an assistant in a medical clinic, he began to do x-ray examina-

Aus dem Radiologischen Institute der Allgemeinen Poliklinik in Wien.

Über traumatische Malazie des Mondbeins
und ihre Folgezustände: Entartungsformen und Kompressionsfrakturen.

Von

Privatdozent Dr. **Robert Kienböck.**

(Hierzu Tafel VII, VIII, IX und X.)

Über die traumatische Erkrankung des Mondbeins sind bisher spezielle Publikationen noch nicht erschienen. Es wurden davon bereits mehrere Dutzend Fälle beschrieben, teils anatomische, teils chirurgisch-operative, teils radiologische Beobachtungen, doch nur gemeinsam mit anderen Verletzungen der Karpalregion und meist nur nebenbei. Wir wollen nun die „Entartungsformen“ und „Kompressionsfrakturen“ des Os lunatum im folgenden ausführlich studieren, und zwar besonders hinsichtlich ihrer Morphologie und Entstehung.

Über das Vorkommen der Frakturen der Handwurzelknochen, speziell der isolierten Fraktur eines Karpales, war vor der Einführung des Röntgenverfahrens fast nichts bekannt, und die spärlichen Beobachtungen, die vorliegen, stammen nicht von Chirurgen, sondern von Anatomen, wie Gruber, Turner, Pfitzner. Aber auch von diesen wurden die Fälle zumeist verkannt, und die isolierten Frakturen der Knochen der Handwurzel wurden in der Regel als Varietäten des Handskeletts aufgefasst. Die Brüche der Karpalien wurden als Naviculare bipartitum und tripartitum, Lunatum bipartitum (Zerfall in zwei etwa gleichgrosse Stücke) und partitum („Entartungsform“ mit Zerfall in kleine, unregelmässige Stücke). Epilunatum und Hypolunatum beschrieben. Nach Pfitzner soll es sich dabei nur ausnahmsweise um traumatische Veränderungen handeln.

Seit Benützung des Röntgenverfahrens erfuhr man, dass die Knochen des Karpus gar nicht so selten brechen, speziell auch eine isolierte Fraktur erleiden. Es war namentlich R. Wolff, der zu zeigen versuchte, dass die sogenannten Varietäten des Handskeletts und die Entartungsformen in der Regel Frakturen sind, ohne Verheilung der Fragmente.

Am häufigsten kommt die isolierte Fraktur des Navikulare vor, demnächst der Bruch dieses Knochens in Kombination mit Fraktur des Radius oder mit Luxation des Lunatum. Oberst konnte (1901) — mit Hilfe der Röntgenuntersuchung unter 1750 Knochenbrüchen 6 Fälle von isolierter Fraktur eines Karpales beobachten (dreimal am Navikulare, zweimal am Lunatum, einmal am Triquetrum); Lilienfeld aber (1905) an einem Krankenkassenmaterial unter 384 Brüchen 13 subkutane, isolierte Frakturen des Navikulare, 5 Luxationen des Lunatum, 1 isolierter Bruch des Mondbeins, und unter 59 Radiusfrakturen waren 5 mit Navikularebruch kombiniert.

Wir wollen nun eine Reihe von Fällen aus der Literatur betrachten, zunächst Fälle von sogenanntem „Epilunatum“ und „Hypolunatum“, welche offenbar mit Unrecht als Varietäten

Robert Kienböck: Über traumatische Malazie des Mondbeins und ihre Folgezustände: Entartungsformen und Kompressionsfrakturen. Fortschr. Geb. Roetgenstr. Nuklearmed., *16*:77–103, 1910. (Courtesy of the National Library of Medicine, Bethesda, Maryland)

tions, and soon other clinics were sending their patients to him. Realizing the importance of this new diagnostic and therapeutic tool, he asked for and was able to obtain a separate department of radiology, with its own personnel and administration.

He was an intense worker, publishing many articles on therapeutic as well as diagnostic radiology, and he became the acknowledged expert in bone and joints. For the last half of his life, he was markedly physically handicapped, having suffered a basal skull fracture from a fall off a horse in 1910. His writings continued, however, and one of his investigations was on the differentiation of Paget's and Recklinghausen's diseases, which up to then were thought to have the same etiology.

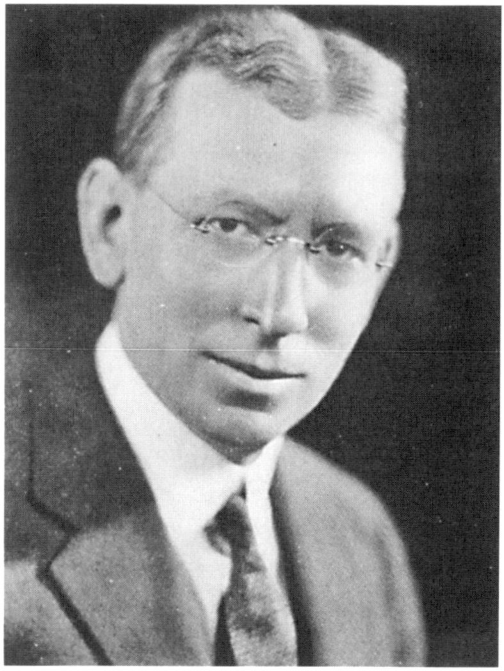

Allen B. Kanavel. (From Memoirs. Ann. Surg., *108*:788–790, 1938. Courtesy of the Library of the College of Physicians of Philadelphia)

He was in his seventies when he published, one volume each year, the eight-volume work, *Radiology of Bones and Joints.* He died at 83, having seen radiology develop from the discovery of Röntgen to a specialty of its own.

In 1912 a book appeared that would be of tremendous significance in the treatment of infections of the hand. **Allen B. Kanavel** (1874–1938) had studied this problem for several years and developed the method of forcible injection into tendon sheaths and fascial spaces in the hand with radiopaque material. These spaces and the extent of the sheaths, of course, were familiar to anatomists, but no one had studied the spread of infection. Kanavel found a definite and constant pattern in the way the material would spread from sheath to space. This finding made it possible, with incisions in the proper place, to drain the areas without damage to important structures. The book has gone through many editions and is a classic.

Kanavel's sign consists of tenderness over the base of the ring finger on the palm side, occurring when an infection of the flexor sheath of the thumb has spread to the ulnar bursa. Kanavel stressed the importance of

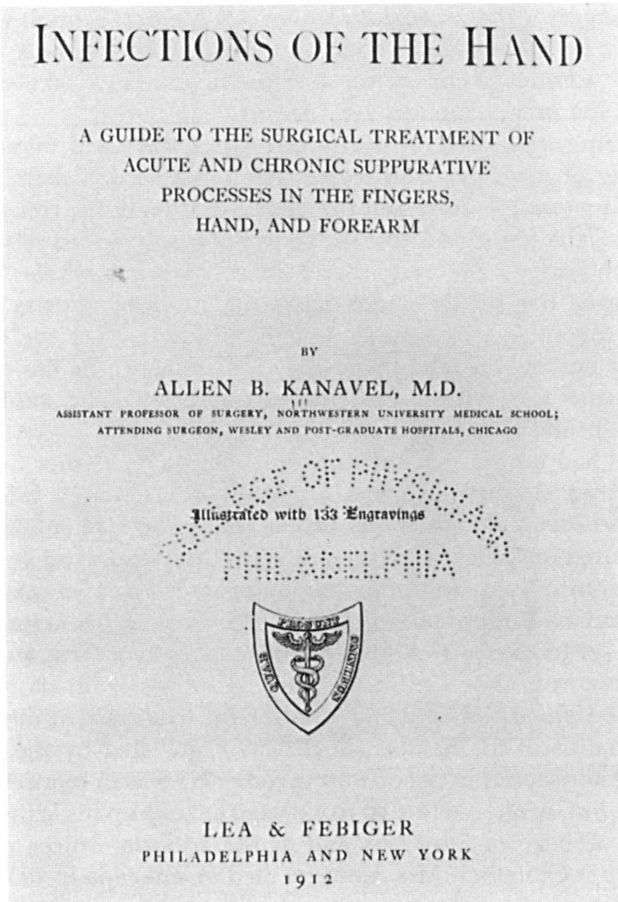

INFECTIONS OF THE HAND

A GUIDE TO THE SURGICAL TREATMENT OF ACUTE AND CHRONIC SUPPURATIVE PROCESSES IN THE FINGERS, HAND, AND FOREARM

BY

ALLEN B. KANAVEL, M.D.

ASSISTANT PROFESSOR OF SURGERY, NORTHWESTERN UNIVERSITY MEDICAL SCHOOL; ATTENDING SURGEON, WESLEY AND POST-GRADUATE HOSPITALS, CHICAGO

Illustrated with 133 Engravings

LEA & FEBIGER
PHILADELPHIA AND NEW YORK
1912

Allen B. Kanavel: Infections of the Hand. ed. 1. Philadelphia, Lea & Febiger, 1912. (Courtesy of the Library of the College of Physicians of Philadelphia)

maintaining the hand in the position of function; Michael Mason, in his review of hand surgery, believed this concept and teaching to be one of Kanavel's greatest contributions.

Allen Kanavel, the son of a Methodist minister, was born in 1874 in a little town on the prairies of central Kansas. He went to Northwestern College and Medical School, graduating in 1899 with honors. He spent 6 months studying in Vienna, where he must have met Kienböck or heard of his work with the roentgen rays, for Kanavel visited the Allgemeine Krankenhaus, which Billroth had made famous. Returning to Chicago, Kanavel interned at Cook County Hospital and then went to the department of surgery of Northwestern University Medical School, where for a whole year he never saw an operation, because he was only allowed to watch the administration of the anesthetic and then take care of the patient in the immediate recovery period.

He became interested in the infections of the hand because of the uncertainty of diagnosis and treatment then accorded them. After the thorough anatomical study and the demonstration of the constant routes of infection, his service became the source of many reports relating to the hand. With Sumner Koch and then Michael Mason, a whole "school" of hand surgery was set up which made the study of injuries as well as infection the subject of studies and publications. (See the section on Mason for studies on tendon repair). His influence in the care of the infected hand was widespread, and his associates and students have carried on in the same tradition.

Kanavel had been a general surgeon, interested in other fields, especially thyroid surgery. He was a good speaker, much interested in people, and especially the young people in training. He enjoyed reading history, biography, and mystery novels. Courteous and considerate, avoiding controversy, and possessing great tact, Kanavel was a giant in our field and made it possible for many others to progress to further goals.

As the years passed, Kanavel limited his work because of two factors—one was the need to get out of Chicago, with its notoriously poor climate which bothered both him and his wife, and the other was the radiodermatitis of his hands, which was aggravated by the scrubbing and use of antiseptics in the operating room. He was in semiretirement at Pasadena, but he often returned to Chicago to keep up his activities at the American College of Surgeons and at the editorial offices of *Surgery, Gynecology & Obstetrics.* Mrs. Kanavel died of leukemia in 1936. Kanavel suffered from severe glaucoma. He died in 1938 as a result of an automobile accident.

Vladimir Petrovich Filatov (1875–1956) was an ophthalmologist, in Odessa, whose primary contributions were in the procedures for corneal transplantation, but his name is included here for a report, in 1917, of the "round pedicle" technique. This tubing of a pedicle of skin was done in a plastic procedure on an eyelid. Although Gillies, who is credited with this technique in the English literature, was not aware of Filatov's report, which appeared in the *Russian Bulletin of Ophthalmology,* he promptly gave Filatov the credit when, some years later, it was brought to his attention.

Filatov, the son of an eye surgeon, was born in central Russia. Immediately after graduating from Moscow University, he spent 2 years in the eye clinic there and another 5 years at the eye hospital, before going to Odessa as house surgeon. Here his research work gained him an

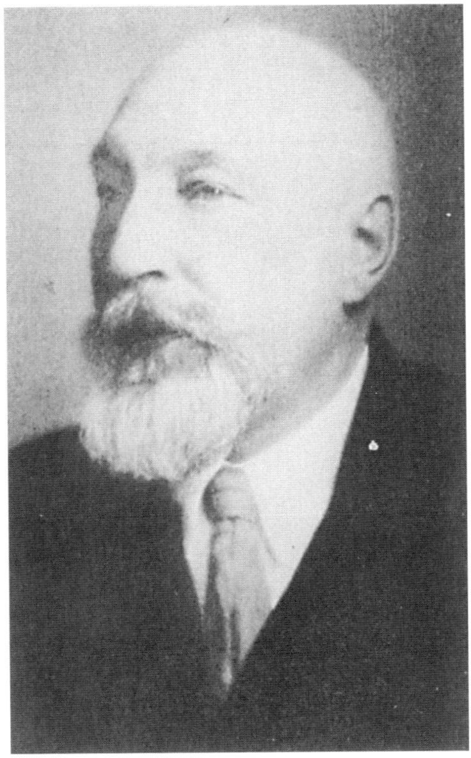

Vladimir Petrovich Filatov. (From Bull. Practical Ophthalmology, *8*[2]:27, 1938. Courtesy of the Library of the New York Academy of Medicine)

appointment as lecturer and an opportunity to travel and study in Berlin, Vienna, Prague, and Munich. From 1911 he was head of the clinic and remained in Odessa until the Second World War, when the Germans overran the Ukraine, and the clinic staff was moved to Tashkent.

His work on corneal grafts was known throughout the world, and he was credited with the introduction of the use of cadaver grafts and the technique of preserving the grafts by refrigeration. Filatov's tubing of a pedicle was an innovation, but Gillies showed us the many uses of this method of delaying a flap, and thus deserves equal credit.

In 1912 a short article in the *Annals of Surgery* described a patient with anterior dislocation of the ulna, treated by subperiosteal resection of the distal end. In 5 weeks the patient had a full range of motion. The author, **William Darrach** (1876–1948), said that he had used this method because in a previous case, an open reduction had resulted in almost complete loss of pronation and supination. It should be noted that his second

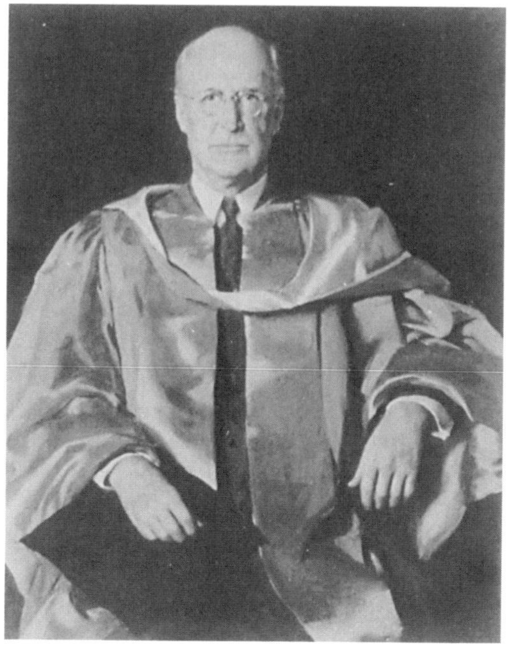

William Darrach. (Courtesy of the Library of the New York Academy of Medicine)

operation was done *sub*periosteally, and the styloid process, which had been broken off, was left in place. Subsequent x-rays showed some regeneration of the lower end of the bone. Ollier, who believed that the periosteum was the mother of bone, had promoted the idea of subperiosteal resection of bone. Currently, we see many patients who have had the lower end of the ulna removed improperly, with persisting symptoms of dislocation of the remaining fragment, and treatment of this is not at all satisfactory. It would be well for surgeons, especially those now so involved in surgery of rheumatoid arthritis, to go back to this simple operation and avoid some of the complications we are seeing. The Darrach operation, properly done, is very useful in restoring pronation and supination, following old, poorly reduced Colles's fractures and other disturbances of the lower end of the ulna.

Darrach was born in Germantown, Pennsylvania, and was educated in private schools and Yale University. He was graduated in medicine from the College of Physicians and Surgeons in New York City in 1901, and he interned at the old Presbyterian Hospital. He became a member of the staff of Roosevelt Hospital and a member of the teaching staff of the medical school. He was a demonstrator in anatomy for 6 years and was later instructor and then professor of clinical surgery. His special interest

ANTERIOR DISLOCATION OF THE HEAD OF THE ULNA.

DR. DARRACH presented a man, 34 years old, who was admitted to the Roosevelt Hospital on July 25, 1911, with the history that six and a half weeks before admission he had caught his left hand in a machinery belt, twisting it in extreme pronation. He went to a hospital, where an X-ray was taken and he was told that his wrist was all right. Since the injury he had been unable to work because of pain and limitation of motion.

On examination, the head of the ulna could be felt half an inch above the palmar crease in the mid-line. Pronation and supination were limited to one-third their normal range; adduction was somewhat increased; extension was normal, and flexion was limited to one-half. There was considerable limitation of motion in all of the fingers. No change of sensation in either the median or ulnar distribution.

William Darrach: Anterior dislocation of the head of the ulna. Ann. Surg., *56*:802–803, 1912. (Courtesy of the Library of the College of Physicians of Philadelphia)

was in fractures. During World War I, he was in a British hospital, and he was director of surgery later in an American hospital.

In 1919, after the war, he was made dean of the faculty, and during this time the Columbia Presbyterian Center was built, an affiliation of the Presbyterian Hospital and the College of Physicians and Surgeons. The many organizational problems were solved, as some say, by his "forbearance, sense of equity, diplomacy and wisdom." He became dean emeritus in 1930. Darrach received many honors, was well liked by his confreres, and served in many offices in the College of Surgeons. He was president of the American Surgical Association in 1944. He died in Greenwich Hospital at the age of 72.

One of the names used commonly today to describe a sign of ulnar palsy is that of **Jules Froment** (1878–1946). He was a neurologist and professor of medicine at Lyon. It was during World War I that he had an opportunity to see a large number of nerve injuries. As Tinel did in Paris at the same time, and as Weir Mitchell had done during the Civil War, Froment made the best of his opportunity and studied the signs and symptoms of peripheral nerve injuries. It was in a nerve unit at Rennes, and then later with Babinski in Paris, that he delineated the signs of various nerve lesions. His sign, also called the newspaper-drawer sign, illustrates the peculiar type of pinch with the thumb when the adductor pollicis is paralyzed.

When a patient is asked to hold a newspaper between the thumb and the index finger and the examiner pulls hard on it, the grip is weak, and only the strongly flexed distal phalanx of the thumb presses against the index to hold the paper. This is in contrast to the normal, when the whole side of the thumb presses against the second metacarpal and base of the

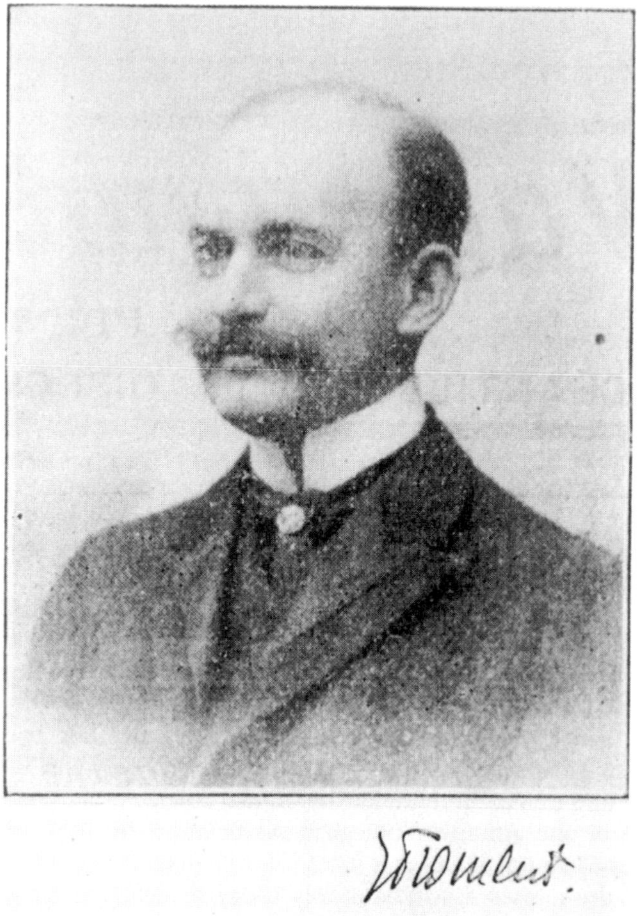

Jules Froment. (From Nouvelles, les nouveaux agrégés. Paris Médical, *7*:507–509, 1913. Courtesy of the Library of the College of Physicians of Philadelphia. Signature courtesy of Dr. Jacques Roullet, Lyon, France)

index to produce a tight grasp. Froment called this deformity the sign of the thumb. Froment did not go into the detailed anatomical or physiological reasons for this deformity; but Lennart Mannerfelt, in his monograph on ulnar palsy, has made a detailed study of the dynamics of this deformity.*

It has long been known that the short abductor of the thumb on the

*Mannerfelt, L.: Studies on the hand in ulnar nerve paralysis. Acta Orthop. Scand. Suppl., *87*:1–176, 1966.

N° 50 LA PRESSE MÉDICALE, Jeudi, 21 Octobre 1915 409

LA PRÉHENSION DANS LES PARALYSIES DU NERF CUBITAL ET LE SIGNE DU POUCE

Par J. FROMENT
Agrégé, Médecin des hôpitaux de Lyon.
(Travail du service du Dr [illegible].)

De tous les troubles moteurs qu'entraine la lésion du nerf cubital, un des plus importants, en pratique, est l'altération du mécanisme de la préhension (consécutive à la paralysie de l'adducteur du pouce). Il nous parait dès lors utile d'attirer l'attention des neurologistes sur un signe objectif nouveau dont la recherche permet, en pareil cas, de dépister rapidement le caractère défectueux de cette fonction, et qui même, dans une certaine mesure, permet d'en apprécier l'importance.

Si l'on fait abstraction des variétés secondaires et accessoires de la préhension (qui tiennent à l'objet que nous avons en main et à l'usage que nous en attendons) et si l'on n'envisage que celle qui se fait entre le pouce et les autres doigts, on peut dire qu'il existe deux modes essentiels de préhension. L'objet que nous saisissons est-il lourd? Est-il nécessaire de le tenir avec fermeté? Le pouce étend sa deuxième phalange, il s'applique fortement contre l'index replié sous lui en crochet et y adhère sur toute sa longueur. L'objet est alors saisi entre les deux branches d'une pince à mors plats qui réalise une préhension énergique. L'objet que nous saisissons est-il, au contraire, petit ou fragile? Craignons-nous de le froisser par une pression trop vigoureuse? Le pouce s'arc-boute, fléchit sa deuxième phalange et se met en contact par la pulpe avec le bord externe de la pulpe de l'index dont les dernières phalanges sont également fléchies. La pince ainsi constituée n'est plus un instrument de résistance, mais bien un instrument de précision. Elle réalise une préhension délicate qui exclut toute force et fait songer, de par ces caractères mêmes, à la pince de Cornet, utilisée en bactériologie pour la manipulation des lames et des lamelles. Dans le premier cas, on dit que nous « empoignons » l'objet et dans le deuxième cas, on dit que nous le « tenons du bout des doigts ». Ces deux locutions courantes témoignent d'une notation populaire très exacte : elles expriment tout à la fois et la modalité et la portée même des deux variétés essentielles de la préhension.

La préhension énergique est réalisée par la contraction de l'adducteur du pouce et de la portion interne du court fléchisseur, innervés par le nerf cubital, à l'exception du chef profond du fléchisseur qu'innerve parfois le médian (Froment[1]; Poirier et Richer, 3 fois sur 30 cas[2]). Ces muscles ne se contentent pas, en effet, de rapprocher le premier métacarpien du second, ils fléchissent la première phalange du pouce qu'ils appliquent ainsi fortement contre les doigts sous-jacents. Ils étendent encore, ainsi que l'a montré Duchenne de Boulogne[3], la deuxième phalange sur la première en raison de l'expansion aponévrotique par laquelle leur tendon s'unit au tendon du long extenseur du pouce. Accessoirement enfin, le court abducteur entre en contraction synergique pour fixer la première phalange à laquelle l'adducteur imprime un mouvement de rotation sur son axe longitudinal (en sens inverse de celui que le court abducteur lui fait exécuter). Mais il s'agit là d'une contraction tout à fait secondaire et, en dernière analyse, l'adducteur est le seul muscle susceptible de réaliser la préhension énergique.

Dans la préhension délicate, l'adducteur par contre n'intervient pas, le pouce et l'index ne s'accolent pas, mais s'opposent simplement par leur extrémité en dessinant une espèce d'ogive. La préhension est ici réalisée à peu près exclusivement par la contraction des fléchisseurs du pouce et de l'index, innervés par le médian.

On conçoit, dès lors, qu'un individu privé de l'adducteur du pouce soit incapable de saisir un objet avec force entre le pouce et l'index. Ce fait n'a pas échappé au remarquable observateur qu'était Duchenne de Boulogne, mais il ne paraît pas en avoir saisi toutes les conséquences pratiques. « Une seule fois, écrit-il, j'ai vu cette paralysie des faisceaux adducteurs parfaitement localisée... Les principaux usages de la main étaient conservés parce que les faisceaux adducteurs du pouce remplissent alors un rôle relativement peu important : ainsi ils pouvaient écrire car les muscles qui président à cette fonction étaient sains, mais ils éprouvaient de la fatigue pour tenir longtemps la plume; ils serraient faiblement les objets qu'on leur plaçait dans la main[1]. » Cette conclusion est beaucoup trop optimiste, pour s'en convaincre il suffit d'interroger les nombreux cas de paralysie du cubital qu'il nous est donné d'observer actuellement ou mieux encore de leur remettre en main les outils de leur profession. Ils s'aperçoivent bien vite, s'ils ne l'ont déjà remarqué eux-mêmes, que la faiblesse de leur pouce apporte un très grand préjudice aux usages industriels de leur main.

Les descriptions classiques de la paralysie cubitale beaucoup moins explicites encore, omettent la préhension comme si ce n'était pas l'acte essentiel de la main et attribuent à la paralysie de l'adducteur des symptômes dont les uns (pouce en abduction, adduction du pouce impossible) sont nettement erronnés et dont les autres (opposition à la base de l'auriculaire) sont pour le moins inconstants.

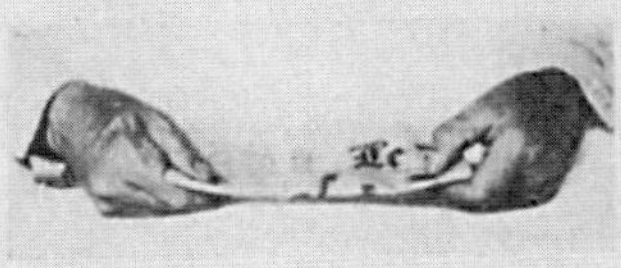

Attitude des pouces dans la préhension énergique chez un blessé atteint de paralysie cubitale gauche.

Pour mettre en évidence le trouble de la préhension, il suffit, cependant, de faire saisir au malade un objet quelconque entre le pouce et les autres doigts, on constate alors deux faits : d'une part la faiblesse de la préhension, d'autre part l'attitude anormale du pouce alors même que rien au repos ne pouvait la faire soupçonner. C'est dans la préhension d'un objet mince que l'attitude vicieuse du pouce apparait le plus nettement. En pratique, nous tendons simplement au blessé un journal plié en lui demandant de le saisir énergiquement avec la main saine, puis avec la main malade, cependant que nous exerçons une assez forte traction[2]. Voici ce que l'on observe. Du côté sain, le pouce adhère fortement par toute son étendue à l'objet saisi, la deuxième phalange est complètement étendue ou à peine fléchie : c'est le type même de la préhension énergique que nous décrivions il y a un instant. Du côté paralysé, le pouce s'arc-boute, fléchit fortement sa deuxième phalange et, quelle que soit la force déployée, n'adhère à l'objet, comme dans la préhension délicate, que par l'extrémité de sa pulpe. Il y a le plus souvent une véritable lucarne entre le pouce et le journal ou, plus exactement, lorsque le journal ne l'oblitère pas, entre le pouce et le bord supérieur de la main. Cette attitude asymétrique des deux pouces apparait très nettement lorsque le malade, saisissant le journal à deux mains, exerce sur les deux extrémités de celui-ci une traction divergente. C'est l'attitude même que reproduit la photographie ci-dessus que nous avons choisie parmi un assez grand nombre d'autres clichés tout aussi démonstratifs.

Le même type de préhension apparait lorsque l'on fait saisir au malade un objet volumineux, un registre par exemple, mais la comparaison entre les deux mains est moins saisissante, l'épaisseur du livre obligeant le pouce sain à s'arc-bouter et à fléchir légèrement la deuxième phalange. Dans l'un comme dans l'autre cas, et plus encore par cette dernière épreuve, on met nettement en évidence la faiblesse de cette préhension « à bout de doigts » des paralysies cubitales. Les objets saisis glissent entre les doigts du malade, entraînés par leur propre poids ou par la traction exercée. La main ne peut les retenir dès que cet acte requiert un peu de force.

Le signe de la préhension ou signe du pouce nous a paru exister dans toutes les paralysies du nerf cubital. Il est plus ou moins accusé suivant le degré de faiblesse de l'adducteur dont il paraît le meilleur mode d'appréciation, l'examen électrique permettant de déceler une atteinte musculaire plus ou moins profonde, mais non pas d'en suivre l'évolution régressive. Il peut être très marqué, alors même que la griffe et l'impotence des quatrième et cinquième doigts sont fort peu accusées ou même négligeables. Mais dans ce cas, il signale toujours une préhension très défectueuse qui compromet gravement les divers usages de la main.

Il est tout à fait distinct de la déformation du pouce étudiée par Jeanne[1]. Dans les cas envisagés par cet auteur, le pouce est fléchi à l'état de repos et il y a, à proprement parler, griffe du pouce. Cette attitude que l'on retrouve d'ailleurs dans un fort beau dessin de Duchenne de Boulogne[2], concernant une paralysie par section du cubital, nous a paru assez rare. Nous l'avons exclusivement observée dans les cas de griffes très accusées des quatre autres doigts avec atteinte simultanée du médian et du cubital. Les deux groupes musculaires, sésamoïdiens adducteurs et opposants, tous deux extenseurs de la deuxième phalange du pouce, sont alors supprimés. La préhension est dans de tels cas si défectueuse, qu'elle mérite à peine le nom de préhension, elle ne parait d'ailleurs ni modifier ni accentuer la flexion phalangienne observée. La flexion du pouce que nous signalons et qui, elle, s'observe à peu près constamment est étroitement corrélative à l'acte de la préhension[3]. Rien ne la fait prévoir dans l'attitude du pouce au repos, il est nécessaire pour la mettre en évidence de faire saisir un objet.

Si nous avons cru utile de mentionner ce nouveau signe, c'est qu'il permet seul de déceler l'importance du trouble de la préhension dans les paralysies cubitales. Ce trouble est assez notable pour gêner les ouvriers dans leur activité industrielle qu'elle rend parfois impossible. La gêne qui en résulte dépend de toute une série de facteurs : intensité de la parésie de l'adducteur, main droite ou gauche, nature de la profession exercée et peut-être encore dispositions anatomo-physiologiques individuelles. Nous nous réservons d'étudier en détail la répercussion industrielle du trouble de la préhension dans les paralysies du cubital. Nous avons voulu simplement le signaler ici et attirer sur lui l'attention des neurologistes. A n'envisager que la griffe cubitale, on risquerait de se faire une idée très inexacte et donc fort injuste, des conséquences qu'une paralysie cubitale va momentanément ou définitivement avoir pour un ouvrier, au moment de la reprise du travail professionnel.

1. FROMENT. *Traité d'anatomie humaine*, p. 513. — 2. POIRIER et RICHER. « Myologie », in *Traité d'anatomie humaine*, t. II, fig. 1, 1912. — 3. DUCHENNE DE BOULOGNE. *La Physiologie des mouvements*, 1867, p. 216.

1. DUCHENNE DE BOULOGNE. *De l'Électrisation localisée*, 3e édit. 1872, p. 977. — 2. Il est nécessaire d'exercer une traction énergique; la préhension avec pouce fléchi n'est pathologique que dans la préhension vigoureuse.

1. JEANNE. « La déformation du pouce dans la paralysie du cubital ». *Bull. et Mém. de la Soc. de Chir. de Paris*, 23 Mars 1915, p. 703. — 2. DUCHENNE DE BOULOGNE. *De l'Électrisation localisée*, 3e édit., 1872, p. 329, fig. 89 (observation de Musset). — 3. Dans un cas récent où nous l'avons vue manquer complètement, l'excitabilité faradique de l'adducteur n'était pas abolie, alors qu'elle l'était pour les interosseux et pour les muscles hypothénars. La préhension était très forte.

Jules Froment: La préhension dans les paralysies du nerf cubital et le signe du pouce. Presse Med., 23:409, 1915. (Courtesy of the Library of the College of Physicians of Philadelphia)

radial side and the adductor pollicus on the ulnar side have fibers of insertion into the extensor apparatus, analogous to those insertions of the interossei muslces into the extensor mechanism of the finger. Some authors induced from this that because in ulnar palsy the function of one, the adductor, would be lost, then the distal joint of the thumb would drop into flexion. Mannerfelt proved the fallacy of this and showed that this hyperflexion of the thumb in ulnar palsy, when a patient attempts to pinch, is due to the fact that the *secondary* adductor of the thumb is the extensor pollicis longus. Thus, the patient with adductor pollicis palsy who attempts to bring into action this mechanism and to improve its efficiency and power, will automatically flex the distal joint of the thumb, thus increasing the effective power of the obliquely passing long extensor tendon of the thumb. Mannerfelt found a patient with a rupture of the extensor pollicis longus and then blocked the ulnar nerve. Froment's sign did not appear. In final analysis, the extensor pollicis longus is a secondary adductor, while the flexor pollicis longus is only a tertiary force, if it functions at all in this maneuver.

Froment directed a Red Cross Hospital after the war and was involved in the serious encephalitis epidemic of 1918 to 1922. In 1926 he was severely injured by an ungrateful patient. (Delpech of Toulouse had been killed by a patient in 1832, but France is not alone in this response to therapy. Verne Hunt, originally from the Mayo Clinic and later a Los Angeles surgeon, was shot and killed by the husband of a patient.)

There are giants among giants, and surgery of the upper extremity can lay claim to having more than its share. The man of whom we write now, **Arthur Steindler** (1878–1959), is best described as being a scholar, and, as this word implies, he was studious, sincere, intelligent, and a lover of truth. He had an indefinable something that draws students, an élan, a spirit of dedication.

Steindler was a Viennese, with all the qualities that that city at the turn of the century encompassed. He was courteous and dignified, a linguist, and a lover of fine music and the arts, and he brought these traits to and maintained them in his adopted country. Iowa City is a small town in the lush farming country of the Middle West, but, because of Arthur Steindler, it became a place where anyone interested in orthopaedics would have to come.

It would be impossible to list the various things he did. Suffice it to say that for surgery of the upper extremity, his book by that title broke new ground. Although we remember him for the one operation of the proximal shift of the flexor origins to gain ability to flex the elbow, he influenced our ideas on all types of tendon and muscle transfers because of his ability to develop the principles of operative procedures. Yet operative surgery to him was the last phase in the study of a patient's problem. The

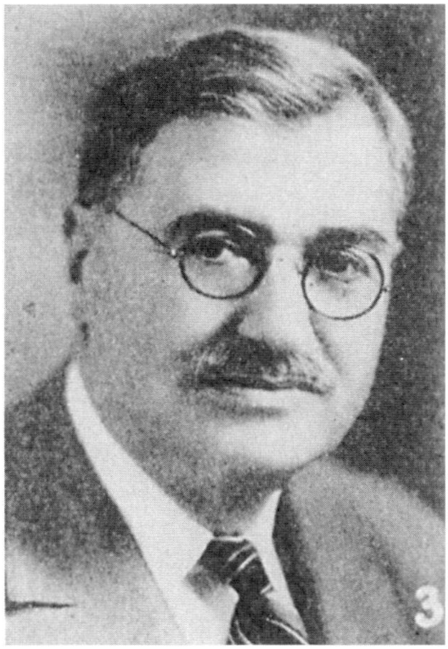

Arthur Steindler. (From Northwest Med., 39:306, 1940. Courtesy of the Library of the New York Academy of Medicine)

history, the diagnosis, and the indications all preceded the specific operative plan. Attention to detail, so characteristic of the German school, was essential to Steindler. He once said, "There are practically no clinical data which can be waved aside as insignificant; anyone may prove to be a valuable landmark for diagnosis."

Steindler was graduated from the University of Vienna Medical School in 1902. (Kienböck had just recently published his first paper on therapeutic radiation.) He trained in Vienna hospitals and emigrated to the United States in 1907. One of his teachers was Adolf Lorenz, the noted orthopaedic surgeon, whose son Konrad, born in 1903, shared the Nobel Prize in physiology in 1973 for his work in ethology.

This period, from 1865 to 1914, produced one of the greatest migrations of peoples in the history of the world. Some 15 million persons entered the United States, and among these were many from central Europe, from Germay, Austria, and Hungary. Because these immigrants tended to group themselves into certain areas, either because of their trade or occupation or because they had relatives who preceded them, the ethnic groupings that we associate with the early years of the 20th century in this country were produced. Generally speaking, this had been true even from the beginning, with the English in Boston, the Dutch in New York,

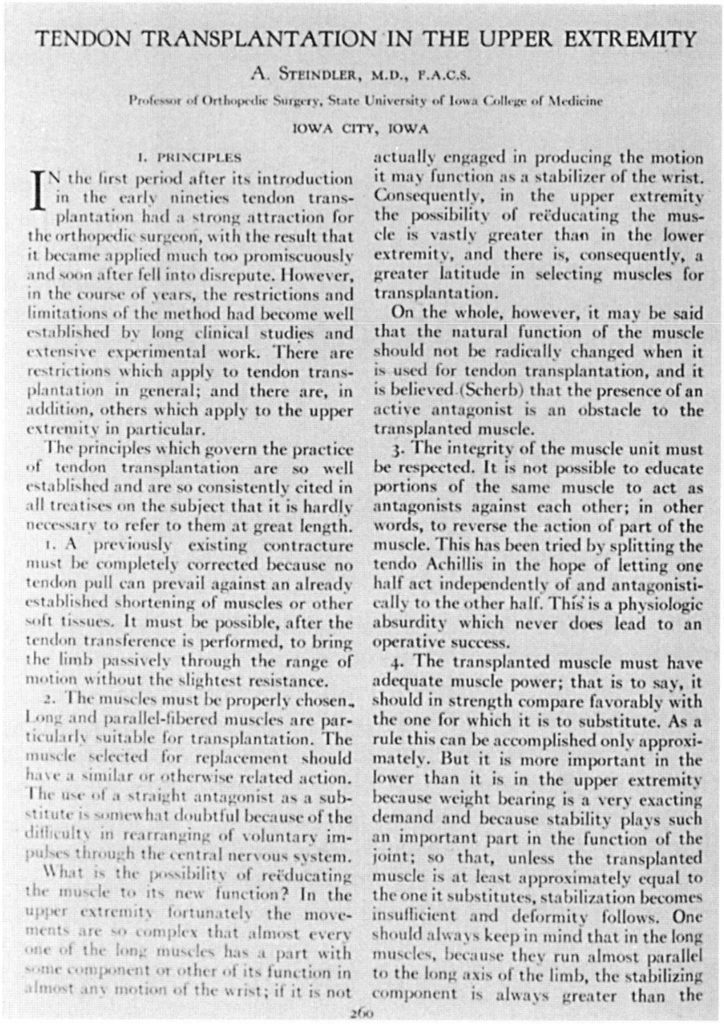

TENDON TRANSPLANTATION IN THE UPPER EXTREMITY

A. STEINDLER, M.D., F.A.C.S.

Professor of Orthopedic Surgery, State University of Iowa College of Medicine

IOWA CITY, IOWA

I. PRINCIPLES

IN the first period after its introduction in the early nineties tendon transplantation had a strong attraction for the orthopedic surgeon, with the result that it became applied much too promiscuously and soon after fell into disrepute. However, in the course of years, the restrictions and limitations of the method had become well established by long clinical studies and extensive experimental work. There are restrictions which apply to tendon transplantation in general; and there are, in addition, others which apply to the upper extremity in particular.

The principles which govern the practice of tendon transplantation are so well established and are so consistently cited in all treatises on the subject that it is hardly necessary to refer to them at great length.

1. A previously existing contracture must be completely corrected because no tendon pull can prevail against an already established shortening of muscles or other soft tissues. It must be possible, after the tendon transference is performed, to bring the limb passively through the range of motion without the slightest resistance.

2. The muscles must be properly chosen. Long and parallel-fibered muscles are particularly suitable for transplantation. The muscle selected for replacement should have a similar or otherwise related action. The use of a straight antagonist as a substitute is somewhat doubtful because of the difficulty in rearranging of voluntary impulses through the central nervous system.

What is the possibility of reëducating the muscle to its new function? In the upper extremity fortunately the movements are so complex that almost every one of the long muscles has a part with some component or other of its function in almost any motion of the wrist; if it is not actually engaged in producing the motion it may function as a stabilizer of the wrist. Consequently, in the upper extremity the possibility of reëducating the muscle is vastly greater than in the lower extremity, and there is, consequently, a greater latitude in selecting muscles for transplantation.

On the whole, however, it may be said that the natural function of the muscle should not be radically changed when it is used for tendon transplantation, and it is believed (Scherb) that the presence of an active antagonist is an obstacle to the transplanted muscle.

3. The integrity of the muscle unit must be respected. It is not possible to educate portions of the same muscle to act as antagonists against each other; in other words, to reverse the action of part of the muscle. This has been tried by splitting the tendo Achillis in the hope of letting one half act independently of and antagonistically to the other half. This is a physiologic absurdity which never does lead to an operative success.

4. The transplanted muscle must have adequate muscle power; that is to say, it should in strength compare favorably with the one for which it is to substitute. As a rule this can be accomplished only approximately. But it is more important in the lower than it is in the upper extremity because weight bearing is a very exacting demand and because stability plays such an important part in the function of the joint; so that, unless the transplanted muscle is at least approximately equal to the one it substitutes, stabilization becomes insufficient and deformity follows. One should always keep in mind that in the long muscles, because they run almost parallel to the long axis of the limb, the stabilizing component is always greater than the

260

Arthur Steindler: Tendon transplantation in the upper extremity. Am. J. Surg., *44*:260–271, 1939. The reader is advised to see a correction to this article in Am. J. Surg., *44*:534, 1939. (Courtesy of the Library of the College of Physicians of Philadelphia)

the French in Louisiana, and the Spanish in New Mexico and the Southwest. In this last period of massive migration, from 1865 to 1914, went the Irish to Boston, the Scandinavians to Minnesota and Wisconsin, the Poles to Pennsylvania, and the Germans to the Midwest. Many were farmers who homesteaded land in this large central plain, of which Chicago was the hub. We do not know what brought Steindler there, but his coming added luster to the country's scientific accomplishments.

Steindler first came to Chicago, where he was associated with Ridlon, and then he became professor at Drake University in Des Moines, Iowa, until 1913. The rest of his life was spent at Iowa City, where he died at the age of 81 of carcinoma.

There are two aspects about Steindler that impressed me. The first was his attendance at meetings, where he faithfully sat through the papers being read, usually in the front row, taking notes. He must have heard much that he already knew or had read about, and he must have shuddered at the style of some of the presentations. He was so accurate in his thinking and so careful in his writing that the modern verbiage must have been a chore for him to listen to; yet there he was, sometimes with Mayer or Bunnell, all intent on what was going on. It always struck me as being comical that here were the masters of orthopaedics sitting there like eager students, while many others, more in need of the instruction, lolled in the back seats like reluctant churchgoers on a Sunday morning.

The other aspect that impressed me was his library in Iowa City, which I visited. Here one can see the books he used; all the writings of the German, English, and Italian schools of orthopaedics. Here was Recklinghausen's works, with marginal notes and well-thumbed pages, and those of Weber and Fick. Steindler was a scholar, and no higher compliment can be made. His library was orderly and neatly labeled and covered every aspect of orthopaedics. More than 900 books, bound volumes of journals, and copies of his own 11 books, along with 85 unpublished manuscripts, filled the shelves and cabinets.

Steindler gave one the impression of being preoccupied. He was not the jovial type; his expression was almost serious. He was not the professor of unapproachable, commanding dignity; he could slide silently into a meeting room and take his seat without expecting anyone to recognize him. He had a humbleness of mien that contrasted to the bumptious actions of many of his confreres. He was courteous in his relations with others, and, when acting as a discussant, he was gracious. He was not partisan and could not stoop to personal attack. He once said, "Certainly, no justice can be done to the case by adopting a partisan standpoint. All opinions are needed and must be heard and explained."

Small-caliber steel wire, with a special point and introduced with a drill, is frequently used in surgery of the hand to fix bony fragments in place or to immobilize a joint. The name given to these wires is that of **Martin Kirschner** (1879–1942), a surgeon and student of Trendelenburg. He first used these wires in 1909, introducing one above and one below a fracture site to maintain the traction and countertraction forces and to prevent overlapping of the bone ends. These wires were thin and would

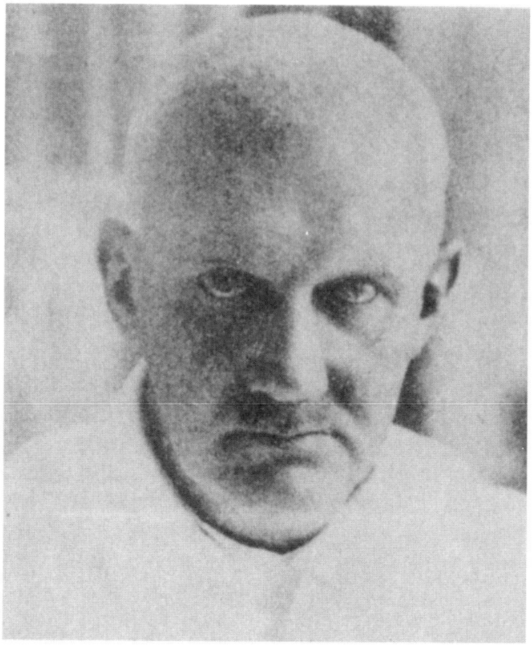

Martin Kirschner. (From Rundschau; Martin Kirschner. Med. Klin., *38*:1103, 1942. Courtesy of the Library of the New York Academy of Medicine)

Ueber Nagelextension.

Von

Dr. Martin Kirschner,

Assistenzarzt.

(Mit 25 Abbildungen.)

Die wenigen bisher bekannt gewordenen Erfolge der Codivilla-Steinmann'schen Nagelextensionsbehandlung stellen es außer Zweifel, daß wir in diesem Verfahren für die Behandlung widerspenstiger und schwer zu reponierender Frakturen ein neues wertvolles Hilfsmittel gewonnen haben. Ich möchte im folgenden zunächst die noch spärliche Kasuistik dieser neuen Methode um einige Fälle bereichern und später einige Verbesserungen kurz besprechen.

1. Ein 20j. gesunder, sehr muskulöser Schnitter brach sich einen Tag vor der Aufnahme in die Klinik beim Sturz vom Fahrrade den l. Oberschenkel zwischen mittlerem und unterem Drittel. Keine Weichteilwunde. — Bei der Aufnahme in die Klinik am 21. V. 09 findet sich eine starke Dislokation der Fragmente, die einen nach innen offenen Winkel bilden. Das distale Fragment weicht typisch nach hinten ab, wesentliche seitliche Verschiebung besteht nicht. Es handelt sich um einen unregelmäßigen Querbruch. Die Verkürzung beträgt 6 cm.

22. V. Unter starker Extension wird in Narkose am v. Bruns'schen Kreuz ein Gipsverband angelegt. Wie das Röntgenbild (Fig. 1) zeigt, wird hierdurch eine nicht befriedigende Verlängerung des Oberschenkels unter

Martin Kirschner: Ueber Nagelextension. Beitr. Klin. Chir., *64*:266–279, 1909. (Courtesy of the Library of the College of Physicians of Philadelphia)

bend, so a tension bow was used to increase the tension in the wire. This was a definite advantage over skin traction or weights and pulley mechanisms. Today the wire is used more as a fixation pin to impale a bony fragment and fix it to the larger fragment; or it is inserted into the metacarpals, where, by passing it into an adjoining stable bone, one may maintain a desired position. Two years later, Fritz Steinmann, in Berne, used the heavy pin called by his name, inserting it into the tibial condyle or calcaneus for traction directly on the skeleton. Kirschner made a point of introducing the wire with a nail starter to prevent it from wandering out, as it does so easily when a high-speed drill is used.

Kirschner was born in Breslau and went to school in Freiburg, Strassburg, Zurich, and Munich, where he graduated in 1904. His father became a high-ranking official in Berlin, and it was there that Kirschner spent 4 years in internal medicine with Renvers. During this time, he was a medical escort to one of the grand dukes on a trip to Ceylon and India, from which came an interesting diary of their travels.

In 1908 he went to Greifswald to work in surgery with Payr, and here he did his first work on the use of fascia lata as a tissue-replacement in tendons and in joints. He went with Payr to Königsberg in 1910. In 1912 he began his experience with wartime surgery, first in the Balkans, then later at the western front, where he became well known for his organizational ability. Apparently, he was capable of planning and carrying out ideas for handling the numerous variety of surgical problems, and of instilling in his co-workers an interest in accurate work based on a careful evaluation of all the factors involved.

When Friedrich, the professor at Königsberg, became ill, Kirschner was recalled to take over the service, and in 1916, after Friedrich's death, he succeeded to the professorship. In the next decade there, his most famous work was the first successful embolectomy of the lung by a procedure devised by his old teacher, Trendelenburg, to whom he gave credit for the procedure and who, in return, credited Kirschner with being able to set up such an efficient system that the operations could be carried out in time to be successful.

In 1927 he was called to Tübingen to succeed Perthes, and there he built a new surgical clinic. In a few years, in 1934, he succeeded Enderlen at Heidelberg, which was the most poorly organized of all the German clinics. He built a new clinic and made it world famous. He was a general surgeon in the widest sense. He made studies on spinal anesthesia, intravenous anesthesia, electrocoagulation treatment of trigeminal neuralgia, extremity surgery, and extension or traction by means of the small wire. Equally versed in abdominal and chest surgery, he also included the genitourinary tract. His surgical technique was based on anatomy, and he was a master. As a general surgeon, he could not see the need for

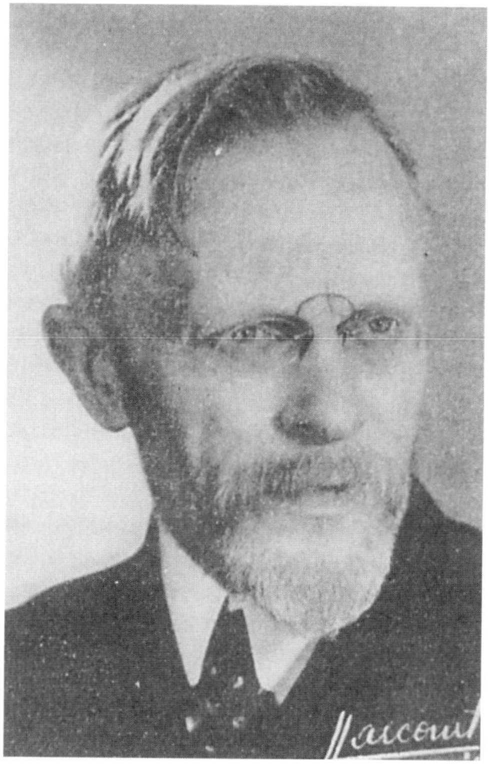

Jules Tinel. (From Ravina, M. A.: Rapport annuel. Bull. Mem. Soc. Med. Hôpitaux Paris, p. 1337, 1952. Courtesy of the Library of the New York Academy of Medicine)

specialization in surgery, and as a leader in German surgery, deplored any attempt to break up surgery into any specialties.

His last years were spent in redoubled efforts at work, trying to overcome the pain and discomfort of a penetrating ulcer of the lesser curvature of the stomach. Only his close friends knew of the problem, and he often appeared to others as being rough, close-lipped, and dejected. When, after 3 years of trouble, an exploratory laparotomy was done, liver metastases were already present, and he died the following year. As no other man did in his era, Kirschner probably encompassed the whole field of surgery as it was then known.

The name of **Jules Tinel** (1879–1952) is frequently used today to describe a sign when a tingling pain occurs on an area of scarred nerve or when a neuroma is percussed. If one reads the original description, it is clear that Tinel distinguished between this pain on pressure over a nerve, or the tenderness present locally at the point of injury, from what he

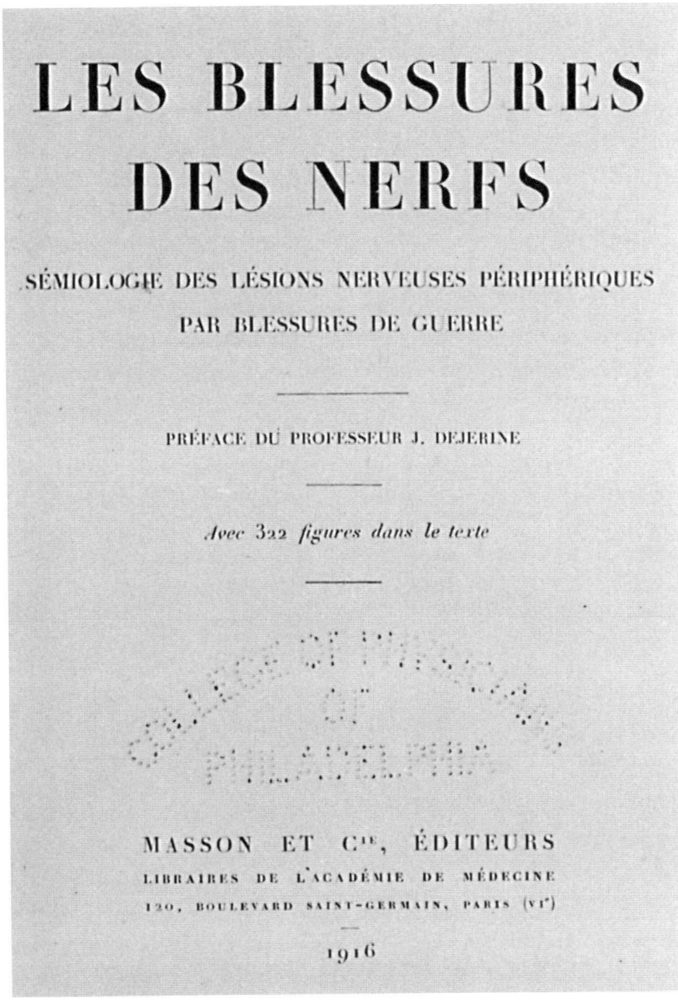

LES BLESSURES
DES NERFS

SÉMIOLOGIE DES LÉSIONS NERVEUSES PÉRIPHÉRIQUES
PAR BLESSURES DE GUERRE

PRÉFACE DU PROFESSEUR J. DEJERINE

Avec 322 figures dans le texte

MASSON ET CIE, ÉDITEURS
LIBRAIRES DE L'ACADÉMIE DE MÉDECINE
120, BOULEVARD SAINT-GERMAIN, PARIS (VIe)

1916

Jules Tinel: Les Blessures des Nerfs. Paris, Masson et Cie, 1916. (Courtesy of the Library of the College of Physicians of Philadelphia)

called his "formication sign." This latter sign is elicited over a nerve trunk distal to the area involved and results in the patient feeling a "creeping sensation," usually compared to that of electricity, in the *cutaneous* region of the nerve. It indicates the presence of newly regenerated axis cylinders. The sign appears 4 to 6 weeks after the wound (or the nerve suture) and persists until the fibers mature. If we use Tinel's formication sign properly, it is a useful diagnostic and prognostic sign for the

76 LES BLESSURES DES NERFS.

Le syndrome de régénération est donc constitué par la réapparition progressive des fonctions d'un nerf, fonction motrice, fonction sensitive, fonction trophique et réactions électriques.

Le début de la restauration après une suture ou une interruption traumatique du nerf, n'est jamais immédiat : les premiers signes de régénérescence n'apparaissent guère avant la 4e ou même souvent la 6e semaine.

C'est qu'en effet toute interruption des fibres nerveuses produit deux ordres de phénomènes. D'une part, elle détermine la dégénérescence de la totalité du segment périphérique, dégénérescence wallérienne. D'autre part, elle provoque en même temps une série de perturbations assez profondes dans le segment central : c'est d'abord une dégénérescence ascendante de la fibre nerveuse au-dessus de la lésion, dégénérescence rétrograde, toujours limitée, qui ne dépasse pas quelques millimètres ; c'est ensuite un retentissement à distance sur la cellule d'origine, que traduit au microscope le phénomène de la chromatolyse cellulaire. C'est seulement après cette courte maladie du nerf que commence la prolifération des cylindraxes du bout central et leur cheminement vers le segment périphérique, et que se manifestent les premiers signes de régénération.

Le retour des fonctions nerveuses se fait parallèlement à la progression des cylindraxes dans le nerf dégénéré ; il suit donc une *marche centrifuge*, c'est-à-dire que la restauration se manifeste d'abord au niveau des muscles et des téguments les plus voisins de la lésion et s'étend de proche en proche, lentement, jusqu'aux muscles et téguments les plus éloignés.

Cette marche n'est du reste pas absolument régulière ; elle se produit assez souvent par poussées, par périodes de quelques jours pendant lesquelles se manifeste l'activité régénératrice, et suivies de périodes de repos. (J. et A. Dejerine et Mouzon.)

En tous cas, la régénération se manifeste à la fois sur le tronc nerveux, sur les muscles, et sur les téguments.

I. — *Signes de régénération du nerf.*

Deux signes de régénération s'observent sur le nerf :

L'apparition du fourmillement provoqué par la pression.

Le retour de la conductibilité électrique.

Le premier est très précoce et très important ; le second est au contraire tardif, presque toujours consécutif au retour de la conductibilité volontaire ; il n'a par conséquent aucun intérêt.

Le *signe important et capital est le fourmillement.* On constate que la pression brusque ou la percussion du tronc nerveux, *au-dessous de la lésion*, provoque une sensation de fourmillement dans le territoire cutané du nerf.

Jules Tinel: Les Blessures des Nerfs. p. 76. Paris, Masson et Cie, 1916. (Courtesy of the Library of the College of Physicians of Philadelphia)

clinician, for one can follow the progress of axis cylinder growth progressively to the hand, as the level at which the sign appears moves farther and farther away from the area of the wound.

Tinel was born in Rouen, the fifth generation of a medical family. His grandfather was a surgeon, and his father was professor of anatomy in the school of medicine at Rouen. He showed a great interest in scientific matters and showed some skill in painting, poetry, and musical composition. In Paris, from 1906 to 1910, he studied with Déjèrine and others and wrote his thesis, "Radiculitis and Tabes." He remained as chief of a service until the First World War, when his regiment was mobilized. Soon he found himself at a hospital at Le Mans. For 3 years he made this a neurological center, and from this came his famous monograph, *Les Blessures des Nerfs,* published in 1916. After 1919 he spent some time in Toulouse, as chief of a neurological laboratory.

In 1922 he reported the first case of paroxysmal hypertension with a suprarenal tumor (pheochromocytoma). He was much interested in encephalitis and the sympathetic nervous system, and later in psychiatric problems.

In 1932 he moved from Charité to Rochefoucauld to set up a laboratory under trying circumstances, in insufficient space, and with meager equipment. There he made many of his apparatuses, particularly one instrument for measuring the intraventricular pressure in an animal by inserting it through a burr hole in the skull. A work on antidromic vasodilatation and the role of the histamines was also done there, and it was in his laboratory that the antihistamine substances were discovered.

He worked at Benjon for 3 years, up to 1940, when the Germans occupied it. He moved to Boucicant and worked with the French underground to hide the downed English and American pilots, who were then guided to the Spanish border by his son, Jacques. Tinel was arrested in May, 1943, and was imprisoned, and his wife was sent to Fresnes for a year. His son, Jacques, was sent to Buchenwald and died of "bad treatment and privations." After the war Tinel returned to the study of the vegetative nervous system and modified Bielschowsky's staining methods of impregnating the neurofibrils.

Tinel was certainly a most distinguished man. A biographer (J. Brincourt, La Presse Medicine, 1952) described him as being a "man of rare grandeur, as much of the heart as the spirit." He was without desire for honors, just as he showed no desire for money. He was known as being devoted and kind to his patients. When he died, a son, Georges Tinel, intern in a Paris Hospital, was left to carry on the Tinel tradition for the sixth generation.

When an occasion arises to use the expression, Tinel's sign, we should recall what he described so clearly and not confuse it with the current incorrect usage. But even if we do not correct this usage, perhaps it is just as well, for we are perpetuating the name of a quiet, dignified, and modest man who loved his country and had the courage of his convictions.

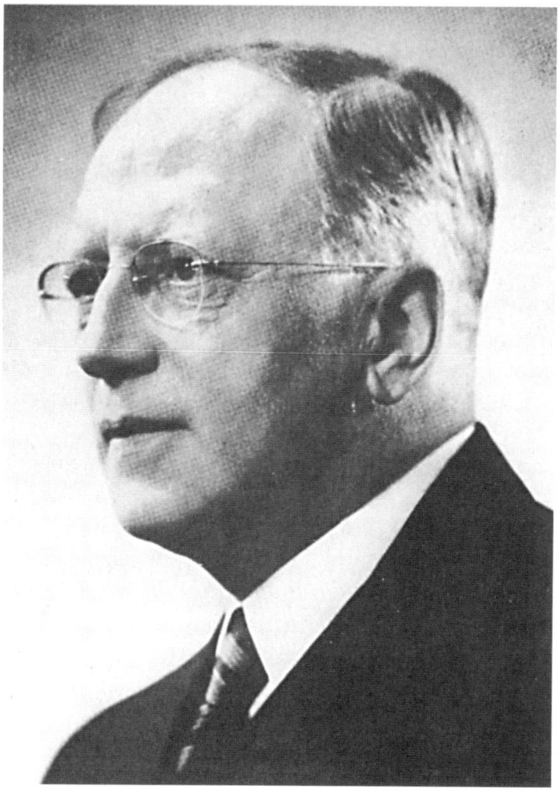

Sterling Bunnell. (From Boyes, J. H.: Bunnell's Surgery of the Hand. ed. 5. Philadelphia, J. B. Lippincott, 1970)

It falls to few men to originate a surgical specialty. **Sterling Bunnell** (1882–1957) did just that for surgery of the hand, although he would deny it and admit only that it was a "field of special interest." He was a general surgeon, in the true meaning of the word, and believed that surgery of the hand was a combination of what the specialties of orthopaedics, plastic surgery, and neurosurgery now cover, as applied to the upper extremity. Although his book is titled *Surgery of the Hand*, he defined the hand as beginning mechanically at the elbow, but dynamically in the opposite hemisphere. It was this concept of the upper extremity as being a unit, to be treated for all its disabilities by one surgeon, that was his greatest contribution, and because of him some of the Army hospitals in World War II were designated as hand centers. (We saw how Robert Jones was able to do this for the orthopaedic cases in World War I, and Gillies, of whom we will deal next, did the same for maxillofacial in-

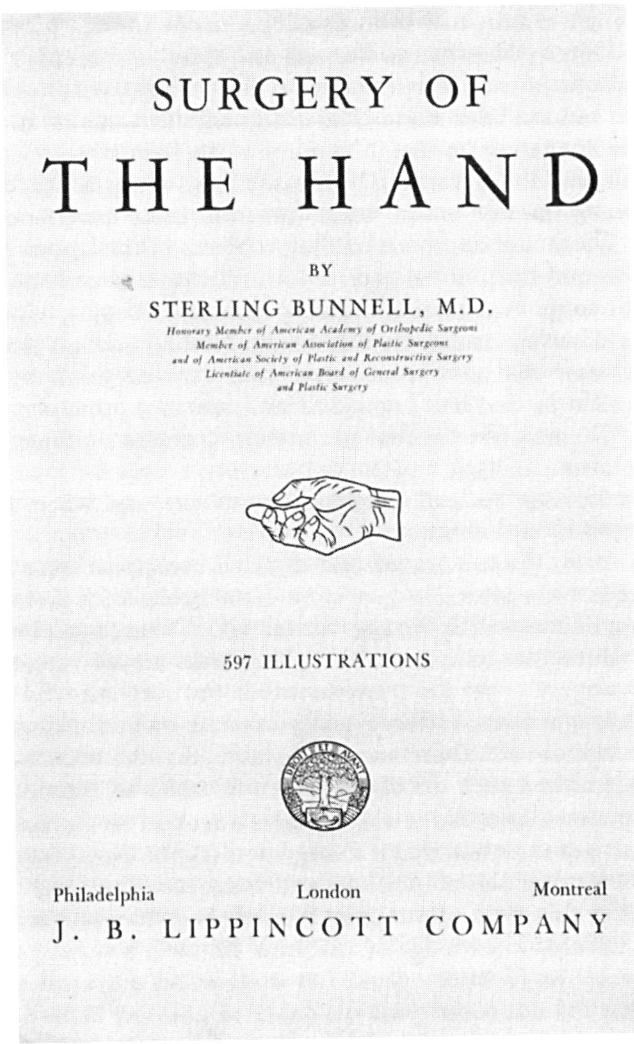

SURGERY OF

THE HAND

BY

STERLING BUNNELL, M.D.

Honorary Member of American Academy of Orthopedic Surgeons
Member of American Association of Plastic Surgeons
and of American Society of Plastic and Reconstructive Surgery
Licentiate of American Board of General Surgery
and Plastic Surgery

597 ILLUSTRATIONS

Philadelphia London Montreal

J. B. LIPPINCOTT COMPANY

Sterling Bunnell: Surgery of the Hand. ed. 1. Philadelphia, J. B. Lippincott, 1944.

juries.) Through Bunnell's influence, surgery of the hand as a special field spread throughout the world.

We use Bunnell's name eponymically for an operation for restoring opposition of the thumb, the first one to use the pulley principle in rerouting a tendon, and for another procedure for overcoming the claw deformity. This latter operation was an extension, on a better anatomical basis, of Stiles' operation. This operation of Stiles developed from one of

Lexer's, which in turn had been developed from an idea proposed, but not carried out, by Nussbaum. Bunnell also is remembered for a method of tendon suture, the development of the pull-out wire technique of inserting a tendon into bone. He designed instruments and splints, which bear his name, for use in surgery of the hand.

All of this was done, working by himself in private practice, during the years between the two world wars, and from these experiences he developed a systematic approach to the problems of the upper extremity. When the opportunity came, and he was called as a consultant to recommend to the surgeon general of the army a means of coping with the large number of disabled hands, he was ready. He had had experience, had tested the methods and procedures, had verified them by detailed follow-up records, and had organized his ideas into principles. As Pliny had said, "No man can become commanding unless a subject suited to his talents presents itself and an opportunity occurs for their development." For 25 years Bunnell developed his talents, and when the opportunity occurred, he was ready.

In book form, the condensed and distilled principles were set down, and examples were given; *Surgery of the Hand* broke forth on the surgical world like a new moon in the sky. Mayer said, "There is no book in any language which can compare with it, for it has actually created a new branch of surgery." Yet the inexperienced, the surgeon who had been trained to carry out some stereotyped procedure by mimicking a preceptor, was disappointed. There were complaints that the book was hard to read, that it lacked such details as where to make an incision (e.g., in tendon transfers), and that it did not have a section on anatomy. I recall that Bunnell's answer was that if a surgeon didn't know anatomy and the basic surgical principles of incisions and tissue handling, then he should not be doing this type of surgery. Bunnell had little use for the man without a detailed knowledge of anatomy. Bunnell, a superb anatomist, knowledgeable in function, could not understand a system of surgical training that did not encompass the study of anatomy as he saw it.

The book was distributed widely, and soon a second edition included specific examples of patients from the various army hand centers. The style remained the same, with terse, short sentences and strong, active verbs, written in what might be called basic English. Bunnell was not a verbose man; as Paget, he never used two words if one would do. If a catch phrase would be of value, he coined it. For example, to express the importance of using a tourniquet and working in a bloodless field, he said, "You can't fix a watch in a bottle of ink." He disliked the style of writing in which so much is in the passive voice, and he used the short, strong, Anglo-Saxon root words, in contrast to the longer, weaker Romance roots. He once described a large dense constricting scar on the forearm, not by listing its measurements, color, and so forth, but by saying that it "girdled" the forearm. He used the term "atraumatic technic" to designate the care and handling of tissues, avoiding damage to the succulent soft tissues. He abhorred the techniques of blunt dissection, preferring sharp knives and scissors. To watch him do a radical neck or an axillary dissection was like a demonstration of anatomy of the parts, sliding along the nerves and vessels with the scalpel, not using a stick sponge for wiping away the areolar tissue, but clearly dividing it and removing the offending mass in a true en-bloc excision.

Motions were not wasted—a plan of operation had been worked out before the surgery began—and with instruments arranged within easy reach, he moved from one step to another with unhurried speed. There was no hit and miss in his surgery, everything was thought out beforehand. If some unusual condition did arise, that also had been planned for. As a commander planning an attack, he always had a way to retreat or another flank to turn in getting to the object of the operation. Bunnell was not an experimental surgeon in the modern sense of the word. True, many of his procedures were unique, but all were based on proven principles applied to the particular problem.

He was a general surgeon, interested in all fields of surgery, except intraocular surgery, which he thought required the ultimate in technical skill. He was an exponent of Böhler's ideas on the treatment of fractures. In the First World War he had served in France on a neurosurgical team, devised a valve for the face mask of the anesthetic machine to allow positive pressure anesthesia for open-chest operations, and preferred perineal to suprapubic prostatectomy because it was a more anatomical procedure. His work on peripheral nerves covered the body, from the first reported repair of the facial nerve in the canal (and also its reconstruction by a free nerve graft) to repair of the sciatic, posterior tibial, recurrent laryngeal, and spinal accessory.

He was most interested in hip surgery because of his own experience. Soon after the First World War, having taken up flying as a hobby in what was then called the Jenny, he crashed while coming in for a landing in the Wawona section of Yosemite National Park. An intracapsular fracture of the neck of the right femur was treated by traction in a Hodgden splint, Whitman spica, and so forth, with resulting nonunion. After a year, Dr. Fred Albee of New York, with Leo Mayer helping, reduced it and transfixed it with an autogenous bone peg from the tibia. For years this hip was almost perfect and stood up to severe use in fishing and hunting trips. Later, changes in the head developed, with increasing pain and discomfort and a noticeable gluteal limp. When the Smith-Petersen nail was devised, Bunnell designed a guide for its insertion that was used on some of the earliest trials of that pin in the San Francisco area.

Bunnell's name is such a part of the field of hand surgery that it is difficult to pick out certain accomplishments that are more properly his own ideas and procedures. The basic concept of surgery of the extremity as a field of activity for one surgeon, who is capable of handling the involvement of all the various tissues, has been described as Bunnell's fundamental contribution. From the more technical aspect, one might say that his pulley operation for opposition of the thumb was original. Here, for the first time, it was pointed out that in median palsy, a transferred tendon should be directed from the area of the pisiform to the metacarpophalangeal joint of the thumb, in order to restore the function of opposition of the thumb. The result is to restore a function, not the action of a single muscle. To do this—that is, to redirect a musculotendinous unit of adequate power from the forearm—he used the pulley principle, comparing it to the omohyoid or abducens pulleys, to redirect the force in the proper direction. All previous operations—and in his paper he reviewed all the known procedures—had failed to obtain the true force in the proper direction. When used with the proper indications (that is, a low median palsy), the results are excellent; but if used with the presence of a combined median and ulnar palsy, or a segmental loss as from poliomyelitis, when adductor function is also lost, the results can be poor. One often finds an operative procedure being blamed for a poor result when the surgeon fails to appreciate the careful study of the patient required and the necessity for following not only the techniques, but the indications for the procedure. One does not blame an architect of a building if a wall cracks or if a door fails to swing properly, but rightly looks to the builder who failed to use the level or the plumb line, as any good workman would do, or to the engineer who failed to consider the stresses and to allow for them.

Wire sutures had been used for many years, but Bunnell devised a method of using a stainless-steel wire suture for tendons that satisfies all the requirements of a good suture and that can then be removed when its usefulness is over. This so-called pull-out wire has widespread use and is adaptable to many conditions. Shortly after he first described it, one of his colleagues in San Francisco reported its efficacy in repairing the anal sphincter.

Bunnell was not one to do some unusual procedure and then rush into print. Priority meant nothing to him. His method of preparing a tubed abdominal pedicle (credited to Gillies and Filatov) was a modification that was not reported until many trials of use and years had passed. I personally saw this procedure in 1935 or 1936 and urged him to report it, but he answered that there were still some technical problems to be solved. Nothing came out about it until it appeared in his book in 1944.

Bunnell used autogenous nerve grafts in the hand, forearm, foot, and face, the donor areas being amputation stumps of fingers or the sural nerve in the calf. In 1936 we were able to study the long-term results.

Bunnell's detailed records of his patients were most impressive, and in my experience were only matched by those of Harvey Cushing in his service at the Peter Bent Brigham.

When one looks back at the giants we have chosen, the most striking characteristics are their knowledge of anatomy, the exquisite detail of their records of the history and findings at examination and operation, and the careful follow-up of the patients for as long as necessary. When these characterisitcs are combined with the integrity of purpose and the quest for the truth that men like Steindler had, and with an innate modesty of their own accomplishments rather than the propagation of some pet idea, they are figures that command our respect and strengthen us in our desire to emulate them. Bunnell was one of these great figures.

Bunnell's family history is like a saga of the Old West. When California became a state of the Union and because of the gold discovered there, a rush of prospectors crossed the plains to seek their fortune. The Wells Fargo Company, with its stagecoaches and banking facilities, became an important enterprise in the booming city of San Francisco. James Sterling Bunnell, a young man from the East, was sent to San Francisco to be an auditor for the company. He brought his wife, who was from an old family, the Mapes, whose forebears had been in the Revolutionary War as well as in the Civil War. A son and daughter were born, and the family moved across the bay to Berkeley before the turn of the century. Sterling Bunnell grew up in this area.

When he was very young, Bunnell showed an intense interest in birds and animals. Who or what drew him to this interest, I do not know. It may be that some contact with someone in this field influenced him. His sister, who was an artist, later married a poet and illustrated her husband's books. She told me that their parents' home was always full of bird skins and mounted specimens. I recall a patient, a retired scientist from the Smithsonian Institution, who had known Sterling Bunnell as a young man. He told me that when Bunnell decided on medical school, the country lost its best potentially world-famous natural scientist.

Bunnell was an accomplished collector of birds before he went to college, and we can only surmise that his study of anatomy and function of birds and mammals found its final goal in the study of human anatomy and function. Bunnell's anatomy was functional and practical; he knew the embryological development and was a firm advocate of the Darwinian School.

He was graduated from medical school in San Francisco and then spent several months at the Crile Clinic in Cleveland, Ohio, the most important result of which was his design of a valve for the mask used in inhalation anesthesia, which permits positive pressure and therefore an open-chest operation.

In these years, hyperthyroidism was being treated surgically, and

George W. Crile was one of the masters. Crile had developed a staged operation, whereby the poles were ligated first and then the gland was removed when the acute phase subsided. When iodine was found to produce a remission, this two-stage operation was no longer necessary; but some patients who were on the medical regimen too long reverted to a hyperthyroid state, which was resistant to all treatment. The culmination was a "thyroid crisis," with hyperthermia, tachycardia, and a very high mortality rate. To handle this problem, an operative procedure of unusual character was developed. The patient was anesthetized, and a rapid subtotal thyroidectomy was done, ligating the bleeders, but not closing the wound. Instead, the wound was packed loosely with gauze, which was sometimes saturated with a solution such as acriflavine. On the following day in the patient's room, under the pretense that a change of dressing was necessary and that it might be uncomfortable, a mask was applied to the patient's face. Quickly from outside the room came the full operating-room setup, and a secondary closure was done. Having been a witness to the success of this method, in contrast to others with higher mortality rates, I can vouch for the relatively smooth convalescence of these very sick patients.

After his time with Crile, Bunnell returned to San Francisco and for a while worked with a surgeon, W. I. Terry, who was well known especially for his thyroid surgery. During the First World War, Bunnell was in France with a neurological team and apparently was interested enough in this field to consider specializing in it in a Philadelphia hospital. After the war, back in San Francisco, he studied the problems of tendon repair, and he soon produced reports of methods of handling the tendons, of new instruments to use, and of the results of various procedures. It was during these years that Bunnell developed a referred practice of general surgery, traveling (as many San Francisco surgeons did) to the surrounding area to see patients, operate, and then return the following week. He took up flying with the tragic result already mentioned.

California, in the meanwhile, taking advantage of the experience of other states, had set up a workmen's compensation law that was quite advanced. Under this law, the employer became responsible for the treatment of injury incurred on the job by any employee, and to protect himself, the employer engaged an insurance company to act for him. The State set up its own company in competition with the private companies, thus setting a pattern of handling the problems. Bunnell's system of recording the findings at examination of such disabilities is the basis for the current form of reporting and evaluating such problems.

In San Francisco, the Presidio, originally a Spanish garrison post, was a famous Army headquarters, where Pershing had been commander when the earthquake and fire of 1906 ravaged the city. On these grounds, just inside the Golden Gate, was Letterman General Hospital, named after the surgeon general of the Civil War who had introduced an ambulance service for the wounded. A young surgeon, one of the first in the Army to specialize in orthopaedics, was stationed there after World War I; a colonel, later Surgeon General Norman T. Kirk, he was an expert on amputations and was familiar with Bunnell's work.

After the United States entered World War II, with the improved treatment of the wounded, a large number of men returned to the United States with severe impairments of the upper extremity. Prompt treatment, well-staffed field hospitals closer to the action, and antibacterial and antibiotic drugs made possible conservative surgery of the extremity rather than amputation. This large group of patients in need of reconstructive surgery presented a problem to General Kirk. He asked Bunnell to make a survey of the base hospitals in the United States and to recommend a plan of treatment. Bunnell left his practice (his two associates, L. D. Howard and Donald Pratt, had already been called to active duty), and from then on, acting as a consultant, Bunnell spent at least one-half of his time in visits and in traveling throughout the country. His plan—finally adopted over the objections of the Army's chief consultant, a general surgeon without any experience in extremity surgery—was to set up a hand service in certain general hospitals, one for each of nine geographic areas known as service commands. Some had already been designated as specialty centers, for vascular work, neurosurgery, or plastic surgery. Often, a combination of plastic surgery and neurosurgery was used; it was in these particular specialty centers that Bunnell insisted on a distinct and separate hand service, with its own staff, to handle the complete care of the extremity. It was this principle of having surgeons who were qualified to do the skin, bone, tendon, and nerve work take charge of the problem, and not shuttling the patient from one service to another, that was Bunnell's greatest contribution. Helping to staff these centers, Bunnell made repeated visits, lecturing, demonstrating, and consulting on the various problems. The men in these centers made up the nucleus of an expanded group that became the founding members of the American Society for Surgery of the Hand. This organization developed toward the end of the war, when it was apparent that many of the men would soon be returning to their civilian practices; they wanted to maintain their interest in this new surgical field. Some were general surgeons, others orthopaedists or plastic surgeons, but all felt a common bond in developing a better knowledge of this most interesting and stimulating field of surgery.

Bunnell was the guiding influence of the society in its early years. He insisted on its membership being restricted to those who had "contributed something worthwhile to surgery of the hand" and believed that a small organization made up of these men could contribute then to the education of others. For this reason, the annual meeting was held just prior to that of the American Academy of Orthopaedic Surgeons, a group which he believed would be most receptive and a specialty which included within its borders about two-thirds of the problems seen in the hand. Despite strenuous objections from some of the general surgeons and plastic surgeons, that pattern has persisted. From a few score at the first meeting, now more than a thousand orthopaedists take time out to spend the extra 2 days to learn what is going on in the field of hand surgery. There are now hand societies throughout the world, and there is an International Federation, which aims to standardize such things as measurements of function, pre- and postoperative evaluation of results, and the classification of congenital deformities. Just as in Bunnell's time the West was opened and a new era begun, so he opened to surgeons a whole new field of endeavor. This is his legacy.

Bunnell was a stoic; he never complained if he was tired, sick, or in pain. His last years must have been quite uncomfortable, with constant pain in his hip and a failing myocardium, but he remained active. Even on the day before he died he was designing a backpack for carrying an oxygen bottle, so he would not miss the annual duck-hunting season. He had one son, Sterling Jr., who took his medical degree at the University of California and practices psychiatry.

Bunnell was an example of what has been defined as a well-informed individual—one who gets all of the facts, adds the results of his own experiences, records his data, and then organizes all into a concept or a principle. Correlating and structuring the experiences into a principle of "law" is not part of the experience itself; this comes from outside, is different and distinct, but is an active part of the knowing process. Bunnell had this quality of condensing experiences into principles, making what some call the "big picture."

He never thought of repairing a tendon or a nerve, but rather looked upon the problem as restoring function to the hand. There is an old story of the man who came upon a building site, where stone masons were laboriously shaping large granite masses into blocks, and stopped to ask one of the workmen what he was doing. The reply was a laconic, "I'm chipping away at this rock." When he asked the next workman the same question, however, he heard the proud reply, "I'm building a cathedral."

Bunnell was born about the time that Koch was discovering the tubercle bacillus and that Pasteur was working on fermentation problems; he was a teenager when Röntgen discovered the x-ray and when the first vascular suture was done. He began practicing in the period before the sulfa drugs and penicillin and before insulin was discovered. If he were to start today, with all our sophisticated aids in diagnosis and treatment, he would still be a pioneer, for he would go back to the fundamentals of surgery—anatomy, pathology, and expert technique—directed by a fertile mind.

Born the same day, month, and year as Bunnell, but half a world away in New Zealand, **Harold Delf Gillies** (1882–1960) was also a pioneer, but in maxillofacial reconstruction. One could hardly find two more different personalities.

Gillies's name is used today in referring to the method of tubing a pedicled skin graft. He wrote about it first in 1920 and again in 1934. He gave credit to Filatov, who had reported it in 1917, saying that he, Gillies, had used it independently the same year. At that time, during the First World War, with the large number of casualties (2,000 patients were admitted to his unit in a 10-day period after the battle of Somme), he had plenty of opportunities to use the method, to broaden its applications,

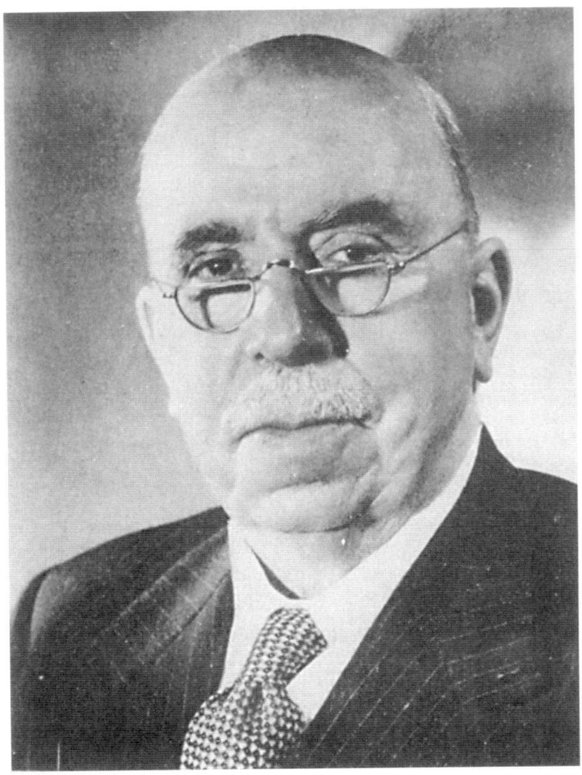

Harold Delf Gillies. (From J. R. Nav. Med. Serv., *45*[1], 1959. Courtesy of the Library of the New York Academy of Medicine)

EXPERIENCES WITH TUBED PEDICLE FLAPS[1]

SIR HAROLD GILLIES, C.B.E., F.R.C.S., F.A.C.S. (HON.), LONDON, ENGLAND
Plastic Surgeon to St. Bartholomew's Hospital, London; the London County Council; the Royal Air Force; St. Andrew's Hospital, Dollis Hill, London, and the North Staffordshire Royal Infirmary, Newcastle-under-Lyme

A TUBED pedicle flap is a type of delayed flap in the form of a tube in which the long edges are sewed together. It is thus completely separated from its bed except at the two attached ends and is not replaced, as is a delayed flap. As for all types of delayed flap the object of the procedure is to induce a blood supply parallel to the long axis of the flap. The tubed flap is different from the other forms of delayed flap in that it prevents any form of granulation or scar tissue formation on its deep surface.

It was first described by Filatoff in 1917 (1), but the idea occurred to me quite independently in the same year (3). Its immense usefulness was immediately recognized by my colleagues in the War at Sidcup. It has since undergone many modifications and its field of usefulness has been extended. In the process its limitations have also been more accurately defined (4).

GENERAL CONSIDERATIONS

The rationale of the flap is to increase its longitudinal blood supply at the expense of the transverse, so that it can survive on the blood supply of one end only. The idea is by no means new and the original Tagliocotian (6) operation was a simple delayed flap. Other forms of delayed flap tend to produce considerable contraction from granulation tissue on the deep surface. The time factor is also different from that of the usual delayed flap as in my own experience I seldom, if ever, trust the blood supply at one end of the flap until a minimum interval of 3 weeks. Lymph stasis in the flap is also one to which consideration should be paid, some of the "tubes" undoubtedly show this condition, and if so, they can be left a further interval of time until the lymphatic circulation is established, their subsequent success as regards viability, adaptability, and cosmetic effect is considerably enhanced. In a long established tubed pedicle, which has had many removes, great liberties can be taken with its blood supply.

ADVANTAGES

Its chief advantage lies in the readiness and safety with which *large quantities of skin* may be transported from a distance. The tubed pedicle having been successfully made, its size can be increased either laterally or longitudinally so that huge quantities of skin can safely be transplanted. It is of particular use where no massive direct flap is available such as is usually used when body skin is transferred directly to the arm or forearm. Another of the characteristics of a tubed pedicle is that when once established its *flexibility* allows it to be twisted and turned in the most liberal manner without causing anxiety as to its viability. It lends itself to temporary attachment through an *intermediate host.*

When the wrist is used as a means of conveying a large abdominal tubed pedicle flap one has given it an additional mobile pedicle whose base may now be considered to be at the shoulder. The flap can therefore be carried to any position of the body from the sole of the foot to the crown of the head or to any intermediate portion. The use of the wrist as an intermediate host is a great step in advance over the caterpillar method. Its *viability* has already been stressed. As a *cosmetic flap* it is at least up to the standard of any other type of flap except in one or two specific restorations.

DISADVANTAGES

The chief disadvantage is the *time factor,* which includes the financial aspect. For example, the shortest time that an abdominal flap can be transported to the neck works out in practice as shown in Table I.

Factors increasing the time. When flaps larger than, say 8 by 3 inches are required or when there are branch extensions of the flap some provision must be made for safeguarding the blood supply of these elongated masses such

[1] Presented before the Clinical Congress of the American College of Surgeons Boston October 15-19, 1934.

Harold Delf Gillies: Experiences with tubed pedicle flaps. Surg. Gynecol. Obstet., *60*:291, 1935. (Reproduced by permission of Surgery, Gynecology & Obstetrics. Courtesy of the Library of the College of Physicians of Philadelphia)

and to study the complications and limitations. It was on October 3, 1917 that he made a large flap on the chest to cover the face, leaving openings for the eyes and mouth, with two side straps from the shoulder area to carry the blood supply, and, apparently without previously planning it, tubed these two side straps, thus closing in the raw areas. Later the idea was carried over to form a tube as a type of delayed flap, promoting a longitudinal blood supply at the expense of the transverse vessels. Tubing the pedicle, of course, cut down the amount of granulation tissue and subsequent contraction. The method allows the transfer of large areas of skin with great facility, for the tube permits some twisting and turning without much danger. For distant parts, an intermediate attachment of one end to the wrist as a carrier permits transfer to almost any part of the body. The idea of tubing the pedicle was undoubtedly a great one, and Filatov gets the credit for first doing it, but Gillies went further and extended its use to delayed flaps, and in unusual situations. Priority did not seem to bother Gillies. He only heard of Filatov's work while on a trip to the United States in 1919, and he quickly acknowledged the work when he verified it; but one of his associates, Aylward, who reportedly tubed a pedicle 15 days after Gillies, bore a grudge against his chief for more than 16 years, when he still claimed the idea of the operation. Gillies made no reply to this. Today Gillies and Filatov share the credit, and our patients benefit from it.

Gillies was born in Dunedin, New Zealand, and was sent to school in England when he was 8, but he returned home to go to college. Athletically inclined, he was captain of the cricket team and was an excellent golfer. When he returned to England for further university work, he already showed traits for which he was later quite famous. Still an athlete, he was on the rowing team, was a top amateur golfer, played the violin, loved a practical joke, and to appearances took life not too seriously.

Why he chose medicine we do not know. He studied at St. Bart's, qualified in surgery, and was house officer to D'Arcy Power and to an ear, nose, and throat specialist named Harmer. Obtaining his fellowship in the Royal College of Surgeons in 1910, he worked with a Mr. Wilson, also in E.N.T. In 1911 he married one of the nurses at the hospital. In the same year, in the French open golf tournament, he was a leader for the first three rounds; however, he was the winner of an important match at Sandwich in 1913.

When World War I began, his whole life was changed. In 1915 he was in France with a Belgian ambulance unit and met a man named Valadier, who, though not a trained dentist, had practiced in Paris, working on jaw injuries and performing bone grafts for these disabling injuries. Gillies became interested in such work, but even more so when he was given

Leidemann's book (in German) on wounds of the mouth and jaw. He then heard of and visited Morestin in Paris, who was at that time France's leading plastic surgeon.

Through friends in higher places, Gillies was sent back to England and organized and developed a center for the care of maxillofacial injuries. His forte was in getting close cooperation with dentists and in having artists assigned to his unit. He even enrolled in a course for artists, to gain experience.

At this time, Gillies's knowledge of the literature of plastic surgery was scant, and when he tried to revisit Morestin in Paris, he was refused. On his own he built up a loyal following. Although all spoke of his unorthodox teaching methods, his indifferent approach to public speaking, and how incorrigible he was in practical jokes, he had a careful, detailed approach to a patient's problem, instilling not only confidence but great respect. His golfing skill was often mentioned, but never with the seriousness that his fly-fishing was. In this there was no thought of joking, such as in a golf game, when he once demonstrated the advantage of using a high tee by driving his golf ball off the top of a beer bottle. McIndoe, who claimed blood relationship with him and who was later his associate, said that his friends praised him for his achievements but damned him for his unpredictability, his incurable lateness in appearing at scheduled operative times, and his fiendish sense of humor. Gillies described McIndoe as a "distant cousin."

Gillies practiced plastic surgery in London with Kilner after the war, and when World War II broke out, he was asked to organize the services of plastic surgery. This he did with great effect, but kept up his golf (+2 handicap) and his fly-fishing and organized the British Society of Plastic Surgery. He died in 1960, recognized by all for his achievements in establishing plastic surgery in England as a specialty in its own right.

In the early years of this twentieth century, three men appeared who would influence the surgery of the upper extremity throughout the world: Steindler, Bunnell, and Mayer. Steindler, the oldest of the three, would come to the central United States in 1907 and in a few years would make his service at Iowa City a mecca for all orthopaedists. His work in the fundamentals of tendon surgery and especially tendon transfers would carry on the Viennese tradition in the center of our country. Bunnell, 4 years younger than Steindler, would make San Francisco known as the birthplace of surgery of the hand, and his wide experience and detailed studies, based on clinical observation, would give us techniques for handling many of the problems in this field. Mayer, the youngest, born in the South but educated at Harvard and Columbia, would, after his original work with Lange in Munich and Bielsalski in Berlin, return to New York and establish the orthopaedic department of the Hospital for Joint Diseases. He would outlive the others.

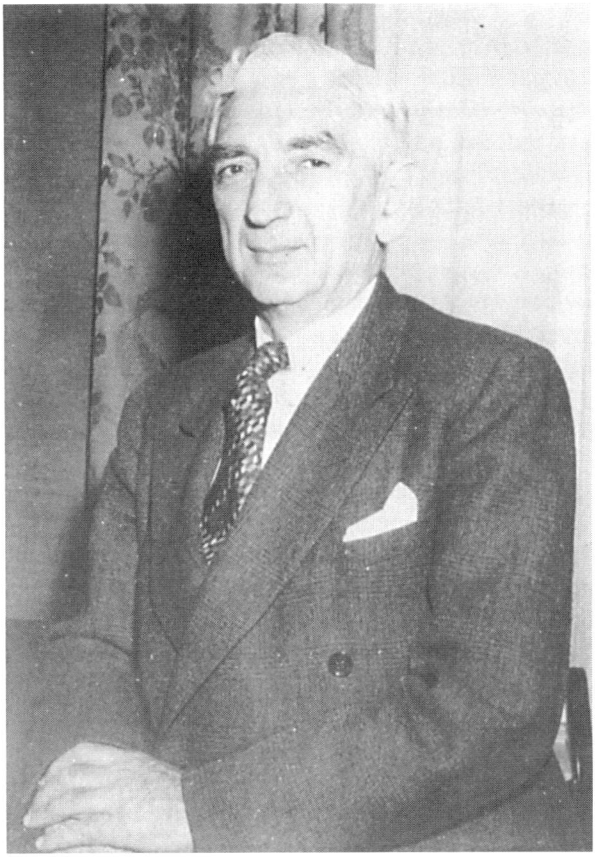

Leo Mayer. (Courtesy of the Library of the New York Academy of Medicine)

All three were surgeons, were members of the American Society for Surgery of the Hand, and were giants. Steindler we have called a scholar; Bunnell, an original thinker and a pragmatist. Mayer was all three.

Leo Mayer (1884–1972), the son of a proprietor of a general store, was born in a small town in Alabama. When his father died, Leo, then age 4, was brought to New York by his mother to live with her family. A strong family relationship, with the loving guidance of a devoted mother, made certain his education on a broad basis in the sciences and the classics. His love of music and poetry was a great source of pleasure to him all his life, and his skill on the violin was more than that of an amateur. Few will forget a dinner meeting, in the early years of the American Society for Surgery of the Hand, when Leo Mayer brought a Stradivarius and demonstrated the clear and beautiful tones of that particular instrument.

Graduating with honors from Harvard, he doubled up on his studies to receive also a master's degree. Sometime during his last year, he decided on medicine as a profession. His medical school years were spent at Columbia University in New York City, where Huntington was professor of anatomy and William Darrach was a young instructor in surgery. In his last year of medical school, Mayer's first contact with orthopaedics under Gibney and Whitman was disappointing, but general surgery was not, and this influenced him to try for a surgical internship at Mt. Sinai Hospital. Here, it was the pathologist, Emanuel Libman, who encouraged him in his review of the German literature and who was responsible for his acceptance as a volunteer in the clinic of Fritz Lange in Munich, where he arrived in January, 1912.

Fritz Lange, Adolf Lorenz, and Albert Hoffa were the originators of orthopaedic surgery in Germany. All had been general surgeons. Lange had been with Madelung, first at Rostock and then at Strassburg. Lange had spent a year with Lorenz in Vienna and had come to Munich in 1896, where he had developed an orthopaedic service and contributed much to the treatment of paralysis, tuberculosis of the spine, congenital hips, and scoliosis. Lange implanted celluloid or metal strips to help stabilize the spine, setting the groundwork for the later operations of Hibbs and Albee. His work on tendons involved all the procedures of shortening, lengthening, and transfer. Both he and Vulpius (Heidelberg) had reported many procedures and carried on a spirited argument as to whether a part of a split tendon could function independently and whether tendon to bone was better than tendon to tendon as a fixation for tendon transfers. Lange's views won out—a muscle with two tendons cannot perform two separate functions, and tendon to bone proved a stronger attachment, as Bielsalski later proved, to everyone's satisfaction.

Lange credited the work of Drobnik and Nicoladoni for some of his ideas on tendon transfer and that of Gluck for his studies in the use of foreign materials for tendon lengthening. There were many problems to be solved, and Lange's clinic was one of the best places to observe the German school of orthopaedics.

Mayer worked here on the problem of adhesions to the transferred tendons, spending many months trying various ways of preventing them. Most of the transfers involved lengthening of the tendon by the use of silk strands, where adhesions formed and spoiled the results. Mayer used various substances to surround the tendon, such as peritoneum, vein, Cargile membrane, and ointments. He also performed the bone growth experiments, disproving Macewen's theory. It was a work of Bielsalski that gave Mayer the idea which he called the physiological method of tendon transfer. Later, when given the opportunity, he went to Berlin and completed and published the book that is still a classic in the field of tendon surgery. Mayer's rule for tendon transfers developed

THE PHYSIOLOGICAL METHOD OF TENDON TRANSPLANTATION[1]

By LEO MAYER, A.M., M.D., New York

Orthopedic Surgeon, Oskar-Helene Home for Crippled Children and Red Cross Military Hospital, Am Urban, Berlin, Germany

I. Historical; Anatomy and Physiology of Tendons

I REFER here not to the free transplanting of a tendon but to the transference of its point of insertion in such a way as to alter the function of a muscle. A rational system of tendon transplantation must be based upon an accurate knowledge of the anatomy and physiology of tendons and muscles. That our present systems are empyric rather than rational is shown by the marked discrepancy in the operative methods of prominent orthopedic surgeons. Thus Lange[2], on the basis of over 2,000 tendon operations, is radically opposed to Vulpius whose experience is almost as great. Lange insists upon the periosteal implantation of the transplanted tendon first advocated by Drobnik, and lengthens the tendon artificially by silk strands. Vulpius maintains the advantages of sewing the transplanted tendon to the paralyzed tendon, the method first advocated in 1882 by Nikoladoni. Lange sutures the tendon under the greatest possible tension, Vulpius under moderate tension, Stoffel without any tension whatever. Lange draws the tendon through the fatty subcutaneous tissues, Vulpius beneath the fascia. The discrepancies in the after-treatment are equally marked. Thus Lange advocates six weeks' fixation, whereas Putti begins to exercise the transplanted tendon several days after the operation.

These divergent views do not concern inconsequential details but the essentials of the operation. It is evident that a tendon transplantation differs radically from a finished surgical procedure, such as a gastro-enterostomy; in the latter, despite slight differences of method, all surgeons are agreed as to the essentials, whereas in the tendon transplantation scarcely a single principle in the operative procedure can go unchallenged.

In these papers I wish to report the result of studies in the anatomy and physiology of tendons, conducted during the past 2 years in the experimental department of the Oskar-Helene Home for Crippled Children, Berlin, and to suggest a series of tendon operations based upon these studies. The essential principle of many of these operations was published in 1910 by Professor Biesalski, the director of the hospital, and it was with his co-operation that the final operative technique has been formulated. I am deeply indebted to Professor Biesalski for his encouragement and for the opportunity to test clinically the practical effectiveness of the operations. The anatomical dissections and the animal experiments were performed in the Pathological Department of the municipal Urban Hospital, Berlin, whose director, Dr. M. Koch, freely placed all the facilities of his department at my disposal.

THE HISTORY AND PLAN OF THE RESEARCH

These studies had their inception during the winter of 1912. Professor Lange of Munich, in whose clinic I was then serving, finding that the results of many tendon transplantations were impaired by post-operative adhesions, urged the need of experimental work to determine the method of preventing these adhesions. I assisted Dr. Henze, of New Haven, in the attempt to solve this problem. We tested successively the effect of ensheathing the tendon operated upon, with fat, fascia, veins, cartilage, vaseline, thin tubes of rolled silver, and Cargile membrane. In all instances except with the Cargile membrane the adhesions proved firmer than where nothing was inserted to prevent their formation. The Cargile membrane, though giving better results than the other substances, did not act effectively to prevent adhesions.

An excellent means, however, proved to be the technique employed by Biesalski: the utilization of the sheath of the paralyzed tendon as a simple physiological means of

[2] See bibliography at end of third paper.

[1] This article is the first in a series of papers on "Tendon Transplantation." The other two articles will appear in subsequent issues.

Leo Mayer: The physiological method of tendon transplantation. Surg. Gynecol. Obstet., *22*:182–197, 1916. (Reproduced by permission of Surgery, Gynecology & Obstetrics. Courtesy, the Library of the College of Physicians of Philadelphia)

out of this work. It states that the proper tension can be determined by approximating the origin and the insertion, and uniting the tendon with zero tension. Mayer became acquainted with Robert Jones during a short visit, after leaving Munich and before going to Berlin. He was much impressed and said later that he counted the friendships of Jones, Bielsalski, and Bunnell as the most important factors in his professional development.

Berlin in 1913 was considered the ultimate goal of German surgeons. Bielsalski was chief; Lange had refused the appointment to succeed Hoffa. Mayer was provided with unlimited anatomical material and animals for experimentation, and when the clinical results were proven reliable, his monograph was published in German.

War broke out in 1914, and Mayer was given the opportunity of caring for many wounded, while Bielsalski took over the organization of a rehabilitation service. Because Mayer was a United States citizen, his position became difficult as Germany and the United States broke off diplomatic relations, but he was asked to continue his work until war was actually declared. Then he and his wife were allowed to return to the United States via Denmark. It is said that he was provided with an honor guard to the train leaving Berlin. What a difference a few years make. Had Mayer been in Berlin in the 1940s, he would have, if lucky, been put in a concentration camp, or, if not, would have been eliminated completely.

The rest of Mayer's professional life was spent in New York City. He worked with Albee at the Post-Graduate Hospital and then started the service at the Hospital for Joint Diseases. Always interested in rehabilitation, he started a society for care of crippled children and later organized the Federation of the Handicapped.

Mayer was an active member of the American Orthopaedic Association, the American Academy of Orthopaedic Surgeons, and the American Society for Surgery of the Hand. His contributions to the surgery of the upper extremity were numerous, among which were a modification of the Steindler flexorplasty and a transfer of the trapezius muscle for shoulder abduction. He was a teacher, and hundreds of men look upon him as respectfully as he did his teachers.

Ischemic contracture of the forearm muscles, as described by Volkmann in 1889, became a well-recognized clinical entity, but a similar process occurring in the intrinsic muscles of the hand was not recognized until years later. In 1920, in the reports of a meeting of the Buenos Aires Surgical Society, an article appeared, titled "Volkmann's Contracture of the Intrinsic Muscles of the Hand," describing a patient with the classical findings. The author was **Ricardo Finochietto** (1888–1962). Because this local journal was not included in the bibliographic indices of the English-speaking countries, the condition went unnoticed until a report was made by Bunnell, Curtis, and Doherty of patients seen among the wounded of World War II. Finochietto's patient, first seen in 1918, was a 17-year-old mechanic whose left hand had been squeezed between an automobile and the pavement some 6 months previously. Immediate pain and great swelling had occurred. A splint and bandage had been applied from the elbow to the tips of the fingers, but they had to be loosened because of the swelling and intense pain, which required morphine for the first 4 days. After a month, massage and baths had reportedly been started, but the persistent swelling hid the underlying deformity.

When the patient was first seen 6 months after the injury, the thumb was held tightly to the index finger, and the index and middle fingers were flexed at the metacarpophalangeal joints. Flexion of the interphalangeal joints was noted to vary with the position of these metacarpophalangeal joints. There was an apparent deformity of the base of the second metacarpal from a healed fracture. There was no involvement of the forearm or of the thenar or hypothenar muscles, and the little finger escaped. Thus this first case illustrated a lesion limited to the adductor, first dorsal interosseus, and the interossei of the second and third clefts. Operative treatment consisted of resection of 1½ to 2 cms. of the contracted interosseus and the adductor muscle and the tendinous insertions into the metacarpals, but with total resection of the first dorsal necessary before the thumb could be abducted. The corrected position was maintained by a splint with traction to extend the finger. Detailed follow-up examinations were made over a 9-month period. In the discussion, Finochietto said that the detailed description of the case had been reported because in the literature available on Volkmann's contracture, he had not found a case where the lesion was limited to the small muscles of the hand. Although some reports had mentioned the involvement of the small muscles of the hand—but without precise data—in none had the hand lesion seemed to require any specific treatment. Finochietto said, in his reported case, that he assumed that the fracture resulted in a hematoma infiltrating the interosseous spaces with their unyielding walls, and thus shutting off the blood supply of the muscle tissue. He also said that the patient had been placed in a tight bandage, as was so often the case in the classical Volkmann's contracture of the forearm. Finochietto's description is clear and explains the abnormal findings on an anatomical basis.

After Bunnell's report, many patients were seen with contractures of these intrinsic muscles, some involving, as did his cases, the thenars and hypothenars as well. There are also a number of patients with typical intrinsic contracture developing after prolonged lying on the hand or forearm, such as in comatose states following heavy drug administration. These usually show the classical findings with involvement of all the small muscles of the hand. But there are minor contractures which may involve only a few interossei, such as those of the index and middle fingers, seen in various diseases or following specific trauma, say to a metacarpal. Therefore, the test for intrinsic contracture, which Finochietto demonstrated but which became better known after Bunnell's detailed description, should be a part of the diagnostic examination of a hand. The test is very simple, but must be done correctly to be meaningful. Based on the anatomy of the interosseous muscle—which takes origin from a metacarpal, passes volar to the axis of motion of the metacarpophalangeal joint, and then inserts into the wing of the extensor mechanism—it is apparent that, if the metacarpophalangeal joint is held in extension, any fixed contracture will restrict the flexion of the proximal interphalangeal joint. Other causes may be present, such as adherence of the extensor tendons to the proximal phalanx, but if the metacarpophalangeal joint is then flexed and the interphalangeal joint now flexes easily and completely, we can localize the lesion to the contracted interosseous muscle. Now anything that will shorten the distance between origin and insertion, such as a subluxation or dislocation of the proximal phalanx, will allow the interphalangeal joint to flex even in the metacarpophalangeal joint appears to be in extension. Similarly, if the index finger is deviated ulnarward, the test will not be positive, for on this digit only the first volar interosseous muscle (i.e., the one on the ulnar side of the index) has a wing attachment, the first dorsal being almost always and entirely a true abductor (with slight flexion) of the index. Thus in performing the test, one must make sure that the proximal phalanx is in proper relationship with the metacarpal, reducing any subluxation and lining up the proximal phalanx with the metacarpal. The test may elicit even minor degrees of contracture by exaggerating or prolonging the distance that the musculotendinous unit has to travel. For example, in the index, placing the finger in radial deviation may demonstrate a slight shortening of the first volar interosseous muscle, which would not be apparent with the finger straight or in ulnar deviation. Similarly, in the long finger, where the second dorsal interosseous muscle has a minimal attachment to the extensor wing, in contrast to that of the third dorsal on the ulnar side, displacing this finger radially will demonstrate a minimal contracture. These signs are often seen in patients with rheumatoid disease of the metacarpophalangeal joints and are always present when ulnar drift has resulted.

Ricardo Finochietto was the younger of two brothers who were born in Argentina of Italian immigrants. As in North America, where many other Europeans migrated to the new world, Argentina was a popular site for

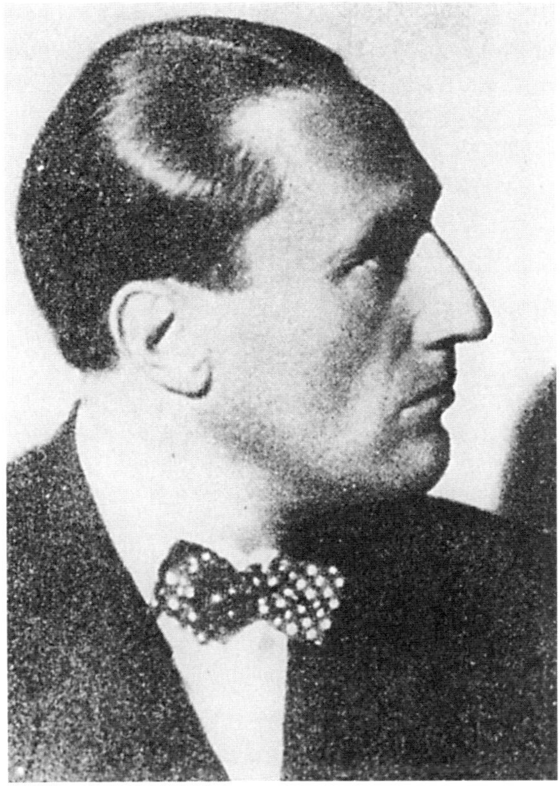

Ricardo Finochietto. (From Doctor Ricardo Finochietto. Nuevo director de La Prensa Médica Argentina. Prensa Med. Argent., 35[12]:473, 1948. Courtesy of the Library of the College of Physicians of Philadelphia)

Italians. In Argentina, where orthopaedics is a well-established specialty, the influence of Putti is very strong. Jose Valls and Carlos Ottolenghi, Vall's associate and successor in the chair, were both trained by Putti, and the Italian hospital is one of the country's leading centers for orthopaedic training.

The Finochiettos, Enrique and Ricardo, were both general surgeons, and although both were great teachers and great surgical technicians, it was Ricardo who was the most renowned, for he was the teacher, fluent and lively and with a skill for explaining and demonstrating the principles he evolved. Their efforts resulted in what has been called the Finochietto School of Surgery, which still carries on at Rawson Hospital, where the department of orthopaedics, traumatology, and surgery of the hand is directed by Eduardo Zancolli.

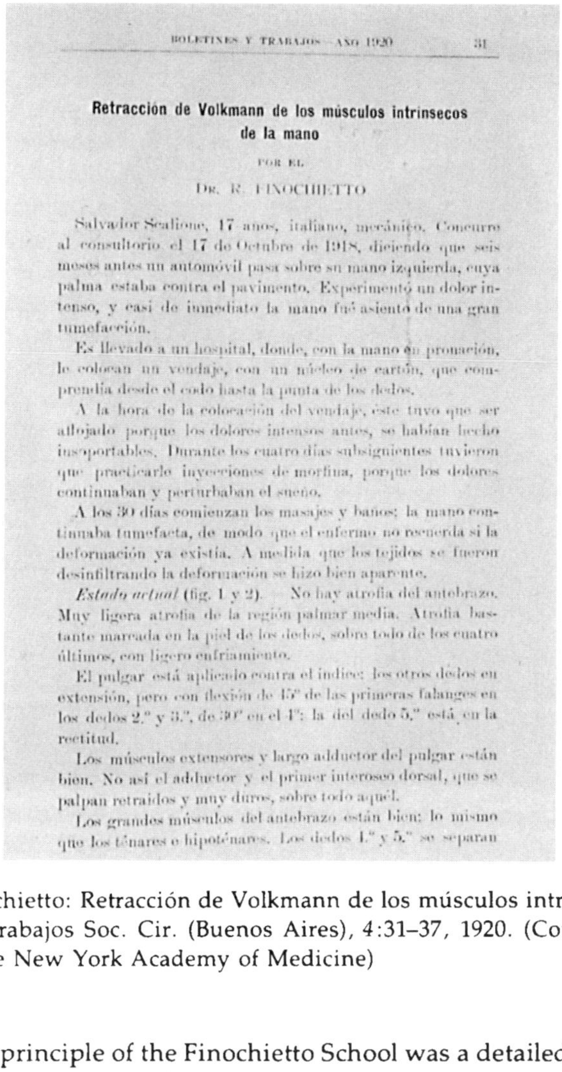

BOLETINES Y TRABAJOS—AÑO 1920 31

Retracción de Volkmann de los músculos intrinsecos de la mano

POR EL

DR. R. FINOCHIETTO

Salvador Scalione, 17 años, italiano, mecánico. Concurre al consultorio el 17 de Octubre de 1918, diciendo que seis meses antes un automóvil pasa sobre su mano izquierda, cuya palma estaba contra el pavimento. Experimentó un dolor intenso, y casi de inmediato la mano fué asiento de una gran tumefacción.

Es llevado a un hospital, donde, con la mano en pronación, le colocan un vendaje, con un núcleo de cartón, que comprendía desde el codo hasta la punta de los dedos.

A la hora de la colocación del vendaje, éste tuvo que ser aflojado porque los dolores intensos antes, se habían hecho insoportables. Durante los cuatro días subsiguientes tuvieron que practicarle inyecciones de morfina, porque los dolores continuaban y perturbaban el sueño.

A los 30 días comienzan los masajes y baños; la mano continuaba tumefacta, de modo que el enfermo no recuerda si la deformación ya existía. A medida que los tejidos se fueron desinfiltrando la deformación se hizo bien aparente.

Estado actual (fig. 1 y 2). — No hay atrofia del antebrazo. Muy ligera atrofia de la región palmar media. Atrofia bastante marcada en la piel de los dedos, sobre todo de los cuatro últimos, con ligero enfriamiento.

El pulgar está aplicado contra el indice: los otros dedos en extensión, pero con flexión de 45° de las primeras falanges en los dedos 2.° y 3.°, de 30° en el 4°: la del dedo 5.° está en la rectitud.

Los músculos extensores y largo adductor del pulgar están bien. No así el adductor y el primer interoseo dorsal, que se palpan retraidos y muy duros, sobre todo aquél.

Los grandes músculos del antebrazo están bien: lo mismo que los ténares e hipoténares. Los dedos 1.° y 5.° se separan

Ricardo Finochietto: Retracción de Volkmann de los músculos intrinsecos de la mano. Bol. Trabajos Soc. Cir. (Buenos Aires), 4:31–37, 1920. (Courtesy of the Library of the New York Academy of Medicine)

The basic principle of the Finochietto School was a detailed knowledge of anatomy as the basis for the surgical procedures to be developed. Every young trainee spent time in the anatomy laboratory and then in experimental surgery on animals. Constant emphasis was placed on good surgical technique and on care and gentleness in handling tissues. Through postgraduate courses, the teaching was spread widely throughout South America.

Enrique died in 1948, remembered principally for a rib-spreading retractor with his name attached, but which was called the Argentine Ambassador. Ricardo kept on working for another 14 years, active to within a few weeks of his death. Although we have no eponym for him, he was a master surgeon, as so many of the giants we have written about, superbly trained in anatomy and capable of using his hands to perform the technical procedures indicated. His name is perpetuated in the school of surgery he founded. One of his students has described him as requiring of them not only the utmost in professional ability but also in conduct and in devotion to the responsibilities of the profession. He was strict in discipline, but patient in explanation, using diagrams and sketches on whatever was available, even a wall or window, to illustrate a point. Knowledgeable in art, literature, and music, he delighted in taking his students to art exhibits. Many have stood on his shoulders to see farther.

A fundamental study of the processes of tendon repair and the rate of tendon healing, presented to the American Surgical Association in 1940, was the work of **Michael Mason** (1895–1963). This work established the rationale for the period of rest after a tendon repair and demonstrated the fallacy of immediate motion of a repaired tendon. An earlier paper, co-authored with Shearon, is one of the classics of the literature of experimental tendon repair.

Mason was born in Illinois of a family of doctors and took his college degree at Northwestern University. The First World War saw him in a hospital unit, but as an orderly in the operating room. After graduating from Northwestern University Medical School and an internship at Cook County Hospital, he spent almost a year in Vienna studying pathology. Returning to Chicago, he became associated with Drs. Allen Kanavel and Sumner Koch.

"Mike," as he was called by practically everyone, was a quiet, soft-

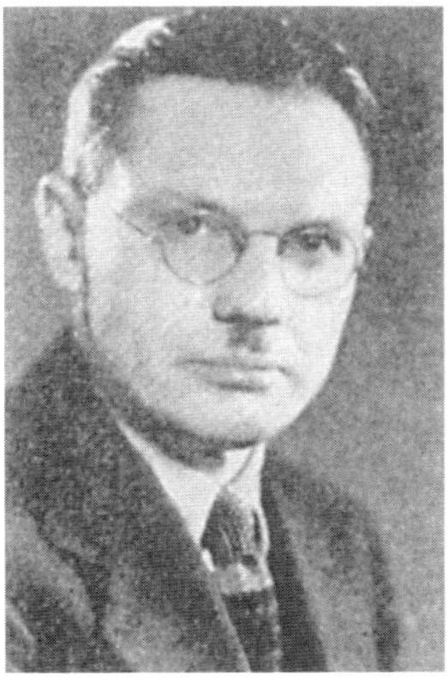

Michael Mason. (From Rocky Mt. Med. J., 37:125, 1940. Courtesy of the Library of the New York Academy of Medicine)

ARCHIVES OF SURGERY

VOLUME 25 OCTOBER, 1932 NUMBER 4

THE PROCESS OF TENDON REPAIR

AN EXPERIMENTAL STUDY OF TENDON SUTURE AND TENDON GRAFT

MICHAEL L. MASON, PH.D., M.D.

AND

CLARENCE G. SHEARON, M.D.

Schweppe Fellow in Surgery, Northwestern University Medical School

CHICAGO

CONTENTS

Historical Data
Experimental Data
  Statement of Problem
  General Outline of Experimental Work
Process of Tendon Repair as Revealed by Experiments with Tendon Suture
  Technic of Experiments
  Protocols of Experiments with Tendon Suture
  The Process of Repair in a Sutured Tendon
Process of Repair as Revealed by Experiments with Tendon Grafts
  Technic of Experiments
  Protocols of Experiments with Tendon Grafts
  The Process of Repair in a Tendon Gap Bridged Across by a Tendon Graft
Résumé of Healing Process of Tendon Grafts
Comment on Results of Experimental Work
  The Importance of the Sheath and Peritendinous Tissues
  The Tendon
Summary
Bibliography

The process of tendon repair and the technic of tendon suture and tendon graft are two of the major problems of present day surgery. The thirty-eighth session of the French Congress of Surgery, 1929, devoted considerable time to the report of Bonnet and Bloch on the repair of tendons of the hand. This, in fact, was one of the three main subjects discussed, the other two being surgical intervention in

From the Department of Experimental Surgery, Northwestern University Medical School.

Dr. Mason worked under a surgical fellowship granted by a friend who desires to remain unknown.

Michael L. Mason, and Clarence G. Shearon: The process of tendon repair. An experimental study of tendon suture and tendon graft. Arch. Surg., 25:615, 1932. (Copyright 1932, American Medical Association. Courtesy of the Library of the College of Physicians of Philadelphia)

spoken man who influenced surgical practice in many ways through his work in the nation's leading surgical societies, as well as in his scientific contributions. Often he was elected secretary and then later president, and he was active on the editorial boards of two of the leading surgical journals. He was an excellent teacher and was admired and respected by his students. He was also an accomplished artist, and his lithographs were seen in many exhibitions.

In 1959 a sudden vascular accident, reportedly a carotid occlusion, left him with an almost complete aphasia and paralysis of the right upper extremity. He never recovered use of his right hand, and 4 years later, in 1963, a rupture of an abdominal aneurysm proved fatal.

We have seen that Kanavel, a general surgeon in Chicago, had called attention to the anatomy of the hand in relation to the course of infections of that part. He and his successors, Sumner Koch, Michael Mason, and Harvey Allen, were responsible for hand surgery in the Middle West. Through their influence on medical education and their intimate contact with Northwestern Medical School and the services at Passavant and Cook County Hospitals, they have taught generations of students, interns, and residents.

Mike Mason's influence in surgery of the hand was that of an accomplished investigator and surgeon. His writings were characterized by a careful delineation of the facts, based on well-done experiments, with logical conclusions. He spoke easily and with obvious sincerity, and because he was an active clinical surgeon, his opinions were respected. His style was not that of the propagandist, burning with a missionary-like zeal to convert everyone to his ideas. Rather he had a low-profile way of explaining what he found and showing his results honestly and completely.

Mike could be brief and to the point when he thought it would make a point. Once having been appointed to a committee whose function was obscure, to say the least, he was asked to give a committee report. His response was, "The committee reports progress."

He was a welcome discussant to a paper. One could always be sure that he would discuss, with courtesy and a mild manner, the salient points and bring up those that the author had not considered. Any criticism was given in an unbiased manner. Many will miss this gentlemanly surgeon from the Windy City.

POSTSCRIPT

Our story of the persons whose names we use as eponyms has covered a period of a little more than 250 years. Each individual was a giant of his time. It is fitting that we honor them by recalling their contributions, but we should not forget that sometimes it was only because of some other person or some other circumstance that they have become eponyms.

They were a varied lot. Some were young when they first did their best work: Pacini was still a student and Klumpke was an intern, and Raynaud described his classic signs in a thesis for his medical degree. But Heberden waited, and, as Paget, made his contributions in his last years. Some were obviously being directed by another. Adams was stimulated while working with Little. Schwann did his best work under Müller's influence; after leaving Berlin, Schwann was responsible for only one major discovery. Others worked alone. Waller, just starting practice, set up a laboratory in his own home, and Ramón y Cajal, with his first microscope and a book of instructions, worked out techniques that made him famous. Duchenne, with his battery and electrodes, overcame innumerable obstacles to become, with Charcot and Marie, one of the triumvirate of French neurology.

Some were scholars, well versed in the classics and fluent in languages. Heberden wrote in Latin, and Volkmann defended his thesis in what was described as "fluent" Latin. Others struggled along with a self-obtained core of practical knowledge. For some, such as Duchenne, speaking before others was impossible; yet Paget was known as the most gifted orator of his day.

Some profited from a development or discovery that provided the opportunity. Erb and Duchenne both benefited from Faraday's discovery of the induced current. The microscope provided the opportunity for Pacini, Waller, Schwann, and Ramón y Cajal, as did Röntgen's x-rays for

Kienböck and Perthes. The Civil War gave Mitchell the material for his classic work, and in Europe the wars of the nineteenth century presented opportunities to Stromeyer, Thiersch, Volkmann, and Esmarch. World War I provided the material for Tinel's and Froment's studies, Stiles's operation, and Robert Jones's and Gillies's skills in organization. World War II afforded Bunnell the opportunity to demonstrate the basic principle of surgery by one surgeon for an entire region, as opposed to the division of surgical care by tissue involvement.

Many, such as Heberden, Garrod, Madelung, and Stiles, are remembered for what was a minor piece of work, whereas their major contributions have gone unnoticed. The names of others are in our memory because chance or fate put them in the right place at the right time. Had Schwann not dined with Schleiden or had Little succeeded as an apothecary and surgeon, we might not have an eponym for the cell theory, or the operation of subcutaneous tenotomy, or the world-renowned Royal National Orthopaedic Hospital. If Belchier, at dinner with his friend, the calico printer, had not been curious about the color of the pork bone, we might have waited years before some other means of study was found.

It is difficult to find a common characteristic among the men and one woman who have been selected for this study. In the main, they were well grounded in the basic knowledge available during their time. If surgeons, they were usually anatomists as well, it being not unusual for both chairs to be held by the same person. Above all, they were curious; this was a common attribute. If they saw something abnormal—implying obviously that they knew the normal—or some unusual pattern of happenings, they recorded their observations clearly and succinctly. "Observe and record"—is that not what Hippocrates advised? This basic dictum, the very foundation of our profession, was their guide. What better advice for the neophyte than, "Know the normal, observe and record the abnormal"?

Index

Numbers in bold face indicate principal discussions; numbers in italics indicate portrait illustrations.

Acrocephalosyndactyly, Apert on, 157
Adams, William, 22, 33, 37, **49–52**, *50*, 62, 64, 212
Addison, Thomas, 24
Albee, Fred, 191, 202, 204
Allen, Harvey, 211
Albinus, Bernhard Siegfried, *9*, 10, 11, 14
Allbutt, Thomas Clifford, 100
Amici, Giovanni Battista, 60, 106
Amputation, Petit on, 15
Anatomy, Bell on, 29
  Bennett on, 117
  Cleland on, 115
  Gruber on, 61
  Guyon on, 104
  von Langer on, 72
  Meissner on, 95
  Merkel on, 125
  Müller on, 47, 59
  of brain, Beevor on, 140
    Klumpke on, 152
  of nervous system, Martin on, 19, 21
  Parona on, 122
  pathologic, Gruber on, 61
    Ramón y Cajal on, 136
  Ranvier on, 113
Andry, Nicolas, 15
Angina pectoris, Heberden on, 16
Ankles, diseases of, Thomas on, 148
Anomalies, Gruber on, 61
Apert, Eugène, **157–159**, *158*
Aran, François-Amilcar, 44
Arterial disease, Raynaud on, 110
Asepsis, Stiles on, 152
  Würtz on, 4
Atrophy, muscular, Duchenne on, 44
Avicenna, 5

Babinski, Joseph, 175
Bailey, Percival, 139, 164
Balfour, Francis Maitland, 68
de Balzac, Honoré, 34, 110
Bandage, elastic, von Esmarch on, 81
    Martin on, 86
Baronio, Giuseppe, 77
Barré, 143, 152
Barton, 117
Basedow, Carl Adolph, 139
Beevor, Charles Edward, **140–142**, *140*
Belchier, J. B., 102, 213
Bell, Charles, **28–30**, *28*, 32, 76
Bell's law, 28
Bell's palsy, 28
Bennett, Edward Halloran, *116*, 117
von Bergmann, Ernst, 38, 39, 51
Bernard, Claude, 70, 90, 106, 114
Bichat, Marie-François-Xavier, 33
Bielsalski, 147, 200, 202, 204
Bielschowsky, 187
Bier, August, 148
Billroth, Theodor, 11, 45, 85, 99, 125, 171
Bladder stone, Camper on, 14
  Heberden on, 16
Bleeding, tourniquets in, Cushing on, 161
    Perthes on, 166

Blood, restriction of flow of, Esmarch on, 81
Martin on, 86
Blood vessels, histological development of, Thiersch on, 78
Bochdalek, 61
Boerhaave, Hermann, 11
Böhler, 191
Bone, growth of, Keith on, 102
Ollier on, 102
Wolff on, 81
Bonnel, Julie, 44
Borges, A. F., 55
Bottini, Albertino, 122, 123
Boyer, Alexis, 33
Brachy-syndactyly, Poland on, 74
Brain, anatomy of, Beevor on, 140
Klumpke on, 152
surgery of, Cushing on, 161
Branca family, 1
Breast, diseases of, Cooper on, 25
Breschet, 104
Bright, Richard, 24, 25
Brown-Séquard, Charles-Édouard, 70
Brunschwig, Hieronymus, 1
Budge, Julius L., 70
Bünger, Christian, 77
Bunnell, Sterling, 147, 148, 152, 181, **188–197**, *188*, 200, 201, 204, 213

Caesarean section, Camper on, 14
Calvé, 166
Camper, Pieter, **12–14**, *12*, 37
Camper's chiasm, 12, 14
Camper's fascia, 12
Cancer, surgical treatment of, Volkmann on, 99
Cazelles, 52
Cell theory, Schwann on, 57
Charcot, Jean-Martin, 41, 42, 118, 139, 142, 212
Charcot-Marie-Tooth disease, 139
de Chauliac, Guy, 1, 5
Chauveau, Auguste, 102
Cheselden, William, 18
Chickenpox, Heberden on, 16
Chiene, 153
Chopart, François, 23
Claw deformity, Stiles on, 152
Cleland, John, *113*, **115–117**
Cline, Henry, 23
Clubfoot, Adams on, 49
Delpech on, 37
Little on, 49
Codman, Ernest, 103
Cohnheim, Julius, 109, 142
Colles, Abraham, **26–28**, *26*, 30
Colles' fascia, 27
Colles's law, 27
Congenital anomalies, Gruber on, 61
Contracture, Cooper on, 52
Dupuytren's, 22, 31, 59
Adams on, 49, 50
Finochietto on, 204
Volkmann, 95, 204, 205
Cooper, Astley Paston, **22–26**, *23*, 30, 31, 33, 52, 76
Cooper, William, 23
Cornil, Victor, 114
Corpuscle, Meissner's, 95
Vater-Pacini, 59
Coxitis, juvenile, Perthes on, 166
Craig, Charles Franklin, 25
Crile, George W., 194
Cruveilhier, Jean, 44
Cushing, Harvey William, **161–165**, *162*, 193
Cuvier, Georges, 65

Darrach, William, **173–175**, *174*, 202
Darwin, Charles, 116
Davis, John Staige, 52
Deformity, of newborn, Apert on, 157
Déjèrine, Jules, 139, 142, 143, 150, 152, 187
Déjèrine-Klumpke, Augusta, 106, 142, 143, **149–152**, *150*, 212
Delpech, Jacques Matthieu, *35*, **37**, 47, 49, 65, 178
Denonvilliers, Charles Pierre, **52–54**, *53*, 55, 104, 115
Desault, Pierre-Joseph, 23, 27
Dieffenbach, Johann Friedrich, 35, 45
Dislocations, Cooper on, 25
Dott, Norman, 164
Dover, Thomas, 165
Drew, A. H., 59
Drobnik, 202
Duchenne, Guillaume, 38, **41–45**, *42*, 76, 93, 118, 119, 142, 149, 150, 212
Duhamel, 102
Dumreicher, 131
Dupuytren, Guillaume, 22, **30–37**, *31*, **44**, 52, 110, 129
Dyschondroplasia, Ollier on, 100

Electricity, Erb on, 119
Enderlen, 183
Epithelial cells, Thiersch on, 77

Erb, Wilhelm Heinrich, 38, **118–121**, *119*, 127, 139, 142, 149, 150
Erb-Duchenne paralysis, 44
von Esmarch, Friedrich, 45, 47, **81–83**, *83*, 85, 89, 115, 125, 162, 213
Esophageal diverticulum, Nicoladoni on, 131
Eulenburg, Hermann, 132
Eustachius, 11
Eye, anatomy of, Merkel on, 126
  disorders of, Horner on, 105

Fabry, Wilhelm, 6
Faraday, Michael, 38, 44, 118, 212
Fasciotome, Adams, 49
Fasciotomy, Adams on, 50
  Delpech on, 37
Fibula, fracture of, Dupuytren on, 32
Filatov, Vladimir Petrovich, 81, **172**, *173*, 192, 197, 199
Fingers, contraction of, Adams on, 51
  ligaments of, Cleland on, 115
  nodes of, Heberden on, 15
  nodules of, Garrod on, 74
Finochietto, Enrique, 207, 208
Finochietto, Ricardo, **204–209**, *207*
First-aid, Esmarch on, 83
Flatt, 158
Flourens, M. J. P., 65, 72
Foix, Charles, 139, 143, 152
Foot, deformities of, Little on, 49
Forrester-Brown, 152
Fracture(s), Bennett on, 117
  Camper on, 14
  Colles on, 26
  Cooper on, 25
  Dupuytren on, 32
  Kirschner on, 181
Fremont, Jules, **175–178**, *176*
Friedreich, 119, 121, 183
Froment, 213
Fulton, John, 164

Galen, 1, 5
Garrison, Fielding H., 38
Garrod, Alfred Baring, **73**, *73*, 213
Garrod, Archibald Edward, 74
Gibney, 202
Gibson, T., 55
Gillies, Harold Delf, 81, 148, 172, 173, 188, 192, **197–200**, *197*, 213
Gluck, 202
Gnudi, Martha, 77
Goiter, de Quervain on, 160
Golgi, Camillo, 134, 135, 136, 152
Goodsir, John, 102, 115
Gout, Garrod on, 74
Gowers, William Richard, 118
von Graefe, Albrecht, 106
von Graefe, Carl F., 77
Grainger, Richard Dugard, 49
Grant, Robert, 47
Gros, Charles, 44
Gruber, Wenzel L., **61**, *62*
Guyon, Felix J. C., 53, *103*, **104**, 123

von Haller, Albrecht, 15, 102
Halsted, William S., 162, 163
Hammond, William Alexander, 90
Hand. See also structures and disorders.
  anatomy of, Bell on, 29
  dorsum of, swelling in, Secrétan on, 142
  infections of, Kanavel on, 170
  nerves of, Martin on, 62
  surgery of, Bunnell on, 188
    Paget on, 64
Harrison, Ross Granville, 68
Harvey, William, 11
Heberden, William, **15–18**, *16*, 73, 99, 212, 213
Heine, Jacob, 44
Heister, Lorenz, 15
Hemochromatosis, von Recklinghausen on, 109
Henle, Jacob, 49, 59, 95, 125, 126, 127
Henoch, Eduard Heinrich, 16
Hernia, Cooper on, 25
Hibbs, 202
Hindu flap method, in reconstructive surgery, 1
Hip, diseases of, Thomas on, 148
  dislocation of, Camper on, 14
  surgery of, Adams on, 49, 50
    Bunnell on, 191
His, Wilhelm, 41, 68, 152
Histology, Ramón y Cajal on, 134
  Ranvier on, 113, 114
Hodgkin, Thomas, 24, 47
Hoffa, Albert, 202, 204
Hooke, Robert, 59
Hoover, Charles, 158
Horner, Johann Friedrich, 56, *105*, **105**
Horner, William E., **55–57**, *55*
Horrax, Golbert, 164
Horsley, Victor, 141, 142, 163
Howard, L. D., 195
Hunt, Agnes, 147
Hunt, Verne, 178

Hunter, John, 16, 19, 30, 37, 102
Hunter, William, 30
Huntington, George Sumner, 202
Hutchison, Jonathan, 150
Hyperthyroidism, Crile on, 194
Hyrtl, Josef, 61

Infections, Kanavel on, 170
Ischemic contracture, Finochietto on, 204
  Volkmann on, 95, 204, 205
Ivy, Robert Henry, 52

Jackson, Hughlings, 141
Jenner, Edward, 45, 87, 88
Joints. See also specific joints.
  anatomy of, von Langer on, 72
  diseases of, Thomas on, 148
  physiology of, Weber on, 41
Jones, Robert, **145–148**, *145*, 156, 188, 204, 213

Kanavel, Allen B., **170–172**, *170*, 209, 211
Kaplan, Emmanuel, 44
Keen, W. W., 90, 93
Keith, Arthur, 81, 102
Key, Charles Aston, 74
Kienböck, Robert, **168–170**, *168*, 171, 179, 213
Kilner, 200
Kirk, Norman T., 195
Kirschner, Martin, **181–184**, *182*
Klumpke, Augusta, 106, 142, 143, **149–152**, *150*, 212
Knee, diseases of, Thomas on, 148
Koch, Robert, 38, 61, 77, 153, 196, 209
Koch, Sumner, 172, 211
Kocher, Emil Theodor, 85, 123, 153, 160, 162
Kölliker, 135
Kraus, Fedor, 78

Laennec, René, 33, 34, 44
Lamarck, Jean-Baptiste, 65
Lambe, William, 69
Landouzy, Louis, 150
Landsmeer, J. M. F., 14
Lane, William Arbuthnot, 102
Lange, Fritz, 129, 147, 200, 202, 204
von Langenbeck, Bernhard R. K., 45, 81, *83*, **84**, 95, 99, 125
von Langenbeck, Konrad J. M., 85
Langenbeck osteotomy, of femur, 50
von Langer, Carl, *70*, **72**
Langhans, 160
de Lapeyronie, François Gigot, **6–9**, *7*
Lawson, 78
Leander, Richard, 99
LeFort, 78
Legg, 166
Leidermann, 200
Lembert, François-Jules, 35
Letterman, Jonathan, 39, 89, 195
Lexer, Erich, 152, 190
Libman, Emanuel, 202
Ligaments, of finger, Cleland on, 115
von Linné, Carl, 19
Lister, Joseph, 38, 39, 50, 67, 78, 83, 99, 102, 123, 153
Listerism, 51, 98, 100, 152
Lithotomy, Cheselden on, 19
  Guyon on, 105
Little, William John, 37, **47–49**, *47*, 52, 57, 62, 76, 95, 118, 125, 212, 213
Locomotor ataxia, duchenne on, 42
Lorenz, Adolf, 179, 202
Lucas, William, 26
Lovett, Robert, 147
Lymphatics, von Recklinghausen on, 107

MacEwen, William, 102, 202
McCurdy, S. L., 55
McIndoe, 200
McNealy, 117
Madelung, Otto Wilhelm, 99, *127*, **128**, 202, 213
Magendie, François, 44
Malformations, Gruber on, 61
Mall, Franklin, 68
Malpighi, Marcello, 15
Mannerfelt, Lennart, 21, 176
Mareschel, 8, 9
Marie, Pierre, 42, 118, *137*, **139**, 212
Marie-Strümpell spondylitis, 139
Martin, Henry Austin, 86–88, *86*
Martin, Peter, 19
Martin, Roland, **19–21**, *19*, 62
Martin-Gruber anastomosis, 19, 61
Mason, Michael, 171, 172, **209–211**, *210*
Maxillofacial reconstruction, Gillies on, 197
Mayer, Leo, 102, 145, 147, 181, 190, 191, 200, **201–204**, *201*
Mayo, William, 147, 156
Meagher, Richard, 164
Meissner, Georg, *93*, **95**, 127
Merkel, Friedrich Sigmund, 59, **125–127**, *125*, 129

Metabolism, Garrod on, 74
Metacarpal bones, fractures of, Bennett on, 117
Microscopy, Amici on, 106
Milford, Lee, 115
Mitchell, Silas Weir, **89–95**, *90*, 175, 213
Moberg, 40, 41
Monsters, Gruber on, 61
Morehouse, George, 90
Morestin, Hippolyte, 200
Morgagni, Giovanni, 15
Moynihan, Berkeley, 147, 156
Müller, Johannes, 47, 57, 59, 63, 125, 134, 212
Murphy, John B., 81
Muscles, anatomy of, Albinus on, 11
  contracture of, Cooper on, 52
    Dupuytren's, 22, 31, 59
      Adams on, 49, 50
    Finochietto on, 204
      Volkmann on, 95, 204, 205
  intrinsic, Beevor on, 140
  movements of, Beevor on, 140
  pectoral, Poland on, 74
  Schwann on, 59
  tensor tarsi, Horner on, 56
Muscle transfers, Steindler on, 178
Muscular atrophy, Duchenne on, 44
Muscular dystrophy, Duchenne on, 42

Nageotte, Jean, 115, 143, 152
Naunyn, Bernard, 109
Nélaton, Auguste, 35
Nerve(s), degeneration of, Waller on, 67
  embryology of, Harrison on, 68
  endings of, Merkel on, 125, 127
    Nicoladoni on, 131
  healing of, Paget on, 65
  injuries to, Mitchell on, 89
    Tinel on, 184
  of Bell, 28
  orbital, Poland on, 75
  paralysis of. See *Paralysis.*
  peripheral, fibromas involving, von Recklinghausen on, 107
    injuries to, Fremont on, 175
      Stiles on, 152
    of hand, Martin on, 62
    Stiles on, 152
    Weber on, 41
  Ranvier on, 113
  regeneration of, Waller on, 70
  repair of, Paget on, 64
    Swan on, 65
  scarred, pain in, Tinel on, 184
  sensations of, Weber on, 39–41
Nerve cell, Ramón y Cajal on, 134
Nerve grafts, Bunnell on, 192
Nervous diseases, Beevor on, 140
  Duchenne on, 44
Nervous system, anatomy of, Martin on, 19, 21
  sympathetic, Budge on, 70
Neurofibromatosis, Von Recklinghausen on, 109
Neurology, Duchenne on, 42
  Erb on, 118
  Froment on, 175
  Klumpke on, 149
  Little on, 47, 49
  Marie on, 139
  Mitchell on, 89
  Ramón y Cajal on, 134
Neurosurgery, Cushing on, 161
Newborn, deformities of, Apert on, 157
Nicoladoni, Carl, *129*, **130**, 147, 202
Nodes, of fingers, Heberden on, 15
  of Ranvier, 113
Nussbaum, Moritz, 190

Oldberg, Eric, 164
Ollier, Louis, X. E. L., 77, 78, 81, **100–103**, *101*
Osler, William, 74
Osteochondritis, Perthes on, 166
Osteotomy, Langenbeck, 50
  subcutaneous, Adams on, 50
Ottolenghi, Carlos, 207
Owen, Richard, 65

Pacini, Filippo, **59–61**, *60*, 134, 212
Paget, James, 49, **62–67**, *64*, 76, 125, 139, 190, 212
Palmar fascia, contracture of, Cooper on, 22
  Dupuytren on, 31, 32
Palsy, Bell's, 28
  brachial, Erb on, 118
    Klumpke on, 149
  radial, Jones on, 146
  ulnar, Fremont on, 175
    Mannerfelt on, 178
Pancoast, Joseph, 77
Paralysis, bulbar, Duchenne on, 42
  Erb-Duchenne, 44
  Erb on, 118
  ischemic, Volkmann on, 97
  of lead poisoning, Duchenne on, 44
  Secrétan on, 142
  tendon transfers in, Stiles on, 152
  ulnar, Mannefelt on, 21
  Volkmann on, 97

Paré, Ambroise, 1
Parona, Corrado, 122
Parona, Ernesto, 123
Parona, Francesco, *121*, **122**
Pasteur, Louis, 39, 57, 196
Pathologic anatomy, Gruber on, 61
  Ramón y Cajal on, 136
Pathology, methods in, Stiles on, 153
  von Recklinghausen on, 107
  Virchow on, 107
Payr, Erwin, 183
Pediatrics, Apert on, 157
Pelletan, 33, 34
Penfield, Wilder, 135
Perthes, Georg, 129, 147, 162, *165*, **166–168**, 183, 213
Petit, Antoine, 19
Petit, Jean-Louis, 15, 81
de la Peyronie, Francois Gigot, **6–9**, *7*
Peyronie's disease, 6
Phalen, George, 139
Physick, Philip, 57
Physiology, Meissner on, 95
Pirogoff, Nikolai, 61
Plastic surgery, Denonvilliers on, 52
  Filatov on, 172
  Gillies on, 197
  Guyon on, 104
  Horner on, 55
  Ivy on, 52
  Wolfe on, 78
Plater, Felix, of Basle, 22
Poland, Alfred, **74–76**, *74*
Poliomyelitis, Duchenne on, 42, 44
Pott, Percival, 18, 32
Pratt, Donald, 195
Prostate, Guyon on, 105
Ptosis, Horner on, 105
Purpuras, Heberden on, 16
Putti, Vittorio, 207

de Quervain, Fritz, 85, 123, **158–161**, *160*

Radiation therapy, Perthes on, 166
Radiology, Keinböck on, 168
  Perthes on, 166
Radius, lower, fracture of, Colles on, 26
Ramón y Cajal, Santiago, **133–137**, *133*, 152, 212
Ramón y Cassasus, Justo, 134
Rand, Carl, 164
Ranvier, Louis Antoine, *111*, **113–115**
Raynaud, Maurice, *109*, **110–113**, 212
von Recklinghausen, Friedrich Daniel, **107–109**, *107*, 113
Remak, Robert, 49, 59, 95
Renvers, 183
Reverdin, Jacques-Louis, 77, 78
Rheumatic disorders, Garrod on, 74
Ridlon, 181
Roentgen, Wilhelm Konrad, 39, 100, 118, 170, 196, 212
Rosenmuller, 41
Roux, Wilhelm, 33

Sanitation, Stromeyer on, 45
Sayre, Louis Albert, 50, 129
Scars. See also *Skin.*
  Denonvilliers on, 52
  depressed, Adams on, 49
Schaudinn, Fritz, 119
Schleiden, Matthias, 38, 59, 102, 134, 213
Schonlein, Johann Lucas, 16, 58
Schwann, Theodor, 38, 49, **57–59**, *57*, 95, 102, 113, 125, 134, 212, 213
Secrétan, Henri François, **142–144**, *143*, 151
Seddon, Herbert, 91, 139
Sensation, Weber on, 39–41
Shaw, Darrel, 73
Shearon, 209
Sherrington, Charles Scott, 135, 162
Simarro, Luis, 135
Skin, Langer on, 72
  Meissner on, 95
  nerve endings in, Merkel on, 125
  transplantation of, Thiersch on, 77
    Wolfe on, 78
Skin flaps, Horner on, 55
  Denonvilliers on, 52
  Filatov on, 172
  Gillies on, 197
  Ollier on, 100
  Reverdin on, 123
  Wolfe on, 78
  Wolfe-Krause, 78, 100
Smallpox, Heberden on, 16
  vaccination for, Martin on, 87
Smellie, William, 13, 14
Smith-Petersen nail, 191
Sorrel-Déjèrine, 152
Spastic disease, Little on, 49
Spiller, William, 143, 152
Splints, Thomas on, 148
Spondylitis, ankylosing, Marie on, 139
Sprengel, Otto, **131–133**, *131*
Steindler, Arthur, 140, 147, **178–181**, *179*, 193, 200, 201
Steinmann, Fritz, 183

Sterilization, von Bergmann on, 51
  steam, Stiles on, 152
Stewart, 153
Stiles, Harold Jalland, 147, **152–156**, *153*, 189, 213
Stokes, William, 28
Strabismus, penile, de Lapeyronie on, 6
Stromeyer, Christian F., 45
Stromeyer, George F. L., 37, **45–47**, *45*, 49, 52, 77, 78, 81, 83, 213
Surgery. See also under anatomic part.
Surgery, aseptic technique in, Wurtz on, 4
  plastic. See *Plastic surgery*.
  reconstructive, Jones on, 145
  subcutaneous, Adams on, 49
Surgical field, bloodless, Esmarch on, 81
  Martin on, 86
Sutures, wire, Bunnell on, 192
Swan, Joseph, 65
Sylvius, Jacobus, 1
Syme, James, 153
Symphysiotomy, Camper on, 14
Syphilis, Colles on, 27

Talbott, 22
Tendon, Achilles, Delpech on, 37
  healing of, Adams on, 49, 50
    Mason on, 209
  injuries to, Bell on, 30
  Little on, 49
  Paget on, 63
  sublimis, transfer of, Stiles on, 152
Tendon sutures, Nicoladoni on, 130
Tendon transfers, Bunnell on, 147
  Jones on, 145
  Lange on, 202
  Merer on, 202
  Nicoladoni on, 130
  Perthes on, 166
  Steindler on, 178
  Stiles on, 152
Tenosynovitis, stenosing, de Quervain on, 158
Tenotomy, Delpech on, 37
  Little on, 49
  subcutaneous, Stromeyer on, 47
Terry, W. I., 194
Thiersch, Karl, 47, *76*, **77**, 83, 85, 89, 98, 100, 103, 115, 166, 213
Thomas, Hugh Owen, 147, **148**, *148*
Thumb, opposition of, Bunnell on, 192
Thyroid, surgery of, Reverdin on, 123
Tinel, Jules, 91, 143, 152, 175, **184–187**, *184*, 187, 213
Tooth, Howard Henry, 139
Tourniquet, pneumatic, Cushing on, 161
  Perthes on, 166
Trendelenburg, Friedrich, 45, 85, 125, 166, 168, 181, 183
Trousseau, Armand, 41, 44, 109
Tumors, of brain, Cushing on, 164

Ulna, dislocation of, Darrach on, 173
Ulnar nerve, paralysis of, Mannerfelt on, 21
Ulnar palsy, Fremont on, 175
  Mannerfelt on, 178
Ureters, transplantation of, Stiles on, 152, 154, 156
Urinary tract, Guyon on, 104

Vaccination, smallpox, Martin on, 87
Valls, Jose, 207
Valsalva, Antonio, 15
Vascular disease, Raynaud on, 110
Vater, Abraham, 59
Velpeau, A.-A.-L.-M., 44
Vesalius, Andreas, 1, 11, 14
de Vigo, Giovanni, 1
Virchow, Rudolph, 108
von Volkmann, Richard, 17, 47, 78, **95–100**, *96*, 100, 107, 132, 204, 212, 213
Vulpian, E.-F.-A., 106, 118, 139, 142, 143, 150, 151
Vulpius, 147, 202

Waller, Augustus Volney, **44**, **67–72**, *68*, 76, 134, 153, 212
Warren, Jonathan Mason, 77
von Wassermann, August, 119
Waterhouse, Benjamin, 88
Watson, Frederick, 147
Weber, Eduard Friedrich, 41
Weber, Ernst Heinrich, **39–41**, *39*, 68
Weber, Wilhelm Eduard, 41
Weber-Fechner law, 40
Weber test, 40
Weber's law, 39
Webster, George, 25
Webster, Jerome P., 77
Weigert, Carl, 38, 142
Weiss, 158
Whitman, 202
Wires, fixation, Bunnell on, 192
  Kirschner on, 181
Wistar, 56
Wolfe, John Reissberg, **78–81**, *79*

Wolff, Julius, 81
Wolfe-Krause graft, 100
Wollaston, William Hugh, 18
Woltman, 139
Wounds, abdominal, Poland on, 75
  Bell on, 30
  Esmarch on, 83
  gunshot, Mitchell on, 90
    Poland on, 75
  resection of, Ollier on, 100
  Stromeyer on, 45
  Würtz on, 4
Wrist, deformity of, Madelung on, 128
  extensors of, Jones on, 146
  Guyon on, 104
Wunderleer, Jan, 11
Würtz, Felix, **3–5**, *3*, 6

X-ray therapy, Keinböck on, 168
  Perthes on, 166

Zancolli, Eduardo, 207
Z-plasty, Denonvilliers on, 55
  Horner on, 55
  McCurdy on, 55